Clinical Sociology: Research and Practice

Series Editor

Jan Marie Fritz, University of Cincinnati, Cincinnati, Ohio, USA
University of Johannesburg, Johannesburg, South Africa

The series explores key research and practice in this rapidly expanding field. Topics include ethical and legal aspects of intervention; the nature of client relationships; methods of intervention and evaluation; and the role of clinical sociology in specific settings. This open-ended series appeals to practitioners, policymakers, students and professors in sociology, social work, community psychology, public health, health education, social policy and counseling.

Harry Perlstadt

Assessing Social Science Research Ethics and Integrity

Case Studies and Essays

Springer

Harry Perlstadt
(emeritus) Department of Sociology
Michigan State University
East Lansing, MI, USA

ISSN 1566-7847
Clinical Sociology: Research and Practice
ISBN 978-3-031-34537-1 ISBN 978-3-031-34538-8 (eBook)
https://doi.org/10.1007/978-3-031-34538-8

This Springer imprint is published by the registered company Springer Nature Switzerland AG
The registered company address is: Gewerbestrasse 11, 6330 Cham, Switzerland

To Tari, my wife and sounding board

Foreword

It is a distinct pleasure to write the foreword for Dr. Harry Perlstadt's book about research ethics, the newest volume in Springer's Clinical Sociology book series. Clinical sociology focuses on the analysis of social situations, and this can include intervention at all levels—individual through global. Analysis can take place without intervention, or it can be connected to an intervention process—research before putting an intervention in place, during the implementation process and/or after an intervention is completed. Research is a basic part of the analysis process and is certainly important for intervention.

I have always admired Dr. Perlstadt's detailed approach to important topics such as applied sociology, healthy cities, health disparities, and ethical research. In this book, he traces the history of research ethics and regulations in the USA. He then provides comprehensive assessments of well-known controversial research in sociology and other social sciences: the Tuskegee syphilis study, the Wichita jury study, Stanley Milgram's research about obedience to authority, Laud Humphrey's study of men's homosexual behavior in "tearooms" (restrooms), Philip Zimbardo's Stanford prison experiment and the studies of the Yanomami. As Dr. Perlstadt notes:

> This volume can serve as a useful reference... It provides the historical-structural context of controversial social science studies, including proposal reviews, replications by other researchers, and any impact on research ethics... By reading this book you may better understand the complex history of social science research ethics and why some studies are so controversial.

It is wonderful to have this important book as part of the Clinical Sociology book series. Indeed, this book is a very, very useful reference.

University of Cincinnati
Cincinnati, OH, USA

University of Johannesburg
Johannesburg, South Africa

Jan Marie Fritz

Preface

This is my story of dealings with my Institutional Review Board (IRB) and how I came to write this book. I was a faculty member in the Department of Sociology at Michigan State University for over forty years and interacted with a series of IRB chairs. Some were very helpful while others were uncompromising. A few left Michigan State to work with the federal Office for Protection from Research Risks (OPRR) or its successor, the Office for Human Research Protections (OHRP).

I was the local evaluator for the Department of Education, Department of Health and Human Services, and Department of Justice's Safe Schools, Healthy Students Initiative to develop and implement violence and substance abuse prevention programs. One suggested strategy encouraged the school district to partner with the county mental health agency to provide counseling for teen parents who had neglected or abused their children.

The county mental health agency used standardized psychological and child rearing instruments at intake and discharge. I requested only summary scores for several measures, along with the ages of the teen parents and children, and their ZIP code to determine which school they were likely to attend. Each family had received a mental health booklet explaining their rights and protections when receiving services. It specified that patient records could be used for research or evaluative purposes provided that all identifiers would be removed from the data records and that the director of the mental health program approved the study and supervised the release of the data. The consent procedure was given orally by a mental health counselor in the presence of a witness.

When my IRB denied approval because I lacked written informed consent, I requested a waiver because I did not need to contact the teen parents since I could get deidentified data. However, the waiver was denied. In desperation, I drafted a report to the three federal departments that concluded with my interim evaluation report, which was a blank page. I sent the draft to the IRB chair who promptly entered into negotiations which allowed me to access the deidentified data without obtaining the written consent of the teen parents.

At MSU, I was required to take online Human Research Protection Tutorials to be a certified researcher. The tutorials would summarize a controversial study like the Wichita Jury or Milgram's Obedience to Authority and then point out its ethical shortcomings followed by a multiple-choice quiz. As a graduate student at the University of Chicago, I had a social psychology class with Fred Strodtbeck. He had worked on the Wichita Jury study and sent his class to a talk given by Stanley Milgram in 1964. This led me to question the tutorials' assessments of these controversial studies.

Starting in 2001, I presented papers on IRBs and research protections at professional meetings. I suggested that the tutorials and handbooks for IRB staff and members did not adequately describe the studies, before pointing out their ethical infractions. One colleague compared the tutorials to Aesop's Fables, in which one paragraph summaries lead to an inevitable moral/ethical conclusion.

As the reader will learn, I strongly support research protections including certification of researchers and IRB members and staff, as well as the accreditation of research institutions. However, the tutorials and handbooks should not retrospectively apply current ethical guidelines and regulations to controversial social science studies conducted before the 1978 *Belmont Report.*

The system should be effective and efficient. I argue that whenever possible, an institution's IRBs should make decisions based on precedent, that is, previous decisions on similar research protocols with identical or similar hypotheses, theories, methods, and/or ethical issues and not on a case-by-case basis. Furthermore, the federal government should adopt an appeal process similar to the 2018 Canadian Tri-Council Policy Statement: Ethical Conduct for Research Involving Humans (TCPS 2) which permits an appeal beyond the researcher's IRBs.

I decided to write a book expanding on my papers on six controversial social science studies: the US Public Health Tuskegee Syphilis Study (Chap. 4), The Wichita Jury Study (Chap. 5), Milgram's Obedience to Authority experiment (Chap. 6), Laud Humphreys' *Tearoom Trade* observational study of homosexuals (Chap. 7), Philip Zimbardo's Stanford Prison Experiment (Chap. 8), and the Yanomami controversy in Anthropology (Chap. 9).

I worked with Ruth Homrighaus of Ruthless Editing and then Caryn O'Connell of Watertight Texts, a developmental editor. Caryn made sure I identified all individuals (who was Kurt Lewin?), clarified examples and explained statistical differences for general readers.

East Lansing, MI, USA Harry Perlstadt

Acknowledgments

I am grateful that MSU grants retirees access to its libraries E-Books & Journals. I am deeply indebted to Jan Marie Fritz, sociology educator, certified clinical sociologist and editor of the book series *Clinical Sociology: Research and Practice* for her support and assistance. I appreciate the efforts of the Springer editors who ensured that in-text citations and references corresponded.

About the Book

Social Science Research Ethics and Integrity provides detailed background information on the history of US efforts to protect human subjects participating in social and behavioral science research. Individual chapters describe the concepts and authors of six controversial studies in the last half of the twentieth century. The six studies are: the US Public Health Tuskegee Syphilis Study, the Wichita Jury Study, Milgram's Obedience to Authority, Humphreys' Tearoom Trade, Zimbardo's Stanford Prison Experiment, and the Yanomami controversy in Anthropology. Each case study explores the social situation that the research will address in an attempt to explain how and why people and groups are more or less likely to act in constructive or destructive ways. Each study's research hypotheses, methods, and findings are presented followed by scientific and non-scientific replications or adaptations. The case studies will point out how ethics have and have not been adequately implemented in the research and the study's impact on social science research ethics.

Contents

1 Introduction 1
- 1.1 History of US Research Ethics 1
- 1.2 Social Science Association Ethics 3
- 1.3 Applied Social Science Association Ethics 4
  - 1.3.1 AACS 5
  - 1.3.2 SfAA 5
  - 1.3.3 AAPC 5
- 1.4 Ethical Research and Practice Principles 6
- 1.5 The Chapters 7
  - 1.5.1 History of US Research Ethics and Regulations 7
  - 1.5.2 IRB Mission and Authority 8
  - 1.5.3 Controversial Case Studies 8
- 1.6 Concluding Comments 12
- References 12

Part I Essays

2 A History of Social Science Ethics and Regulations in the United States 17
- 2.1 Introduction 17
- 2.2 The Evolution of Medical Research Ethics 18
  - 2.2.1 Lesser Harms 19
  - 2.2.2 The Nuremberg Code 20
  - 2.2.3 The Declaration of Helsinki 21
- 2.3 Developing US Biomedical and Social Science Research Ethics 21
  - 2.3.1 Concerns About Biomedical and Social Science Research 22
  - 2.3.2 The USPHS Tuskegee Syphilis Study 23
  - 2.3.3 The Codification of Research Ethics in the United States (1973–1994) 23

2.3.4 The National Commission and *Belmont Report* . . . 24
2.3.5 The Common Rule (*45 CFR 46*) . . . 26
2.3.6 The Canadian Tri-Council Policy Statement . . . 28
2.4 Revising the Common Rule (45 *CFR 46*) 1995–2018 . . . 28
2.4.1 The Inspector General's Report . . . 29
2.4.2 The NBAC . . . 30
2.4.3 The National Research Council (NRC) 2003 . . . 32
2.4.4 Advance Notice of Proposed Rulemaking (ANPRM) 2011 . . . 33
2.4.5 Notice of Proposed Rulemaking (NPRM) 2015 . . . 34
2.4.6 The Revised Common Rule (*45 CFR 46*) 2018 . . . 34
2.5 Conclusion . . . 35
References . . . 36

3 IRBs and Police Power: The Intersection of Law and Ethics . . . 41
3.1 Introduction . . . 41
3.1.1 IRBs . . . 42
3.2 Folkway, Mores and Laws . . . 45
3.2.1 Types of Law . . . 46
3.3 Police Power . . . 49
3.3.1 Bureaucracies of Virtue . . . 52
3.3.2 A Collegial IRB . . . 53
3.4 Limiting IRB Excesses . . . 54
3.4.1 Public Policy . . . 55
3.4.2 Accreditation and Certification . . . 56
3.4.3 Appeal Process . . . 59
3.4.4 The Revised Common Rule 2018 . . . 62
3.5 Conclusion . . . 63
References . . . 64

Part II Case Studies

4 The US Public Health Tuskegee Syphilis Study: A Sociological Perspective . . . 71
4.1 Introduction . . . 71
4.1.1 Syphilis . . . 72
4.1.2 Syphilis Becomes a Public Health Problem . . . 73
4.1.3 Race-Related Differences in Disease . . . 74
4.2 Background and Context of Syphilis Study . . . 75
4.2.1 Julius Rosenwald's Legacy for the African American Community . . . 75
4.2.2 Macon County in the 1930s . . . 76
4.2.3 Prevalence Surveys . . . 77
4.2.4 Developing the Study . . . 80
4.2.5 The Initial Study . . . 83

4.2.6 The 1936 Report . . . 85
4.2.7 The Chicago Syphilis Control Program . . . 86
4.3 The USPHS Tuskegee Longitudinal Study . . . 87
4.3.1 Penicillin . . . 88
4.4 The Exposé . . . 90
4.4.1 Sociology of Whistleblowing . . . 90
4.4.2 USPHS's Early Internal Critics . . . 91
4.4.3 External Critics . . . 91
4.4.4 The Whistleblower . . . 93
4.5 After the Exposé . . . 95
4.5.1 The Ad Hoc Advisory Panel . . . 95
4.5.2 The Institutionalization of Research Ethics . . . 96
4.5.3 The Class Action Lawsuit . . . 97
4.5.4 The Legacy Committee . . . 98
4.6 Discussion and Conclusions . . . 98
4.6.1 Ethical Research . . . 99
4.6.2 Moral Responsibility . . . 99
4.6.3 Racism and Health . . . 101
References . . . 102

5 The Wichita Jury Study: Violating a Sacred Trust . . . 107
5.1 Introduction . . . 107
5.2 The Chicago Jury Project . . . 108
5.2.1 The Mock Jury Studies . . . 109
5.2.2 Access to Actual Jury Deliberations . . . 111
5.2.3 Taping Jury Deliberations . . . 113
5.2.4 Presenting Preliminary Findings . . . 114
5.3 The Scandal . . . 115
5.4 Subsequent Studies . . . 117
5.4.1 Entertainment and Jury Consulting . . . 119
5.5 Discussion and Conclusion . . . 120
5.5.1 Research Ethics . . . 120
5.5.2 Research and Jury Integrity . . . 122
5.5.3 Ownership of Data . . . 124
5.5.4 Conclusion . . . 125
References . . . 125

6 Obedience to Authority: A Whirlwind of Controversy . . . 129
6.1 Introduction . . . 129
6.2 Background . . . 130
6.2.1 Developing Obedience to Authority . . . 132
6.2.2 The Grant Proposal . . . 133
6.3 The Controversy . . . 135
6.3.1 Diana Baumrind . . . 136
6.3.2 Milgram's Reply . . . 138

6.3.3 Gina Perry in the Milgram Archives 138
6.3.4 Credibility of the Cover Story 140
6.3.5 Our Moral Compass 141
6.3.6 Scientific Replications 142
6.4 Nonlaboratory Replications 143
6.4.1 The Experiment as Entertainment 144
6.4.2 Prank Calls 147
6.5 Discussion and Conclusions 148
6.5.1 Ethics 148
6.5.2 Theoretical Explanations 150
6.5.3 The Holocaust 151
6.5.4 The Importance of Milgram's Experiments 153
References 154

7 *Tearoom Trade*: The Ethics of Studying Social Problems 159
7.1 Introduction 159
7.2 Study Background and Description 159
7.2.1 Study Design and Methods 161
7.2.2 Creating Samples 162
7.3 The Ethics Controversy 164
7.3.1 The Moralizers 166
7.3.2 Humphreys' Postscript 169
7.4 Related Participant Observation Studies of the Period 170
7.4.1 Personal and Professional Ethics 171
7.4.2 Ethics of Journalism and Social Sciences 172
7.5 Humphreys' Impact on Ethics 173
7.5.1 Interpreting and Implementing Research Ethics 176
7.6 Discussion and Conclusion 177
References 178

8 The Stanford Prison Experiment: The Power of the Situation 183
8.1 Introduction 183
8.2 Preliminary Experiments 184
8.2.1 The NYU Deindividualization Experiment 184
8.2.2 Research on Liberating Behavior Through Hypnosis 185
8.2.3 The Stanford Student Project 187
8.3 From Application Through Prisoner Rebellion 188
8.3.1 Constructing the Mock Prison 190
8.3.2 Creating a Total Institution 191
8.3.3 The Prisoners Rebel 192
8.4 Who's Who in the SPE 193
8.4.1 The Prisoners 193
8.4.2 Prison Guards 199
8.4.3 Father McDermott 201
8.4.4 Carlo Prescott 201

8.4.5 A Psychology Dcpartment Colleague and Wife 203
8.4.6 Prisoner 1037's Parents 203
8.4.7 Christina Maslach 204
8.5 Discussion and Conclusion 205
8.5.1 Ethical Issues 205
8.5.2 Should the Prison Experiment Be Replicated? 207
8.5.3 Research on Evil Practices 207
8.5.4 Conclusion 208
References 209

9 The Yanomami: A Case of Retrospective Ethics 211
9.1 Introduction 211
9.1.1 James Neel 213
9.1.2 The Genetics of Primitive Societies 214
9.1.3 The Measles Outbreak 214
9.2 Napoleon Chagnon 215
9.2.1 Chagnon, Anthropology Outcast 216
9.2.2 The Gold Rush 217
9.3 The Acrimonious Debate 220
9.3.1 Getting to El Dorado 220
9.3.2 The Controversy over *El Dorado* 221
9.3.3 The 2000 AAA Annual Meeting 223
9.3.4 The Task Force Investigates the Controversy 224
9.3.5 The Referendum 225
9.4 Ethical Issues 227
9.4.1 Yanomami Blood Samples 227
9.4.2 International Ethics Research Codes 228
9.4.3 Protecting Indigenous Peoples 228
9.4.4 Professional Codes of Ethics 229
9.5 Conclusion 230
References 231

Index 235

About the Author

Harry Perlstadt learned to report on events and write critically on the University of Michigan student newspaper, *The Michigan Daily*. He earned his PhD in Sociology at the University of Chicago and MPH in Health Planning and Administration at the University of Michigan. He was professor in the Michigan State University Sociology Department and director of the Bioethics, Humanities, and Society Program in the College of Human Medicine. He conducted evaluations for the W.K. Kellogg Foundation, the Michigan Department of Community Health, and the World Health Organization/Europe. His publications include a chapter Ethics and Values in Sociological Practice in *Doing Sociology: Case Studies in Sociological Practice*. He received the American Sociological Association's Distinguished Career Award for the Practice of Sociology. His email address is hphd2023@yahoo.com

Chapter 1
Introduction

Research means that you don't know, but are willing to learn.—Charles Kettering

This chapter introduces social science research ethics, related concepts, important themes and a summary of the book's contents. The first section covers the history of social science research ethics in the United States from the early 1960s including its relationship with biomedical research ethics. It describes the major social science disciplines followed by a discussion of social science professional ethics which are based on ethical practice rather than the principles of ethical research found in the *Belmont Report*. The next section contains a summary of the book's chapters. Chapters 2 and 3 are essays on the history of US research ethics and the mission and authority of Institutional Review Boards (IRBs). The remaining chapters explore six controversial social science studies in chronological order.

1.1 History of US Research Ethics

The United States Federal Government's interest in research ethics began in 1963. James Shannon, the director of the National Institutes of Health (NIH), appointed a committee to report on the problems of inadequate participant consent and relying on researchers to self-scrutinize the adequacy of research proposals submitted to NIH for funding. The committee decided that the NIH should not attempt to shape the educational foundations of medical ethics. Shannon and Surgeon General Luther Terry then asked the National Advisory Health Council (NAHC) to discuss the possibility of developing guidelines for the conduct of human experimentation in its extramural project grants program (Katz, 1987, p. 3).

The NAHC's 1965 report concluded that the US Public Health Service (USPHS) should require researchers to submit extramural grants to a collegial group at their institution before submission for federal funding. This group would provide an independent judgment concerning the risks and potential medical benefits and

H. Perlstadt, *Assessing Social Science Research Ethics and Integrity*, Clinical Sociology: Research and Practice, https://doi.org/10.1007/978-3-031-34538-8_1

adequate informed consent of subjects and concerns. This "prior review" requirement was the first federal requirement for nongovernment IRBs (Schrag, 2009, p. 6).

On December 12, 1966, the Public Health Service announced that investigations in the behavioral and social sciences would have to undergo the same vetting as medical experiments (Schrag, 2009, p. 8). However, only the riskiest projects would require "thorough scrutiny." Many social and behavioral science research studies involve no more than observing or collecting information about the subject's status, by means of administration of tests, inventories, questionnaires or surveys of personality or background. Usually, these procedures should not require the fully informed consent of the subjects or even their knowledgeable participation (Schrag, 2009, p. 8).

Also in 1965, a House Government Operations subcommittee held hearings on the Minnesota Multiphasic Personality Inventory (MMPI) and other psychological tests used for hiring and evaluating federal employees. Although witnesses noted that some questions were of a personal or intimate nature, participation was voluntary. Four Congressmen requested the PHS ensure that personal privacy was protected.

NIH Director Shannon reaffirmed that this was an existing policy. Apparently referencing the Kinsey Reports on sexual behavior, he would later write:

> It's not the scientist who puts a needle in the bloodstream who causes the trouble. It's the behavioral scientist who probes into the sex life of an insecure person who really raises hell. (Schrag, 2009, pp. 6–7).

Meanwhile, social psychologist Stanley Milgram (1963) published his initial findings from his experiments on Obedience to Authority. He was able to convince 65 percent of the subjects to administer what they may have believed to be lethal electric shocks to a fellow subject. A year later clinical and developmental psychologist Diana Baumrind (1964) published an ethical critique of Milgram's experiment, starting a decades-long controversy.

In 1966, Surgeon General William Stuart specifically included the behavioral and social sciences in his statement requiring prior review of PHS extramural grants (ACHRE, 1995, p. 190; Schrag, 2009, p. 6). In April 1971, the Department of Health, Education, and Welfare (HEW) applied the PHS prior review requirement to all department sponsored research. This included questionnaires and surveys. In December 1971, HEW distributed *The Institutional Guide to HEW Policy on Protection of Human Subjects* (Schrag, 2009, p. 9).

The National Commission for the Protection of Human Subjects of Biomedical and Behavioral Research (National Commission, 1979a) published the *Belmont Report* which contained ethical principles and guidelines for the protection of human subjects. Several social scientists were concerned that social science research was being held to the same standards as biomedical research which had higher risks. These concerns resurfaced in 1991 when 15 federal departments and agencies agreed to follow the Department of Health and Human Services (HHS) federal regulations at *45 CFR 46* which became the *Common Rule*. It would take social science ethics over 50 years to crawl out from under the restrictive shadow of biomedical research ethics to emerge in 2018 under favorably revised federal regulations.

1.2 Social Science Association Ethics

The Social Sciences are areas of academic and scientific learning and research that explore human behavior in its social and cultural aspects at a variety of levels and perspectives. The five main social science disciplines are Anthropology, Economics, Political Science, Psychology and Sociology. Human Geography and some areas of History are also considered to be social sciences. At some universities, programs such as African-American Studies, Latinx Studies, Women, Gender and Sexuality Studies may be included as social sciences. The term "behavioral science" is often used by those who favor a stronger connection with the physical and biological sciences (Greenfeld & Nisbet, 2021).

Anthropology is subdivided into cultural anthropology, biological/zoological physical anthropology, the study of human diversity, evolution and the interactions between humans and the animals they live and work with, archaeological study of the human past using material remains that people created, modified, or used and linguistic anthropology.

Since anthropologists work in different cultural and national settings, they may find themselves subject to more than one code of ethics that may not be compatible. As a result, the AAA Code of Ethics provides a framework and guidelines for making ethical choices when conducting research, teaching, advising or consulting. The AAA code of ethics "does not adjudicate claims for unethical behavior" (AAA, 1998) and has no provisions for addressing any reported violations or known offenses.

In contrast, the ethical codes in psychology (APA, 2016), political science (APSA, 2020) and sociology (ASA, 2018) have procedures for reviewing ethics complaints against members and imposing sanctions including termination of association membership. The Society for Applied Anthropology (SfAA, 1991) promotes the investigation of the principles of human behavior and the application of these principles to contemporary issues and problems.

Sociology studies values, norms, traditions and interactions at the micro, mezzo and macro level of analysis. The micro level comprises the social psychology of individuals and families; the mezzo level, neighborhoods, schools and work organizations; and the macro level, state and national governments and regional areas of the world as well as international political, health, economic and cultural systems. Some clinical and applied sociologists are in private practice, have academic appointments and/or work for government agencies or consulting firms. They conduct needs assessments, interventions and/or evaluations to avoid, reduce or solve problems and improve life situations at all three levels (Fritz, 2021, p. 36).

Clinical and applied sociologists conduct their research while observing the research ethics requirement of their principal investigator, employer or funder. The common rule (45 CFR 46 §104) exempts research from IRB review if "benign behavioral interventions are brief in duration, harmless, painless, not physically invasive, not likely to have a significant adverse lasting impact on the subjects, and the investigator has no reason to think the subjects will find the interventions offensive or embarrassing" (HHS, 2018). In addition, the participants in the intervention or research are protected and should not be identified in the data, findings and/or publications.

Microeconomics studies individual people and businesses while macroeconomics focuses on economies as a whole at the global, national and local levels. Economists may apply their knowledge and skills in international organizations like the World Bank and Catholic Relief Services, government agencies that develop and implement budgets and economic policies, as well as commercial and investment banks and insurance agencies. Others do independent consulting.

Political Science focuses on domestic politics and government, comparative politics, international relations, and political theory as well as the applied areas of public policy and administration. Some political scientists work as consultants for political candidates and parties.

Psychology includes scientific experimental researchers and clinicians providing services to individuals, groups and organizations. Major research areas are personality and social psychology, developmental psychology, quantitative and qualitative methods, psychological study of social issues, experimental psychology and cognitive science, behavioral neuroscience and comparative psychology.

Areas of applied or practicing psychology are clinical psychologists working directly with patients to diagnose and treat mental and behavioral issues. Industrial and organizational psychologists help with recruitment, hiring, training, productivity and performance of employees or members. Forensic psychologists work with attorneys, judges and other law professionals to understand the psychological elements in legal cases as well as jury selection and witness credibility. Sports psychologists help teams and individual athletes train and mentally prepare for competitions.

1.3 Applied Social Science Association Ethics

Some social scientists are not employed by academic institutions but work as independent consultants and/or as members of a consulting firm, business or government agency. They may belong to organizations such as the Association for Applied and Clinical Sociology (AACS), the American Association of Political Consultants (AAPC) and the SfAA. Both the AACS and the AAPC explicitly mention "ethics," while the SfAA statement describes itself as simply "a guide to professional behavior," not a code of ethics.

1.3.1 AACS

The AACS was formed in 2005 when the Society for Applied Sociology and the Sociological Practice Association merged. Its members are applied and clinical sociologists as well as public sociologists. Applied sociologists use sociological ideas, concepts, theories and models when conducting program assessment and evaluation research for workplaces, community groups or organizations.

Clinical sociologists seek to improve, prevent or ameliorate social conditions using analysis and research to see what an intervention needs to include and then evaluating the processes and outcomes of the intervention. They work with individual, group, organizational or community clients. Public sociologists engage with nonacademic audiences to address policy issues of concern such as institutional racism and health disparities.

Ethics is an important concern for AACS. Laue and Cormick (1978) point out that ethical principles guide an intervenor's decision-making and subsequent actions. In addition, someone who wishes to be certified either as a Certified Applied Sociologist (CAS) and Certified Clinical Sociologist (CCS) has to submit an ethical statement and address ethics as part of her or his required demonstration session (Lehnerer, 2023, p. 120).

1.3.2 SfAA

Members of the SfAA (1991) promote the investigation of the principles of human behavior and the application of these principles to contemporary issues and problems. They work in academia, business, law, health and medicine in the public and government sectors. The Society's statement is a guide to professional behavior toward the peoples and communities they study, their colleagues students, and employers and other sponsors.

1.3.3 AAPC

The AAPC sets the standard for American political campaigns. Members craft effective strategies and employ best practices so their clients win at the ballot box and in the halls of government. AAPC's (n.d.) Professional Code of Ethics sets standards for campaign and business practices to promote integrity and confidence in the American political system.

1.4 Ethical Research and Practice Principles

Research Ethics concerns how investigators ought to conduct research on human beings by applying ethical principles when designing and carrying out their research. Most researchers are familiar with the three principles of Beneficence, Respect for Persons and Justice in the *Belmont Report* (National Commission, 1979a). The three principles are restated to clarify their meaning and describe what investigators and IRBs should apply when reviewing study proposals.

Beneficence is the obligation not to harm by deciding when it is justifiable to seek certain benefits despite the risks involved. It requires researchers and IRBs to balance risks versus benefits usually through a risk–benefit analysis. They must also weigh the benefits and risks to the study participants against the benefits from the findings for individuals or groups that are not part of the study.

Respect for Persons is the obligation to treat individuals who are recruited for and participate in research as capable of making decisions about their actions based on information that they consider to be accurate. Researcher and IRBs develop informed consent statements which explain the study's objectives and procedures, which can be a medical or social intervention, a laboratory experiment, a survey or questionnaire, or the direct observation of the subject in a public or private area. The potential subject will learn about their likely risks and benefits if they choose to participate, and how their privacy will be protected during the study and in any publications or presentations. In most cases, they are asked to sign the consent form, although verbal consent is permissible in telephone and other surveys or face-to-face observations. However, children, persons with mental illness and prisoners may not have the ability or autonomy to make such decisions or can be easily coerced to participate. Potential subjects and IRBs must decide whether or not they should be included in the research.

Justice is the obligation to ensure that the benefits and risks of research are distributed fairly but not necessarily equally. This requires investigators and IRBs to ensure that subject election is inclusive by not limiting their recruiting to individuals who could benefit from the research or who justify a convenience sample. A convenience sample consists of research subjects who were easily recruited. Historically, most medical research was conducted on lower class or indigent patients in public or charity hospitals or on prisoners who would volunteer in exchange for money or access to some form of medical care.

Kitchener and Kitchener (2009, pp. 9–10, 68–71, 82) have adjusted the *Belmont Report*'s (National Commission, 1979a) three basic ethical principles of Respect for Persons, Beneficence and Justice so that they can serve as the foundation for guiding psychologists, counselors and by extension clinical sociologists. They sought to ground the American Psychological Association (APA) Code of Ethics in an adequate philosophical theory, e.g., Principlism.

They renamed beneficence as nonmaleficence to emphasize that psychologists and clinical sociologists should not harm the individuals, groups or organizations with which they are working, rather than primarily focusing on the promised benefits of the intervention. Respect for Persons became Autonomy to ensure clients can make informed decisions about the proposed intervention methods and outcomes. They added Fidelity as a fourth principle to avoid unnecessary deception when informing clients, and assessing or evaluating the intervention.

Justice was unchanged and states that the distribution of benefits and burdens of research ought to be distributed fairly between research participants and nonparticipants.

According to Beauchamp and Rauprich (2016), the three ethical principles are respect for autonomy, justice and, like Kitchener and Kitchener (2009), nonmaleficence, the obverse of beneficence. Principlism subsumes a global ethics that is universally applicable and acceptable in all societies. However, legitimate differences may exist in the ethics of medical research and practice. This implies that social science research and practice ethics may differ from biomedical ethics. Furthermore, research ethics may differ from practice ethics, since the latter are based on professional values and qualities which vary in specificity by professions.

While professional practice ethics are designed to assist individual level decision-making and give people from diverse fields a straightforward set of moral standards, the principles of research ethics are useful for making policy type decisions in government and research institutions as well as legitimating the policy to individual researchers and IRB members and administrators (Evans, 2005, pp. 230–231). The relationship between the *Belmont* Principlism approach to research and the professional ethics approach to practice merits further discussion.

1.5 The Chapters

This volume is divided into two parts: Essays and Case Studies. Chapters 2 and 3 are essays. The first essay (Chap. 2) provides a historical overview of research ethics on human subjects with a focus on the United States. The second essay (Chap. 3) explores the delegation of authority from the federal government to research institutions and their IRBs. The remaining six chapters are case studies of controversial research in chronological order: The 1934 Public Health Service Tuskegee Syphilis Study (Chap. 4), The 1954 Wichita Jury Study (Chap. 5), Milgram's 1963 Obedience to Authority (Chap. 6), Humphreys's 1968 Tearoom Trade (Chap. 7), Zimbardo's 1971 Stanford Prison Experiment (Chap. 8) and the 2000 *Darkness in Eldorado* Yanomami Controversy (Chap. 9).

1.5.1 History of US Research Ethics and Regulations

The first essay (Chap. 2) recounts how social science research and interventions became regulated in the United States. Concerned about medical experiments conducted without the patient's consent, the director of the NIH called for an impartial peer review of the risks and rights of research subjects. In 1971, the Department of Health Education and Welfare (HEW) published guidelines for protecting human subjects and three years later required IRBs to approve research proposals before submission for funding. In 1991, 15 US departments and agencies agreed to adopt the Department of Health and Human Service (HHS) regulations in the Code of Federal Regulations (45 CFR 56) known as the *Common Rule*.

Meanwhile, in 1979, the National Commission for the Protection of Human Subjects published the *Belmont Report* identifying three ethical principles that underlie research with human subjects: respect for persons, beneficence and justice. The Commission had no members who were social scientists, and some questioned the application of the *Belmont Report* to the social sciences. As IRBs started to enforce 45 CFR 46, a firestorm slowly emerged in the social science research community. The Common Rule (45 CFR 46) was finally amended in 2018 to address many of the concerns of social scientists. Nevertheless, some IRBs may be rather inflexible with social science protocols.

1.5.2 IRB Mission and Authority

The second essay (Chap. 3) explores police power, the delegation of decision-making and enforcement authority over the protection of human subjects in research from the federal government to universities and their IRBs. IRBs were expected to be collegial, with several IRB members drawn from an institution's scientists and researchers, in order to facilitate a culture of trust. The National Commission for the Protection of Human Subjects published recommendations concerning IRB performance and its review process. It recommended that HEW research regulations be adopted by other federal departments. This was achieved in 1991 with the Common Rule (45 CFR 46). It also called for the accreditation of IRBs and the education of IRB members and staff.

IRBs usually make decisions on a case-by-case basis rather than applying a set of principles or precedents from the IRB's previous reviews of similar proposals. The local control over human research protection programs has led to inconsistent and uneven application of federal research policies within and across institutions. Some IRBs have become bureaucracies of virtue, with the head of the IRB making the key decisions as the first among equals. Other IRBs are viewed as ethics police.

1.5.3 Controversial Case Studies

The six studies of controversial cases in chronological order are: Public Health Service Tuskegee Syphilis Study (Chap. 4), Wichita Jury Study (Chap. 5),

Obedience to Authority (Chap. 6), Tearoom Trade (Chap. 7), Stanford Prison Experiment (Chap. 8) and Yanomami Controversy (Chap. 9).

1.5.3.1 Public Health Service Tuskegee Syphilis Study

The 1972 exposé of 40 years of inhumane treatment of subjects in the Public Health Service Tuskegee Syphilis Study (Chap. 4) led to regulations to protect human research participants, a successful class action lawsuit and a Presidential apology.

Although a key word in the study's title, the Tuskegee Institute itself lacked any substantial decision-making authority. In 1929, the USPHS asked the Julius Rosenwald Foundation to fund a joint project dealing with syphilis among African Americans. When the Foundation ended its support in 1932, the USPHS then developed a longitudinal study to observe untreated syphilis and conduct autopsies to determine the effects of the disease on vital organs. The study recruited 600 African-American men comprised of 399 men with syphilis and a control group of 201. All were given medical examinations, general health care and burial insurance. Although penicillin was not effective on late-stage syphilis, it was not administered to men in the comparison group if they contracted syphilis.

1.5.3.2 The Wichita Jury Study

In 1952, the University of Chicago Law School received a grant from the Ford Foundation to learn if juries followed the judge's instructions. It involved audio taping mock juries and taping actual jury deliberations (Chap. 5).

A lawyer contacted the law school, suggesting that they tape record actual juries in Wichita. The lawyer prepared a detailed set of procedures resembling a research protocol. The District Judge did not want the jurors to be informed that their deliberations would be recorded. The Chicago researchers did not listen to any of the Wichita deliberations until all possible appeals had been resolved for the case in question.

However, at the 1955 Judicial Conference, a portion of a jury deliberation was played.

A few months later the *Los Angeles Times* broke the story on this eavesdropping on juries. The result was a law which prohibited anyone not a member of the jury from recording the proceedings of a federal jury while it is deliberating or voting.

The main ethical issue at stake in this study was that the jury members did not consent to the taping. The threat of harm was to the jury system itself since the taping violated an unwritten norm.

1.5.3.3 Obedience to Authority

The ethical issues in Milgram's *Obedience to Authority* (Chap. 6) are deception and the stress experienced by the participants during and after the experiment. The experiment prodded subjects to obey an order to administer what appeared to be dangerous electric shocks. During the experiment, the probability of stress was beyond what would be expected in everyday life.

Milgram's initial finding that 65 percent of 40 subjects administered all 30 shocks made national headlines. In his first article, Milgram failed to mention that the research involved 24 experimental conditions which resulted in many fewer subjects administering all 30 shocks. One condition was moved from the Yale laboratory to a rundown office building in a downtown shopping district. In another variation, only women were subjects.

Milgram was able to pressure 65 percent of his subjects to administer all 30 shocks in only 5 of 23 (21.7 percent) conditions.

Diana Baumrind, a developmental psychologist, disapproved of his use of deception. However, Milgram's experiments have been replicated in various forms in the United States and other countries. A nonlaboratory replication of Milgram's experiments involved nurses following doctors' orders. His impact extended to imaginative representations on television, plays and movies as well as prank telephone calls from someone claiming to be an authority figure.

1.5.3.4 Tearoom Trade

Tearoom Trade (Chap. 7), Laud Humphreys' observational study, was designed to gain insight into the lifestyle and behavior of homosexuals. In 1966, Humphreys began hanging around restrooms in public parks with nearby parking used by men for homosexual activities.

He talked with some men away from the restrooms, known as tearooms, and one suggested that Humphreys assume the role of "lookout," or "watch queen," to warn if police were approaching. He created a nonrandom sample of 100 men by copying license plates and obtaining the car owners home addresses. He then interviewed the men at their homes.

After his dissertation defense, the sociology department belatedly filed a newly required human protections form because Humphreys had a National Institute of Mental Health's (NIMH) predoctoral research fellowship. The NIMH wrote the Washington University Chancellor that Humphreys' research purpose was not a problem.

However, the *St. Louis Post Dispatch* published a story that included references to Humphreys' dissertation. Two years later, a *Washington Post* journalist asserted that the information collected could be used for blackmail and/or extortion and without the knowledge of the people involved.

Humphreys kept the master list under lock and key, and later had them burned. He concealed all identifiers in his dissertation and publications.

1.5.3.5 Stanford Prison Experiment

Philip Zimbardo's Stanford Prison Experiment (Chap. 8) was designed to investigate deindividualization when an individual in a group participates in antisocial behavior. A review committee approved his proposal. It would document how the student study participants adjusted to prison life over two weeks.

Zimbardo recruited college students through newspaper ads. Students were randomly assigned to be guards or prisoners. The guards wore uniforms and no name tags, which deindividualized them. They could act arbitrarily and create some degree of fear. Guards on each of three shifts lined up prisoners for a "count." When prisoners arrived on Sunday at the Stanford Psychology Building, they were given a smock with numbers on the front and back to individuate them. A guard reads them the prison rules prisoners and guards were required to follow.

Having been awakened twice early the next day, the sleep-deprived prisoners rebelled. The prisoners asked for less physical abuse and requested religious services. Zimbardo asked a Catholic priest to play prison chaplain.

On Wednesday, Zimbardo created a parole board headed by Carlo Prescott, an actual ex-convict. Prescott, who had been denied parole several times, was hard on the Stanford prisoners. On Thursday evening, Zimbardo's former teaching assistant was shocked to see a chain gang of prisoners. She convinced him to end the experiment on Friday.

1.5.3.6 The Yanomami: A Case of Retrospective Ethics

The Yanomami controversy (Chap. 9) centered on Patrick Tierney's claims that James Neel made a measles epidemic worse and that Napoleon Chagnon exaggerated the level of violence in Yanomami society. The Yanomami live in about 300 villages along rivers in Venezuela and Brazil. Neel, a pioneer in human genetics, hoped to learn if hunter-gatherers developed immunity to pathogens. He and anthropologist Chagnon collected blood samples which revealed that many Yanomami villages lacked measles antibodies. On arriving in Brazil, Neel immediately began inoculating Yanomami with Edmonston B vaccine and administered Gamma Globulin once it arrived.

In *Science,* Chagnon (1988) reported that Yanomami claimed that men who have killed have more wives and offspring than men who have not. This generated debate among cultural anthropologists, who believe that culture alone shapes human behavior. Just before the 2000 AAA meetings, the *New Yorker* published Tierney's negative views on Chagnon. The association held two extraordinary sessions on Tierney's claims.

The AAA Executive Board appointed an El Dorado Task Force to explore the issues of contention. In 2005, a referendum rescinded the Task Force Report because the inquiry did not follow the AAA policy prohibiting ethics adjudications.

1.6 Concluding Comments

This chapter has presented an overview of the history of social science research ethics in the United States and the powers of IRBs, and has examined six controversial social science studies. In 1963, the NIH became concerned about inadequate participant consent in human research studies and relying on individual researchers to assess the ethical adequacy of their research proposals. This led to the 1971 Department of Health Education and Welfare (HEW) policy on protection of human subjects and the 1974 regulations requiring the creation of IRBs to approve all research proposals before they could be submitted for funding. In 1991, the HHS regulations were incorporated into the Code of Federal Regulations (45 CFR 56) and became known as the *Common Rule*.

Following US Senate hearings on the Wichita KS wiretapping jury scandal, Congress created and charged the National Commission for the Protection of Human Subjects of Biomedical and Behavioral Research to identify the basic ethical principles that underlie biomedical and behavioral research, and to develop guidelines for observing those ethical principles. Its conclusions were published in the National Commission (1979a) *Belmont Report* which described the principles of respect for persons, beneficence and justice. The National Commission (1979b) also published a set of recommendations concerning IRB performance and its review process.

This volume can serve as a useful reference for those interested in an in-depth examination of social science research ethics. This includes clinical and applied sociologists and psychologists as well as students, professors, researchers, IRB members and staff and clinical and applied social scientists in the social sciences and humanities. It provides the historical-structural context of controversial social science studies, including proposal reviews, replications by other researchers and any impact on research ethics. This goes beyond online tutorial accounts that briefly describe these studies in a paragraph or two and then list their shortcomings, such as lack of documented informed consent or deception about the purposes and methods of the study.

By reading this book, you may better understand the complex history of social science research ethics and why some studies are so controversial. Current standards and interpretations will inevitably change over the coming years. Hopefully, you will be able to comprehend proposed changes and feel comfortable adding your perspective to the ongoing discussion.

References

AAA. (1998). *American Anthropology Association*. Code of Ethics of the American Anthropological Association. Available at: AAA Code of Ethics (PDF) - Amazon S3. Retrieved January 11, 2023, from https://s3.amazonaws.com › pdfs › issues › upload

ACHRE. (1995). *Advisory Committee on Human Radiation Experiments: Final Report*, Washington DC: Superintendent of Documents, U.S. Government Printing Office. October

1995. Advisory Committee on Human Radiation Experiments: final report. United States. Advisory Committee on Human Radiation Experiments: Free Download, Borrow, and Streaming: Internet Archive. Retrieved December 26, 2020

APA. (2016). American Psychological Association. *Ethical principles of psychologists and code of conduct*. Available at: Ethical principles of psychologists and code of conduct. Retrieved January 16, 2023, from apa.org

APSA. (2020). *American Political Science Association Ethics Final Principals*. Retrieved January 16, 2023, from https://www.apsanet.org/Portals/54/diversity%20and%20inclusion%20prgms/Ethics/Final_Principles%20with%20Guidance%20with%20intro.pdf?ver=2020-04-20-211740-153

ASA. (2018). American Sociological Association Code of Ethics. Available at: asa_code_of_ethics-june2018.pdf (asanet.org) Accessed 30 Nov 2023

Baumrind, D. (1964). Some thoughts on ethics of research: after reading Milgram's "Behavioral study of obedience"

Beauchamp, T. L., & Rauprich, O. (2016). Principlism. In H. ten Have (Ed.), *Encyclopedia of global bioethics*. Springer International Publishing. ISBN 978-3-319-09482-3.

Chagnon, N. A. (1988). Life histories, blood revenge, and warfare in a tribal population. *Science, 239*(4843), 985–992. https://doi.org/10.1126/science.239.4843.985

Evans, J. H. (2005). Max Weber meets the *Belmont Report*: Toward a sociological interpretation of principlism. In J. F. Childress, E. M. Meslin, & T. Shapiro (Eds.), *Belmont revisited: Ethical principles for research with human subjects* (pp. 228–243). Georgetown University Press.

Fritz, J. M. (2020). Clinical sociology: A global perspective. In T. Uys & J. M. Fritz (Eds.), *Clinical sociology for Southern Africa* (pp. 85–104). Juta and Company (Pty) Ltd.

Fritz, J. M. (2021). History of international clinical sociology. In J. M. Fritz (Ed.), *International clinical sociology* (2nd ed., pp. 35–56). Springer.

Greenfeld, L., & Nisbet, R. A. (2021, October 22). *Social science. Encyclopedia Britannica*. Retrieved May 27, 2022, from https://www.britannica.com/topic/social-science

HHS. (2018). Department of Health and Human Services. *Exemptions 2018 requirements*. Accessible at: Exemptions (2018 Requirements) | HHS.gov. Retrieved January 17, 2023.

Katz, J. (1987). The regulation of human experimentation in the United States: A personal Odyssey. *IRB: Ethics & Human Research, 9*(1), 1–6. https://doi.org/10.2307/3563644

Kitchener, K. S., & Kitchener, R. F. (2009). *Social science research ethics: Historical and philosophical issues*. Retrieved May 19, 2022, from https://www.researchgate.net/publication/288882077_Social_science_research_ethics_Historical_and_philosophical_issues

Laue, J., & Cormick, G. (1978). The ethics of intervention in community disputes. In G. Bermant, H. Kelman, & D. Warwick (Eds.), *The ethics of social intervention*. Halstead Press.

Lehnerer, M. (2023). Certification: Validating the work of sociological practitioners. *Clinical Sociology Review, 18*(1), 118–130.

Milgram, S. (1963). Behavioral study of obedience. *Journal of Abnormal and Social Psychology, 67*, 371–378. https://doi.org/10.1037/h0040525

National Commission. (1979a). *The Belmont Report: Ethical principles and guidelines for the protection of human subjects of research*. DHEW Publication No. (OS) 78-0013. U.S. Government Printing Office, Washington, D.C. Retrieved February 10, 2020, from https://www.hhs.gov/ohrp/regulations-and-policy/belmont-report/read-the-belmont-report/index.html

National Commission. (1979b). *Report and recommendations. Institutional Review Boards*. DHEW Publication No. (OS) 78-0008. U.S. Government Printing Office, Washington, D.C. Retrieved June 15, 2022, from https://repository.library.georgetown.edu/bitstream/handle/10822/778625/ohrp_institutional_review_boards_1978.pdf#page=1

Schrag, Z. M. (2009). How talking became human subjects research. The Federal Regulation of the Social Sciences, 1965–1991. *Journal of Policy History, 21*(1), 3–37.

Society for Applied Anthropology. (1991). *About the SfAA*. Retrieved January 19, 2023, from https://www.appliedanthro.org/about

Part I
Essays

Chapter 2
A History of Social Science Ethics and Regulations in the United States

Thou shalt not sit with statisticians nor commit a social science.—W. H. Auden "Under Which Lyre"

2.1 Introduction

Social science is feared. Its subject matter deals with our everyday lives, groups, organizations and cultures. Since most people consider themselves knowledgeable about such matters, they may question or deny findings that are counterintuitive or do not correspond with their experiences. By its very nature, social science may threaten our traditional beliefs and values and criticize our established institutions and organizations (Francis, 1959). Theories, experiments, surveys and media analyses reveal that we are susceptible to manipulation and have limited free will.

Some research findings even conclude that the use of social engineering can resolve problems or transform society. In one of the twentieth-century's most well-known examples, the Third Reich adopted work in applied and rural sociology to expel or annihilate certain populations from newly conquered territory (Klingemann, 1992). Sociologist Jonathan Turner (2001, pp. 100–102) pointed out that sociologists themselves distrust social engineering. One reason is a disconnect between theory, research and practice. He thought that sociological theories may support or criticize social ideologies rather than explaining how the world works.

The issue at stake with research in the social sciences is not whether proposed social behavioral science research should be reviewed from an ethical perspective. Both social behavioral and biomedical research should maximize possible benefits and minimize possible harms to research subjects. Both should provide sufficient information in an informed consent statement about the research to enable a potential research subject to freely decide whether or not to participate. But social behavioral researchers have argued that their research is sufficiently different from biomedical research that the regulations should not be identical in detail. The degree of harm in

H. Perlstadt, *Assessing Social Science Research Ethics and Integrity*, Clinical Sociology: Research and Practice, https://doi.org/10.1007/978-3-031-34538-8_2

social behavioral research is less than the life and death risks in some biomedical research.

This chapter will explore how both biomedical and social science research and interventions became regulated.

According to Max Weber (1978, pp. 24–37; 212–254), when irrational traditional values and activities are challenged, some changes are made to written rules, codes and/or laws that are overseen and enforced by a bureaucracy of officials with expert training. This bureaucracy of virtue (Bosk, 2007, pp. 197–1980) draws upon a set of value-rational (*Wertrational*) ethical principles to guide biomedical and social science research. These are then interpreted and implemented by IRBs and Ethics Committees at universities and hospitals.

Standards are the result of a great deal of hard work with the goal of ordering human behavior. Ethical codes are initially developed in response to horrific biomedical or social behavioral experiments. Over time, new techniques and discoveries need to be incorporated into existing standards. In addition, ethical standards requiring estimates of risk and benefits raise questions about the efficacy of existing standards. In the case of research ethics, these questions may include unintended consequences that actually do harm, either to the researcher or the participants (see Citro, 2013, p. 7; Busch, 2011, pp. 70, 247). It should not be surprising that it takes years to develop, implement, evaluate and revise ethical research standards.

Two early ethical statements were the Nuremberg Code (1947) and *Declaration of Helsinki* (1964). In the United States, concerns about biomedical and social science research began in 1963 with Milgram's Obedience to Authority experiments (see Chap. 6) and became a public issue with the 1972 exposé of the USPHS Tuskegee Syphilis Study (see Chap. 4). Congress passed laws that led to the codification of research ethics and established a national commission to identify ethical principles for biomedical and behavioral research. In 1991, given the methodological advances in such areas as biogenetics, personal and ethnic history and evaluation and survey research, 15 federal departments and agencies agreed to follow the Department of Health and Human Services (HHS) research regulations, which became the Common Rule (*45 CFR 46*).

By 2001 both biomedical and social science professional organizations had raised concerns about the appropriateness of the Common Rule. Ten years later, in 2011, HHS published an advance notice requesting comments on proposed changes to the Common Rule. Revised rules were finally promulgated in 2018 and became effective over the next two years. However, despite these revisions, some IRBs continue to be rather inflexible with social science protocols (Babb, 2020, p. 92).

2.2 The Evolution of Medical Research Ethics

Medicine's concern for ethics is well-known. The Hippocratic Oath requires physicians and surgeons to abstain from doing harm. They are expected to act in their patient's best interest when they diagnose and treat medical conditions. They also promise not to disclose things which they learn about the lives of their patients. This assumes a virtuous physician who will consciously act morally and ethically with respect to her or his patients. However, physicians in the eighteenth and ninetieth centuries conducted experimental treatments for small pox, scurvy and venereal diseases on slaves, sailors and prisoners who could not refuse to participate. Some heroically tested their treatments on themselves. In 1803, Thomas Percival published *Medical Ethics* for the professional conduct of physician and surgeons. He recommended that they should first seek the opinions of their peers when testing a new medication on patients (Sierra, 2011, p. 395). Researchers in England and France developed medical research ethics in the mid nineteenth century.

At the end of World War II, the victorious allies convened a series of war crime trials in Nuremberg, Germany, including a trial of Nazi doctors who had committed atrocities in the name of medical science. Almost 20 years later, in 1964, the World Medical Association (WMA) issued the *Declaration of Helsinki*, which consisted of ethical principles for medical research. Neither had a direct impact on German or American national law on medical research.

2.2.1 Lesser Harms

Sociologist Sydney Halpern (2004, p. 9) noted that individuals are rarely unilateral moral actors. They are embedded in communities with norms and traditions that guide them when confronting moral problems. In the case of medical research, these communities are the social and professional networks of the physician-researchers and the organizations that sponsor human research experiments. The question became how to address the risks of clinical experiments compared with the risks of letting a disease take its natural course. As we will see in Chap. 4, the Tuskegee Study refused to treat syphilis even when penicillin became available.

In the first half of the nineteenth century, physicians began to rely on medical laboratory sciences.

Some used laboratory reports for diagnosis and treatment while others considered it a threat to the knowledge they gained through years of clinical practice (Löwy, 2011, p. 117). Pierre Louis was a pioneer practitioner who, in Paris in the 1820s and 1830s, conducted both controlled experiments on hospital patients with pneumonia and called for the systematic evaluation of medical therapies using empirical observation, autopsies, experimental controls and statistical comparisons (Halpern, 2004, p. 4; Simmons, 2002, pp. 75–79).

For lesser harms, Halpern (2004, pp. 41–42) offers the example of the moratorium on conducting vaccinations for polio on humans. In 1934, two American research teams had developed an immunizing agent and began tests on humans. A moratorium on polio research was imposed by a group of leading researchers after reports surfaced that several recipients had contracted paralytic polio and a few had died. The moratorium held until the early 1950s, when Jonas Salk and Albert Sabine produced their vaccines.

Interestingly, Salk conducted the first human trials on former polio patients and on himself and his family (History.com Editors, 1953).

2.2.2 *The Nuremberg Code*

In 1946–1947, the United States convened a series of war crime trials in Nuremberg, Germany. The Doctors' Trial accused 23 German physicians and administrators of conducting unethical medical experiments in concentration camps holding Jews, Poles, Russians and Roma (Gypsies). The experiments were conducted without the consent of the subjects and did not allow them to voluntarily leave the experiment. These experiments sought to facilitate the survival of military personnel in the field, to develop and test drugs and treatment methods for injuries and illnesses of military and occupation personnel and to advance Nazi racial and ideological goals (Holocaust Museum, n.d.; Gardella, 1999).

The physicians asked to be judged under the 1931 Guidelines for Human Experimentation that had been passed by the German parliament (*Bundestag*) before the Nazis came to power and were still in effect (Grodin, 1992, p. 129; Ghooi, 2011; AHRP, 2015). The Guidelines appear to be among the first national regulations governing medical research. They covered both therapeutic and nontherapeutic research and required mandatory informed consent, including disclosure of the purpose, justification and manner in which the research will be carried out. They prohibited exploitation of patients who were poor or socially disadvantaged (ACHRE, 1995, p. 148).

The Nazi doctors' request was countered by Dr. Leo Alexander, a psychiatrist and neurologist, who had taught at Harvard and Duke Universities. He was the chief medical officer to Telford Taylor, Chief of Council for War Crimes. In April of 1947, Alexander submitted a memorandum defining legitimate research containing six points. These were expanded to ten and included in a section of the verdict entitled "Permissible Medical Experiments." This became the Nuremberg Code. It called for voluntary consent, avoiding all unnecessary physical and mental suffering and injury and permitting human subjects to bring the experiment to an end, and it mandated that researchers terminate an experiment if it is likely to injure, disable or cause the death of the experimental subject. However, these points were not included in the verdict and thus failed to establish the legal force of the Code (Holocaust Museum, n.d.). Sociologist Robert Dingwall (2008, p. 2) suggests that the Allies did not take the Nuremberg Code very seriously in applying it to themselves. He argues that the Code became a creation myth to legitimize the institutionalization of ethical regulations and enable traditional research elites to retain their power and influence.

2.2.3 *The Declaration of Helsinki*

The next milestone in human research protections was the *Declaration of Helsinki* (WMA, 1964). It took the WMA 17 years to develop this international agreement on ethical principles for medical research involving human subjects. According to Susan Lederer (1995, pp. 209–210), the WMA had to reconcile human research practices across nations, the biomedical research needs of the US pharmaceutical industries and the question of whether to include or exclude children and/or persons in mental hospitals, prisons and reformatories. It is a set of recommendations guiding doctors in clinical research that focuses on clinical studies and therapeutic experiments with their patients as subjects. It has no standing under international law.

In the *Declaration,* nontherapeutic medical research on human subjects was included under general processes to ensure that ethical principles would be followed. But these processes were intended for research physicians. For example, Point 23 stated that when obtaining informed consent for the research project, the physician should be particularly cautious if the subject is in a dependent relationship with the physician or may consent under duress. Point 31 read, "The physician should fully inform the patient which aspects of the care are related to the research. The refusal of a patient to participate in a study must never interfere with the patient–physician relationship."

Regardless of the nature of the research on human subjects, Point 13 required a clearly formulated experimental protocol, which should be submitted to a specially appointed ethical review committee, which in turn was given the right to monitor ongoing trials, and obligates the researcher to report any serious adverse events. Regarding publication of results, Point 27 recommended that only reports of experimentation in accordance with the principles laid down in the Declaration should be accepted for publication. The *Declaration* at the time of its publication did not mention, and still does not mention, social and behavioral science research on health and illness, health services or health promotion and prevention.

2.3 Developing US Biomedical and Social Science Research Ethics

While the WMA was drafting the *Helsinki Declaration*, the United States took its first real steps toward regulating research on human subjects. It began in the USPHS and NIH and, by early 1966, led to requiring prior review of research proposals submitted to the USPHS for extramural grants. A few months later the *New England Journal of Medicine* published a landmark article by Henry K. Beecher (1966) that brought greater attention to questionable clinical research. In 1972, the revelations of the Tuskegee Syphilis Study sullied the reputation of the PHS and called for federal action on research ethics (see Chap. 4).

2.3.1 Concerns About Biomedical and Social Science Research

Shortly before the WMA adopted the Helsinki Declaration, the USPHS and the NIH asked the NAHC to discuss the possibility of developing guidelines for the conduct of human experimentation in its extramural project grants program (Katz, 1987, p. 3).

In late 1963, NIH director James Shannon became concerned about a research program at the Jewish Chronic Disease Hospital in Brooklyn, in which researchers injected cancer cells into noncancerous patients without their consent. He appointed a committee to investigate the problems of inadequate consent and of relying on the self-scrutiny of the researchers for research protocols and procedures for contracted research. The committee concluded that the NIH should not attempt to address the ethical issues underlying inadequate consent and researcher self-scrutiny.

Shannon and Surgeon General Luther Terry then met with the NAHC. Shannon called for an impartial prior peer review of possible risks to research subjects and a review of the protection of the rights of subjects. In its 1965 final report, the Council agreed that USPHS should require researchers applying for extramural grants to submit to prior review by institutional associates. This collegial group would provide an independent judgment that informed consent was appropriately obtained, including the risks and potential medical benefits of the study. It did not recommend any substantive guidelines, noting that both the Nuremberg Code and *Declaration of Helsinki* were too rigid and did not address public health research and concerns (ACHRE, 1995, pp. 174–1975; Katz, 1987, p. 3). This was implemented in early 1966 by US Surgeon General William Stewart when he specifically included the behavioral and social sciences in his statement requiring prior review for USPHS grants (ACHRE, 1995, p. 190; Schrag, 2009, p. 6).

While the original focus had been medical and clinical research, the social and behavioral sciences were included because of concerns over invasions of privacy. In 1965, Congressman Cornelius Gallagher (D-NJ) and a House Government Operations subcommittee held hearings on the use of the MMPI and other psychological tests for evaluating federal employees and job applicants. During the hearings, a witness told the committee that some mental health research sponsored by the PHS contained questions of a personal or intimate nature, but that participation was entirely voluntary and that invasion of privacy was not an issue.

Gallagher and three other Congressmen requested the USPHS to ensure that protecting personal privacy was a paramount concern. NIH director Shannon assured Congress that this was the policy.

Probably referring to the *Kinsey Reports* on sexual behavior, as readers will recall, he later stated, "It's not the scientist who puts the needle in the bloodstream who causes trouble. It's the behavioral scientist who probes into the sex life of an insecure person who really raises hell" (Schrag, 2009, pp. 6–7).

In April 1971, the Department of Health, Education, and Welfare (HEW) applied the USPHS prior review requirement to all department sponsored research. When a review committee member brought up the question of behavioral and political science research, department representatives insisted that questionnaires are definitely subject to the Department's policy. In December 1971, the department created and distributed a pamphlet, *The Institutional Guide to HEW Policy on Protection of Human Subjects,* known by its cover as the *Yellow Book* (Schrag, 2009, p. 9).

2.3.2 The USPHS Tuskegee Syphilis Study

In July 1972, most major newspapers carried an article about the USPHS Tuskegee Syphilis Study. In 1932, the PHS began a longitudinal study of syphilis in Macon County, AL, with medical examinations and procedures carried out at the John A. Andrews Memorial Hospital of the Tuskegee Institute. They enrolled 399 poor black men with syphilis and 201 without syphilis as controls. The men were told they were being treated for "bad blood." They were given free medical exams and free burial insurance. However, they were not given penicillin, a treatment for syphilis, after it became generally available in 1953 (see Chap. 4). The study raised a host of questions relating to social injustice and racism that remain of abiding interest to social scientists and researchers.

2.3.3 The Codification of Research Ethics in the United States (1973–1994)

An Advisory Panel Report (HEW Report, 1973) recommended that the USPHS Tuskegee study be stopped immediately and that the remaining subjects be given necessary medical care resulting from their participation. The Report also recommended that Congress establish a permanent body with the authority to regulate all federally supported research involving human subjects (ACHRE, 1995, p. 180).

Facing fast track legislation, and in an attempt to prevent Congress from writing mandatory ethical standards governing federally sponsored research or setting up a regulatory agency to oversee the NIH, the Secretary of Health, Education and Welfare, Caspar Weinberger, waived all the usual clearances for regulations. Those HEW agencies that customarily commissioned social science or educational research and the normal HEW clearance points for the issuance of regulations including public comment, were either bypassed or given extremely brief deadlines (Tropp, 1982, pp. 931–932; McCarthy, 2001, 2004). Primarily drafted by the health side of HEW, a set of regulations was produced based on the 1971 *Institutional Guide to HEW Policy on Protection of Human Subjects.*

On May 22, 1974, Weinberger signed the Protection of Human Subjects regulation that made existing NIH guidelines a departmental policy. The regulations required the formation of what became known as IRBs to approve all research proposals before they could be submitted to HEW for funding consideration. These committees were to review, among other things, the safety (risks and potential benefits) of the proposed research and the adequacy of the informed consent obtained from each subject prior to participation.

Two months later, in July 1974, Congress passed the National Research Act (PL 93-348) which officially gave HEW the authority to establish regulations, and incorporated them as title 45 of the Code of Federal Regulations (CFR) part 46 (*45 CFR 46*) Protection of Human Subjects under United States Law. The law specifically limited the scope of the regulations to biomedical and behavioral research. For example, some research conducted in schools such as assessing and evaluating regular and special education instructional strategies, techniques or curricula are exempt from IRB review.

2.3.4 The National Commission and Belmont Report

The 1974 National Research Act also established the National Commission for the Protection of Human Subjects of Biomedical and Behavioral Research. Congress charged the Commission with the task of identifying the basic ethical principles that underlie biomedical and behavioral research and to develop guidelines to assure that investigators conducting research on human subjects would adhere to those ethical principles. Specifically, it was to address issues of informed consent, risk and benefit assessment and subject selection—all issues that had been raised by the USPHS Tuskegee Syphilis Study. The National Commission for the Protection of Human Subjects of Biomedical and Behavioral Research (1979) published its ethical principles and guidelines for the protection of human subjects in the *Belmont Report.*

The 11-member commission consisted of three physicians, three attorneys, a bioethicist, a Christian ethicist, a behavioral-biologist, a physiological-psychologist and the president of the National Council of Negro Women (*Belmont Report*, 1979). Noticeably missing were members representing any of the major social science research disciplines: anthropology, economics, political science, psychology and sociology.

The Commission had a small professional staff that included, among others, philosopher Tom L. Beauchamp, psychologist Miriam Kelty and sociologist Bradford H. Gray, along with two special consultants, physician Robert J. Levine and philosopher-historian Stephen Toulmin. Kelty (2004) was a psychologist trained in clinical psychology and was head of the Office of Scientific Affairs at the APA. When she joined the Commission staff, she was head of the APA Office of Scientific Affairs where she tracked federal legislation. She met with the Consortium of Social Science Associations (COSSA), a nonprofit advocacy organization which serves as a united voice for social and behavioral sciences in federal policy making.

She also worked on a large national public opinion survey on attitudes toward advances in biomedical and behavioral research technology and alternative policies to deal with them (Kelty, 2004; *Federal Register*, May 25, 1979). At that point in time, Kelty was advocating for self-regulation before the government would impose regulations on social and behavioral science research. Twenty-five years after the report, Kelty thought that the empirical approach, based on observed, concrete and verifiable evidence, rounded out the Commission's philosophical papers and discussions.

When he joined the Commission staff, Gray had just published his doctoral dissertation in which he reviewed the deliberations of a university peer-review committee on proposed biomedical research and interviewed participants in two of the studies (Gray, 1975). He found that although the participants had signed a consent form, 39 percent of 51 women who participated in a drug trial for inducing labor did not know they were part of a research project until he interviewed them. Furthermore, poor, uneducated, nonwhite clinical patients were more apt to be recruited than private patients. He concluded that despite the university review committee's rather strict interpretation of the existing rules, the overall structure of the research situation did not facilitate informed consent.

Gray (1975) noted that the Commission was not staff-driven. The staff edited meeting transcripts into drafts that the commissioners could review before their next monthly meeting. In addition, the staff arranged for the writing of background papers requested by the Commission, organized hearings and site visits and planned and oversaw empirical research in support of the commission's deliberations.

However, as Beauchamp (2004) recalled, Gray often argued on behalf of social and behavioral research in staff meetings, and sometimes in front of the Commission, but very little attention was paid to social and behavioral research and few of the models considered by the commission pertained to it.

Gray (1980, p. 12) wrote that although the Commission did not recommend an appeal process, the idea of an appeal process had its merits and deserved further consideration. The Commission recommended that IRBs notify investigators in writing of the basis for its decision and that investigators be given the opportunity to respond in person or in writing. But Gray noted that no independent appeal process exists if an injustice occurs.

The Commission's final statement, *The Belmont Report* (1979) began with a review of writings and discussions on research ethics, asking, "What are the basic ethical principles that are used to judge the ethics of human subject research?" This led to the three *Belmont Report* principles of respect for persons, beneficence and justice. Respect for persons includes both respect for the autonomy of human subjects and the importance of protecting vulnerable individuals, e.g., children and people with mental disabilities. Beneficence is the duty of researchers to both promote the well-being of subjects and to maximize the benefit-to-harm ratio for individual subjects and for the research program as a whole. Justice requires that subjects are not systematically recruited for a study because of their easy availability within social institutions (e.g., prisons, schools), or are inclined to participate for small monetary or other rewards, or are from groups unlikely to be among the beneficiaries of subsequent applications of the research.

Furthermore, justice demands that the benefits or applications of the research should not be limited to those who can afford them.

When Beauchamp (2004) joined the staff, one of his first questions was, "What do these three principles mean?" He was told to figure it out by talking to the commissioners and other members of the staff. The principles were then defined and applied to the issues at hand: informed consent, assessment of benefits and risks and selection of human subjects. The *Belmont Report* noted that the assessment of risks and benefits was closely related to the principle of beneficence. A beneficent assessment necessitates gathering systematic and comprehensive information about the proposed research. This information enables a review committee to determine whether the risks to study participants are justified. It also allows prospective subjects to decide whether to participate. Benefits refer to something of positive value related to health or welfare. A benefit/risk assessment is concerned with weighing anticipated benefits against the probabilities and magnitudes of possible harm.

Among those unhappy with the *Belmont Report* was MIT political science professor Ithiel de Sola Pool. He was aware that the National Commission had no social scientists on it, though two social scientists, Bradford Gray and Miriam Kelty, were on its staff. In early January 1979, de Sola persuaded Pulitzer Prize winning journalist Anthony Lewis to raise questions about the *Belmont Report* in his *New York Times* column (Schrag, 2010, p. 104). Lewis argued that IRBs should review biomedical or similar research but not social science work with competent adults. Pool then formed an emergency committee of prominent social scientists to protest the application of the *Belmont Report* to the social and behavioral sciences. Richard Tropp, who had worked in the office of the HEW Secretary and written a background paper for the *Belmont Report* (Tropp, 1978), remarked that as IRBs started to enforce *45 CFR 46*, a firestorm was slowly emerging in the social science research community (Tropp, 1982, pp. 391–392).

*2.3.5 The Common Rule (*45 CFR 46*)*

Researchers conducting historical work were also placed under scrutiny at this time. For example, the Oral History Association acknowledged the ethical obligations of historians and others who systematically collect autobiographical documents or interview people about stressful events they have experienced, (Moyer, 1999), e.g., the Holocaust or the 1960s civil rights movement. Some IRBs feared respondents may experience trauma from recalling and reliving bad experiences. Other IRBs did not approve of open-ended questions or recommended limiting opportunities to ask spontaneous follow-up questions. Still other IRBs could prescribe anonymity by requiring that those conducting oral research not identify their sources or reveal who was involved in certain events.

While this may shield innocent victims and protect them from possible repercussions for past mistakes or misdeeds, it creates an incomplete and unverifiable historical account (Jones, 2007). In such cases, social behavioral researchers are more constrained than journalists, who undertake investigative reporting on the same topics with the same sources but have more discretion in whether to withhold names. Ethicist Kelly McBride (2007) suggested that the naming question is best answered on the basis of its effect on three principles: reporting the truth as fully as possible, remaining independent and minimizing harm.

Sociologist Jerome Skolnick (1968) noted that when law is considered to be a tool for educating people or achieving social order, it can readily become an instrument to promote a state-endorsed morality. In such cases, moral entrepreneurs, who favor a particular value system, work for the creation and enforcement of rules and laws that delineate what they consider to be proper behavior and then label as deviant those who do not conform (Becker, 1973; Erikson, 1966). I suggest that this assessment can apply to IRBs, which have become instruments for not only implementing, but indoctrinating researchers in federally developed and approved research ethics. Some efforts to protect human participants go well beyond their original intentions, for example, by expecting researchers to serve as positive role models to counter the mad scientists of popular culture, e.g., Dr. Frankenstein, Dr. Jekyll and Dr. Strangelove.

Charles R. McCarthy served as staff director of the Secretary of HEW's Ethics Advisory Board from 1978 through 1980 and as director of the Office for Protection from Research Risks (OPRR) from 1978 through 1992. He stated that the group that drafted the 1981 federal regulations on the protection of human subjects asked itself: "What were the indignities to subjects that it felt needed attention?" Its answer was:

> The Wichita jury bugging case [see Chapter 5], the tearoom trade research [see Chapter 7], . . .and our own unpleasant memories of Psychology 101 and Sociology 102, when we felt we had better humor our professors so we volunteered as research subjects rather than risk grade discrimination!" (McCarthy, 1984).

Ten years earlier, Stanley Milgram, who conducted the obedience to authority experiments (see Chap. 6), essentially agreed, writing that "subjects more commonly respond with distaste to the empty laboratory hour, in which cardboard procedures are employed and the only possible feeling is that one has wasted time in a patently trivial and useless exercise" (Milgram, 1974, p. 237).

A year later, sociologist Donald Warwick (1982) presented a "deliberately one-sided," wide-ranging taxonomy of potential harms arising from social science research, in order to provide a framework for a more careful analysis of the issues at stake. He illustrated them with a variety of real and hypothetical examples. Zimbardo's Stanford Prison Study (see Chap. 8) exemplified the risk of physical abuse and injury in his taxonomy, while Milgram's Obedience to Authority experiment exemplified the risk of psychological abuse or injury. He used Humphreys' Tearoom Trade (see Chap. 7) as an example of an experiment that provoked anxiety and placed participants in legal jeopardy, since at the time homosexuality was a crime.

Warwick also pointed out that Milgram and Humphreys both employed deception that not only harmed research participants, but could harm society and the social science disciplines. Deception undermines the trust necessary for the positive functioning of the social order, from friendships to democracy. In particular, the Wichita Jury Study violated the sanctity of the jury. The revelation of the secret recordings created public outrage that had the potential to negatively affect future jury deliberations, and led to a federal law banning taping federal court proceedings and jury deliberations.

In an effort to promote uniformity and compliance with federal human subject protections, 15 US departments and agencies agreed to adopt the 1991 revisions to the Department of Health and Human Services (HHS) rules and regulations, which covered biomedical and behavioral research involving human subjects in the CFR (*45 CFR 46*). This made *45 CFR 46* the Common Rule for these departments and agencies. As of 2018, 20 departments and agencies agreed to follow the revised Common Rule as amended.

2.3.6 The Canadian Tri-Council Policy Statement

In 1978, the year the *Belmont Report* was issued, the Canadian Medical Research Council (MRC), now the Canadian Institutes of Health Research (CIHR), first produced ethics guidelines which were followed by the Social Sciences and Humanities Research Council in 1981. They were joined by the Natural Science and Engineering Research Council (NSERC) in 1998, with the adoption of the Tri-Council Policy Statement (TCPS) Ethical Conduct for Research Involving Humans. The guiding ethical principles of the policy are Respect for human dignity, Concern for welfare and Justice. The TCPS was revised and updated in December 2011, resulting in the 2nd edition (TCSP2). As a condition of funding, the councils require that researchers and their institutions, as a minimum, apply the ethical principles and the articles of the policy.

The TCPS2 covers Research Ethics Boards (REBs), the equivalent of IRBs and their review procedures. But unlike US IRBs, Canadian REBs are allowed to consider appeals from researchers, although this is neither a substitute for REBs and researchers to work closely together nor a way to seek a second opinion (TCP2, 2018: Article 6.19).

2.4 Revising the Common Rule (45 *CFR 46*) 1995–2018

The 1991 Common Rule (45 CFR 46) was only a milestone on the road to addressing the concerns of social scientists. A government agency must follow an established process to revise federal regulations. The first step is often a response to an accident, an unexpected death or a scandal. For instance, in 1999, Jesse Gelsinger died in a human therapy experiment. He had a mild version of a rare metabolic disorder which he managed on a regimen of nearly 50 pills a day. He went to the University of Pennsylvania where he was 18th person to receive a modified virus that was being used as part of a treatment plan. Four days after receiving the shot Jesse was declared brain dead and taken off life support (Rinde, 2019). The National Institute of Health (NIH) and the Office for Human Research Protections (OHRP) responded by requiring all people conducting or overseeing human subjects research to have training in research ethics.

The agency also considers findings from government reports. In 1998, the HHS Inspector General's report revealed that that the long-established system for protecting human research subjects had weaknesses and was not as effective as it could be. In 2001, the National Bioethics Advisory Commission (NBAC) noted that researchers in the social sciences and humanities believed that some IRBs had imposed requirements that were inappropriate for nonbiomedical research. The Commission supported the certification of individuals involved in conducting, reviewing or monitoring human research, as well as the accreditation of the universities, hospitals and research institutions in which the work was carried out.

2.4.1 The Inspector General's Report

In June 1998, the Inspector General of the Department of Health and Human Service (HHS) published *Institutional Review Boards: A Time for Reform*. It concluded that "the long-established system for protecting human research subjects has vulnerabilities that threaten its effectiveness" (Brown, 1998, p. 1). For example, in the 1980s, most studies took place at only a single site, but since then multisite studies have increased, as well as research involving databases, the Internet and biological specimen repositories. New types of research require highly specialized areas of expertise and raise issues of informed consent. It found that IRBs review too much too quickly and conduct minimal review of approved research.

Among the Inspector General's recommendations were that research institutions have programs for educating its investigators and IRB members about human subject protection, and that they require the registration of IRBs (Brown, 1998, pp. ii–iv). Under *45 CFR 46* subpart E, research institutions would be required to register all IRBs with HHS if they planned to be engaged in nonexempt human subjects research conducted or supported by HHS. The institution could then receive a Federalwide Assurance (FWA) committing to comply with *45 CFR 46*.

While generally accepted, the human research protection system has faced continuing criticism, particularly from behavioral and social scientists who believe that it has inappropriately applied biomedical research standards to behavioral and social research and that some IRBs are insufficiently knowledgeable about the behavioral and social sciences (O'Hara, 2005; Jones, 2008). *The Illinois White Paper* (Gunsalus et al., 2007) found that IRBs have undergone mission creep by expanding their responsibilities to the point that they are imposing an unreasonable burden of inappropriate regulation and restriction on social and behavioral research. IRBs have been asked to check for potential financial conflicts of interest, methodological soundness, scientific merit and health-record privacy. In addition, local control over human research protection programs has led to inconsistent and uneven application of HHS policies within and across institutions (Jones, 2008).

2.4.2 *The NBAC*

In October 1995, President Bill Clinton created the NBAC to examine topics including cloning, human stem cell research and research involving human subjects. The NBAC published its final report in August 2001 and made 30 recommendations. Like the HHS Inspector General, it found that:

> The current system for protecting human participants in research is in need of reform. It does not protect all research participants, and where protection is offered, it is often burdened by excessive bureaucracy, confusing or conflicting interpretations of rules, and an inability to respond to emerging areas of research (NBAC, 2001, p. vii).

The NBAC was well aware that investigators in the social sciences and humanities believed that IRBs with primarily biomedical members sometimes imposed unreasonable requirements that are inappropriate for nonbiomedical research. The NBAC (2001, p. 63) noted that IRBs were required to possess the professional competence necessary to review specific research activities since scientific expertise is to a large extent discipline specific. Appropriate expertise and experience are essential both for the protection of participants and the promotion of ethical research.

To meet these objections, the NBAC recommended certification of individuals involved in conducting, reviewing or monitoring research on human subjects as well as the accreditation of organizations in which they work. Certification means that an individual investigator, IRB member or IRB staff has successfully completed training in research ethics and is competent and skilled in their role. Accreditation means that an organization that conducts or reviews research involving human subjects has received the approval of a recognized accrediting agency after the agency has reviewed the organization's procedures with respect to human research protection and determined that it meets existing standards.

This would include colleges and universities, hospitals, medical research institutions and entities that fund human research (NBAC, 2001, p. 63). Colleges and universities, it further recommended, should include research ethics in curricula related to research methods.

The NBAC (2001, p. xii) recommended that institutions should develop internal mechanisms to ensure IRB and investigator compliance with regulations, guidance and institutional procedures. One such mechanism would create a place for reporting noncompliance to all relevant parties. I suggest that this could be accomplished through a compendium similar to *Law Reporters*, a series of volumes that contain selected judicial opinions from state and federal courts. For research ethics, this would include IRB decisions that could serve as models or precedents for other IRBs as well as appealed decisions, if that were allowed.

The composition of IRBs was an issue of concern. For example, an IRB should not consist wholly of members from one profession. This suggests that large research institutions could have IRBs for different types of research, e.g., one for biomedical research and one for social behavioral and educational research.

The NBAC (2001, pp. xvii–xviii) addressed some aspects of informed consent that are of interest to social and behavioral researchers. IRBs should be flexible with respect to the form and wording of the informed consent document. Some required elements of informed consent are appropriate for clinical research but are nonsensical for behavioral and social science or historical research, for example, requiring a disclosure of appropriate alternative procedures or course of treatment (NBAC, 2002, p. 100). Requiring signed informed consent forms in some cases might threaten respondent confidentiality and IRBs should allow investigators to use other means of verifying that they have obtained informed consent. IRBs should be able to waive informed consent in studies using identifiable or observational data. In such instances, the IRB must determine that all components of the study involve minimal risk or that any component involving more than minimal risk must also offer the prospect of direct benefit to participants. Furthermore, the benefits from the knowledge to be gained from the research study must outweigh any future harm (NBAC, 2001, pp. xvii–xviii).

Multisite studies were also considered by the NBAC. Such sites provide large, diverse samples with sufficient statistical power to detect significant differences. Their findings are more generalizable than studies from a single research site. When research is conducted at more than one institution, it is often reviewed by all relevant IRBs. These IRBs may differ in their requirements for informed consent for initial surveys and follow-up contacts or interviews. For example, one IRB may require a single page signed consent form which is separated from a returned survey, while another may require that the survey's introductory page define the consent process and state that returning the survey constitutes the responder's consent to participate in the study (Morahan et al., 2006). A proposed change to a consent form by one IRB could trigger a round of negotiations among all the collaborating IRBs, increasing costs and creating time delays (NBAC, 2001, p. 118).

To gather direct feedback from diverse research stakeholders, the NBAC received public and expert testimony at a series of meetings between 1996 and 2001 in the DC metropolitan area, as well as San Francisco, Salt Lake City, Madison, WI, Cleveland, Atlanta, and Miami, FL, among others. At these meetings, it learned that often the reason an IRB turned down a protocol was rarely for a local factor, but rather because it found some aspect of the study design, such as the incentive to participate, i.e., cash, a gift card or course credit, unacceptable (NBAC, 2001, pp. 118–119). It therefore recommended that federal policy should permit a central or lead IRB to review a multisite study, provided that participants' rights and welfare are rigorously protected (NBAC, 2001, p. vii).

2.4.3 The National Research Council (NRC) 2003

The NRC produces reports to inform public policy and advance the pursuit of science, engineering and medicine. Political scientist Constance Citro, psychologist Daniel Ilgen and sociologist Cora Marrett compiled the NRC's report, *Protecting Participants and Facilitating Social and Behavioral Sciences Research* (NRC, 2003; Citro et al., 2003). The report recommended that committees or commissions created to provide advice to the federal government on human research protections should include members who represent the range of social, behavioral and economic sciences (SBES). It strongly encouraged the development of detailed guidelines with clear examples on what qualifies as SBES research and which types of SBES research IRBs should be exempt from review or subject to an expedited review procedure (Recommendations 6.1, 6.4, 6.5, 7.2).

The report (NRC, 2003, pp. 26–28) briefly described six types of SBES harms: physical, psychological, social, economic, legal and moral. Failure to provide adequate informed consent or use of deceptive techniques in SBES research may occur when participants are encouraged to behave unethically or harmfully toward others. However, informing potential participants that they may feel distress, anger or embarrassment during an experiment may not protect everyone from these psychological harms. To give another example, disclosure that one is participating in a study of gang violence may lead to physical harm if gang members retaliate. Outside knowledge of an individual's participation in health behavior or substance abuse studies may result, for instance, in the social harm of stigmatization, the economic harm of loss of insurance or employment, or the harm of arrest, conviction, incarceration and civil lawsuits.

In its review of IRBs, the NRC concluded that IRB reviews varied considerably. Specifically, this variability was much more likely to affect the type and nature of minimal-risk research compared with research that was more than minimal-risk (NRC, 2003, p. 35). Sociologist Lawrence Busch (2011, pp. 28, 239) argued that standards are about power and that organizations set rules researchers must follow, just as they often establish a limited range of acceptable research topics and/or procedures. The NRC (2003, p. 174) considered the desirability of recommending that a formal appeal process be added to the Common Rule. This would provide recourse to an investigator who believed the required changes would harm the scientific integrity of the proposed research but not provide additional participant protection. Such a process would not be needed if researchers received clearer guidance from IRBs and, in turn, if IRBs had more explicit guidance from the OHRP.

2.4.4 Advance Notice of Proposed Rulemaking (ANPRM) 2011

Eight years after the NRC report, the Office of the Secretary of the Department of Health and Human Services (HHS) issued an Advanced Notice of Proposed Rulemaking (ANPRM, 2011) on Human Subjects Research Protections. The HHS OHRP was considering changes to the Common Rule because of the sizable increases in the volume of multisite studies and health services and social science research (OHRP, 2011). It acknowledged that the risks to subjects in certain types of survey and interview research is low and such research may be over-regulated and may distract from social and behavioral research projects that do pose threats to the welfare of subjects (*Federal Register*, 2011, p. 54413).

The ANPRM requests public participation in the formulation of a regulatory change, including research institutions, professional associations, individual researchers and anyone interested in human research protections. It listed 75 questions including several that specifically mentioned or were of interest to social and behavioral sciences (*Federal Register*, 2011, pp. 44517–44529). For instance, Question 17 asked under what circumstances, if any, should a social or behavioral research study qualify for the excused category if the study involves a form of deception (and if so, how should deception be defined).

Concerning multisite research, Question 30 requested comments on the advantages and disadvantages of mandating, as opposed to simply encouraging, a single IRB of record for domestic multisite research studies, and Question 32 asked if eliminating local IRB reviews in multisite research would affect a research institution's regulatory and legal liability. With respect to international research, Question 74 sought comments on the advisability of all Common Rule agencies having one set of guidelines, and if this would adequately address human subjects protections in diverse populations and across biomedical, national security, education and social behavioral research.

The ANPRM request for comments also addressed the 1996 Health Insurance Portability and Accountability Act (HIPAA), which established standards for identifiable and deidentified data of health information. HIPAA Rules allow subjects to authorize researchers to disclose their identities if the investigator wishes to publicly recognize their subjects in published reports. Questions 54 and 59 asked if these standards are appropriate for use in social and behavioral research, and, if not, what standards would be more appropriate. Question 68 noted that some data must be reported to the Federal Government in order to gather information on the effectiveness of the human subjects protection system. Should this requirement apply to biomedical intervention studies only or to all types of human subjects research including behavioral and social science research?

2.4.5 Notice of Proposed Rulemaking (NPRM) 2015

Having reviewed public comments received after the 2011 ANPRM, the Department of Health and Human Services on behalf of 16 federal departments and agencies issued an NPRM in August 2015 to better protect human subjects involved in research under the Common Rule (*45 CFR 46*). The NPRM (*Federal Register*, 2015, p. 53954) noted that most IRB reviews of social and behavioral research effectively protects subjects from psychological or privacy and informational risks. Overregulating social and behavioral research in general may result in insufficient attention being paid to social and behavioral research that poses ethical challenges and may therefore merit significant oversight.

The NPRM identified activities that will not have to satisfy any regulatory requirements and will not undergo any type of prior review process. It explicitly exempted the following:

> Oral history, journalism, biography and historical scholarship activities that focus directly on the specific individuals about whom the information is collected (NPRM, 2015, p. 53948).
>
> Survey procedures, interview procedures or observation of public behavior (including visual or auditory recording) uninfluenced by the investigators, provided that that human subjects cannot be identified, directly or through identifiers and that disclosure would not reasonably place the subjects at risk (NPRM, 2015, p. 53951).
>
> Conducting quality assessment and improvement activities, including outcomes evaluation and development of clinical guidelines, provided that the primary purpose is not health research to obtain generalizable knowledge (NPRM, 2015, p. 53946).
>
> Benign interventions with the collection of data from adult subjects if the subject prospectively agrees to the intervention and collection of data. These interventions would be brief, harmless, painless and not likely to have significant adverse lasting impact on the subjects. Deception would be permissible if the prospective agreement informs the subject that he or she will be unaware of or misled regarding the nature or purposes of the research (NPRM, 2015, p. 53960).

2.4.6 The Revised Common Rule (45 CFR 46) 2018

The 2018 Common Rule revisions included the above-mentioned changes. However, it did not address issues of international research and an appeal process. The University of Washington (n.d.) recommends that researchers in the United States who plan to conduct research at an international site are expected to submit their proposals to their home institution's IRB as well as an ethics review entity in one of 133 countries. They may also need the approval of university or research entities where they plan to be based and/or have coinvestigators, research assistants, etc. The rules for providing research subjects with gifts or monetary compensation varies by country and researchers should consider the average daily wages in both US and foreign currency to prevent inappropriately high or low levels of compensation.

Finally, a researcher may need approval of both United States and other ethics review entities to modify or make major changes prior to implementing the changes.

Although some research institutions have a process that allows investigators to appeal their IRBs decision to an IRB panel composed of that institution's IRB members who did not serve on the original IRB, or to an IRB at another institution, the revised Common Rule did not require every institution to provide an appropriate appeal mechanism. The need for an appeal process is examined more in Chap. 3.

2.5 Conclusion

The Common Rule (*45 CFR 46*) was revised in 2018 to address the concerns of social and behavioral scientists and clinicians. That was almost 40 years after Ithiel de Sola Pool organized an emergency committee to protest the application of the *Belmont Report* to the social and behavioral sciences. While it takes time and effort to revise a federal standard like the Common Rule, social science professional associations have revised their codes of ethics more frequently in response to the changing research environment. As influential social theorists have proposed, the difference in the length of time needed to make changes broadly reflects the fundamental difference between sacred and profane values (Mauss, 1975, pp. 23–25; Durkheim, 1964, pp. 41, 53). Sacred values have historically been enduring and unquestionable, although they may become obsolete before laws are changed.

Those who challenge existing research ethics may be viewed as troublemakers and politely ignored. Authority is delegated to local IRBs, some of which may choose to more strictly enforce the rules against social behavioral researchers. Those IRBs and investigators who bring sacred values to bear on their evaluations can be considered a part of the moral community of ethical researchers.

From a sociological perspective, an individual's moral compass is set within his or her sociocultural milieux and reinforced by religious, occupational and political communities. Though it is not always obvious, ethical research standards emerge from traditional belief systems and practices and are incorporated in laws and codes which are then monitored and enforced by a bureaucracy of experts trained in the intricacies of human research protection.

In order to change the CFR, a government agency must follow an established process. The agency is spurred into action by a public scandal, tragedy or series of complaints about the need to take into account new techniques and discoveries as well as the rise of multisite research among universities, hospitals and government institutes. The agency may need to consult with other agencies as well as seeking expert and public opinions of what changes are needed and why. The agency then must review and report on its proposed changes and respond to any feedback before announcing proposed new rules. All this takes time. It took 27 years from 1991, when the Common Rule was promulgated, until it was revised in 2018. The revisions addressed the concerns of the social behavioral sciences and treated them differently from the biomedical sciences.

References

ACHRE. (1995). *Advisory Committee on Human Radiation Experiments: Final Report*, Washington DC: Superintendent of Documents, U.S. Government Printing Office. October 1995. Advisory Committee on Human Radiation Experiments: final report. United States. Advisory Committee on Human Radiation Experiments: Free Download, Borrow, and Streaming: Internet Archive. Retrieved December 26, 2020.

AHRP. (2015). *1931: Germany: "Guidelines for Human Experimentation"*. Alliance for Human Research Protection. Retrieved November 4, 2020, from https://ahrp.org/1931-germany-guidelines-for-human-experimentation/

ANPRM. (2011). *Advance Notice of Proposed Rulemaking (ANPRM) on human subjects research protections: Enhancing protections for research subjects and reducing burden, delay, and ambiguity for investigators 76 Fed. Reg. 44521* (July 2016).

Babb, S. (2020). *Regulating human research: IRBs from peer review to compliance bureaucracy*. Stanford University Press.

Beauchamp, T. L. (2004). Interview with Tom Beauchamp, Ph.D. *Belmont Oral History Project*. Retrieved January 25, 2020, from https://www.hhs.gov/ohrp/education-and-outreach/luminaries-lecture-series/belmont-report-25th-anniversary-interview-tbeacham/index.html

Becker, H. S. (1973). *Outsiders: Studies in the sociology of deviance*. The Free Press.

Beecher, H. K. (1966). Ethics and clinical research. *New England Journal of Medicine., 274*, 1354–1360.

Belmont Report. (1979). *The Belmont Report: Ethical principles and guidelines for the protection of human subjects of research*. The Government Printing Office HEW Publication No. (OS) 78–0012. Retrieved January 26, 2020, from hhs.gov/ohrp/humansubjects/guidance/belmont.html

Bosk, C. L. (2007). The new bureaucracies of virtue or when form fails to follow function. *PoLAR: Political and Legal Anthropology Review, 30*(2), 192–209. https://doi.org/10.1525/pol.2007.30.2.192

Brown, J. G. (1998). *Institutional review boards: A time for reform*. Department of Health and Human Services, Office of the Inspector General. Retrieved March 28, 2022, from https://oig.hhs.gov/oei/reports/oei-01-97-00193.pdf

Busch, L. (2011). *Standards: Recipes for reality*. MIT Press.

Citro, C. F. (2013). Workshop on Proposed Revisions to the Common Rule in Relation to the Behavioral and Social Sciences, Washington, DC, March 21, 2013. Retrieved January 17, 2021, from https://www.nap.edu/read/18383/chapter/3

Citro, C. F., Ilgen, D. R., & Marrett, C. B. (2003). *Protecting participants and facilitating social and behavioral sciences research*. The National Academies Press.

Dingwall, R. (2008). The ethical case against ethical regulation in humanities and social science research. *21st Century Society, 3*(1), 1–12. https://doi.org/10.1080/17450140701749189

Durkheim, E. (1964). *The elementary forms of the religious life* (J. W. Swain, Trans.). George Allen & Unwin Ltd. Retrieved March 30, 2022, from https://www.auro-ebooks.com/wp-content/uploads/downloads/Emile-Durkheim-The-Elementary-Forms-of-the-Religious-Life.pdf

Erikson, K. T. (1966). *Wayward puritans: A study in the sociology of deviance*. John Wiley & Sons.

Federal Register. (2011). Advance notice of proposed rulemaking (ANPRM). 76(143:44512-44531 Tuesday, July 26, 2011.

Federal Register. (2015). Notice of proposed rulemaking. (NPRM)/ 80(173): 53933-54061. Tuesday, Sept. 8, 2015.

Francis, R. G. (1959). Social science education. In J. S. Rouček (Ed.), *The challenge of science education* (pp. 305–318). N.Y. Books for Libraries Press.

Gardella, J. E. (1999). The cost-effectiveness of killing: An overview of Nazi 'Euthanasia'. *Medical Sentinel, 4*(4), 132–135.

Ghooi, R. B. (2011). The Nuremberg Code-A critique. *Perspectives in Clinical Research, 2*(2), 72–76. https://doi.org/10.4103/2229-3485.80371

Gray, B. H. (1975). *Human subjects in medical experimentation: A sociological study of the conduct and regulation of clinical research*. Wiley-Interscience.

Gray, B. H. (1980). Social research and the proposed HEW regulations. *IRB, 2*(1), 1–5, 12.

Grodin, M. A. (1992). Historical origins of the Nuremberg Code. In G. J. Annas & M. A. Grodin (Eds.), *The Nazi doctors and the Nuremberg Code: Human rights in human experimentation* (pp. 121–145). Oxford University Press.

Gunsalus, C., Bruner, E., Burbules, N., Dash, L., Finkin, M., Goldberg, J., Greenough, W., Miller, G., & Pratt, M. (2007). The Illinois White Paper: Improving the system for protecting human subjects: Counteracting IRB Mission Creep. *Qualitative Inquiry, 13*(5), 617–649. https://doi.org/10.2139/ssrn.902995

Halpern, S. A. (2004). *Lesser harms: The morality of risk in medical research*. University of Chicago Press.

HEW Report. (1973). Final Report of the Tuskegee Syphilis Study Ad Hoc Advisory Panel, Department of Health, Education, and Welfare (Washington, D.C.: GPO, 1973). Available at FINAL REPORT of the Tuskegee Syphilis Study Ad Hoc Advisory Panel (1973) (lsu.edu). Retrieved December 20, 2020

History.com Editors. (1953, March 26). Dr. Jonas Salk announces polio vaccine. Retrieved March 25, 2022, from https://www.history.com/this-day-in-history/salk-announces-polio-vaccine

Holocaust Museum. (n.d.). *Nazi Medical Experiments*. US Holocaust Memorial Museum. Retrieved November 11, 2020, from https://encyclopedia.ushmm.org/content/en/article/nazi-medical-experiments

Jones, A. (2007). Letter on Expedited Review to Office for Human Research Protections from the American Historical Society Dec 20, 2007. Retrieved January 27, 2020, from https://www.historians.org/publications-and-directories/perspectives-on-history/february-2008/aha-statement-on-irbs-and-oral-history-research

Jones, A. (2008). Letter to the federal Office of Human Research Protections (OHRP) from the American Historical Society Sept 29, 2008. http://blog.historians.org/profession/618/training-discernment-and-oral-history-review

Katz, J. (1987). The regulation of human experimentation in the United States: A personal odyssey. *IRB: Ethics & Human Research, 9*(1), 1–6. https://doi.org/10.2307/3563644

Kelty, M. (2004). Oral History of the *Belmont Report* and the National Commission for the Protection of Human Subjects of Biomedical and Behavioral Research. Interview August 26, 2004. Retrieved January 9, 2022, from https://www.hhs.gov/ohrp/education-and-outreach/luminaries-lecture-series/belmont-report-25th-anniversary-interview-mkelty/index.html

Klingemann, C. (1992). Social scientific experts – No ideologues: Sociology and social research in the Third Reich. In D. Kasler & S. P. Turner (Eds.), *Sociology responds to fascism* (pp. 127–154). Routledge.

Lederer, S. E. (1995). *Subjected to science: Human experimentation in American before the second world war*. Johns Hopkins University Press.

Löwy, I. (2011). Historiography of Biomedicine "Bio," "Medicine," and in between. *Isis, 102*(1), 116–122.

Mauss, A. L. (1975). *Social problems as social movements*. J.B. Lippincott Co.

McBride, K. (2007). *Duke Lacrosse Case: Should We Name the Accuser?* The Poynter Institute Poynter Online Jan 29, 2007 http://www.poynter.org/content/content_view.asp?id=116123

McCarthy, C. R. (1984). Introduction: The IRB and social and behavioral research. Chapter 3. In J. E. Sieber (Ed.), *NIH readings on the protection of human subjects in behavioral and social science research. Conference proceedings and background papers*. University Publications of America.

McCarthy, C. R. (2001). Reflections on the organizational locus of the office for protection from research risks. In National Bioethics Advisory Commission (Ed.), *Ethical and policy issues in research involving human participants Volume II*. Washington, D.C. Retrieved November 4, 2006, from http://www.georgetown.edu/research/nrcbl/nbac/pubs.html

McCarthy, C. R. (2004). Interview with Charles R. McCarthy. *Belmont Oral History Project*. Available at http://www.hhs.gov/ohrp/docs/InterviewMcCarthy.doc

Milgram, S. (1974). *Obedience to authority: An experimental view*. Harper and Row.

Morahan, P. S., Yamagata, H., McDade, S., Richman, R., Francis, R., & Odhner, V. C. (2006). New challenges facing interinstitutional social science and educational program evaluation research at academic health centers: A case study from the ELAM Program. *Academic Medicine, 81*, 527–534.

Moyer, J. (1999). *Step-by-step guide to oral history*. Available at http://dohistory.org/on_your_own/toolkit/oralHistory.html#WHATIS

National Commission for the Protection of Human Subjects of Biomedical and Behavioral Research. (1979). *The Belmont report: Ethical principles and guidelines for the protection of human subjects of research*. U.S. Department of Health and Human Services. https://www.hhs.gov/ohrp/regulations-and-policy/belmont-report/read-the-belmont-report/index.html

NBAC. (2001). National Bioethics Advisory Commission. *Ethical and Policy Issues in Research Involving Human Participants. Vol. 1 Report and Recommendations*. 288 p.

NBAC. (2002). National bioethics advisory commission. Research involving persons with mental disorders that may affect decision-making capacity. *Journal International de Bioethique, 13*(3–4), 173–179. PMID: 12747354.

NPRM. (2015). Notice of Proposed Rulemaking. In the *Federal Register* 80(173):53933-54061. Tuesday, Sept. 8, 2015.

NRC (National Research Council). (2003). *Protecting participants and facilitating social and behavioral sciences research*. The National Academies Press. https://doi.org/10.17226/10638

O'Hara, P. (2005). Report on an International Conference on Ethical Issues. In *Behavioural and Social Sciences Research: Forum for Institutional Review Boards (IRBs)/Research Ethics Boards (REBs) in Canada and the United States (FOCUS)*. Montreal, Quebec, Canada — June 3–4, 2005. http://www.ncehr-cnerh.org/english/international/focus/focus_2005_report_e.pdf

OHRP. (2011). Office of human research protections. *Guidance on reporting incidence to OHARP*. Washington, DC. US Dept of Health and Human Services.

Rinde, M. (2019). The Death of Jesse Gelsinger, 20 years later. *Science History*. Retrieved February 13, 2023, from https://www.sciencehistory.org/distillations/the-death-of-jesse-gelsinger-20-years-later

Schrag, Z. M. (2009). How talking became human subjects research: The Federal Regulation of the Social Sciences, 1965–1991. *Journal of Policy History, 21*(1), 3–37.

Schrag, Z. M. (2010). *Ethical Imperialism: Institutional Review Boards and the Social Sciences, 1965–2009*. Johns Hopkins University Press.

Sierra, X. (2011). Ethics in medical research in humans: A historical perspective. *Actas Dermo-Sifiliográficas, 102*(6), 395–401. https://doi.org/10.1016/j.adengl.2011.03.002

Simmons, J. G. (2002). *Doctors and discoveries: Lives that created today's medicine*. Houghton Mifflin Harcourt.

Skolnick, J. H. (1968). Coercion to virtue: The enforcement of morals. *Southern California Law Review, 41*(3).

TCPS-2. (2018). Canadian Institutes of Health Research, Natural Sciences and Engineering Research Council of Canada, and Social Sciences and Humanities Research Council of Canada, *Tri- Council Policy Statement: Ethical Conduct for Research Involving Humans*, December 2018. Retrieved January 12, 2022, from https://ethics.gc.ca/eng/documents/tcps2-2018-en-interactive-final.pdf

Tropp, R. A. (1978). What problems are raised when the current DHEW regulation on protection of human subjects is applied to social science research? In the *Belmont Report* Appendix vol II. 18: 1–16.

Tropp, R. A. (1982). A regulatory perspective on social science research. In T. Beauchamp, R. R. Faden, R. J. Wallace, & L. Walters (Eds.), *Ethical issues in social science research* (pp. 391–415). Johns Hopkins University Press.

Turner, J. H. (2001). Social engineering: Is this really as bad as it sounds? *Sociological Practice, 3*(2), 99–120. https://doi.org/10.1023/A:1011526902178

University of Washington. (n.d.). *International Research*. University of Washington, Seattle, Human Subjects Division. Retrieved January 10, 2022, from https://www.washington.edu/research/hsd/guidance/international-research/

Warwick, D. P. (1982). Types of harm in social research. In T. Beauchamp, R. R. Faden, R. J. Wallace, & L. Walters (Eds.), *Ethical issues in social science research* (pp. 101–124). Johns Hopkins University Press.

Weber, M. (1978). In G. Roth & C. Wittich (Eds.), *Economy and society: An outline of interpretative sociology*. University of California Press.

WMA. (1964). World Medical Association. *Declaration of Helsinki*. Ethical Principles for Medical Research Involving Human Subjects. Available at Declaration of Helsinki - World Health Organization. Retrieved January 8, 2021

Chapter 3
IRBs and Police Power: The Intersection of Law and Ethics

Have them serve as judges for the people at all times, but have them bring every difficult case to you;
the simple cases they can decide themselves.
That will make your load lighter, because they will share it with you.—*Exodus* 18:20

3.1 Introduction

Operating under federal regulations for the Protection of Human Research Subjects (45 CFR 46), IRBs are charged with the protection of the rights and welfare of individuals who are the subjects of biomedical and social behavioral science and education research. IRBs review and approve, modify or deny applications from scientific investigators to conduct such research. They may even suspend or terminate the research.

Most IRBs follow rules and regulations based on guidelines derived from the three basic principles identified in the *Belmont Report* (1978) of the National Commission for the Protection of Human Subjects of Biomedical and Behavioral Research. As readers will recall, the three principles are: (1) Respect for persons: individuals should be treated as competent to make decisions about participating in research, and those with diminished competence are vulnerable and should be protected; (2) Beneficence: The benefits of those who participate in the research should be maximized to protect their well-being; and (3) Justice: individuals should have the same chance of being included in research studies. Those who are eligible to benefit from the research should not be excluded without a good reason or be undeservedly exposed to a higher risk than others.

Robert Klitzman (2011, 2015) interviewed 46 chairs, administrators and members of 34 IRBs. He noted that one of his first interviewees told him that the IRB tries not to be the "Ethics Police." He became interested in how IRBs are perceived and their effectiveness. His 2011 article was titled, "The Ethics Police? IRBs' Views

H. Perlstadt, *Assessing Social Science Research Ethics and Integrity*, Clinical Sociology: Research and Practice, https://doi.org/10.1007/978-3-031-34538-8_3

Concerning Their Power," and his 2015 book, *The Ethics Police? The Struggle to Make Human Research Safe.*

Klitzman was not the first to write on the possible police power of IRBs. Over 20 years earlier, Robert J. Levine, who was on the staff of the National Commission, became concerned that IRBs were at times performing police functions when monitoring and auditing research protocols. He thought that human protection regulations were based on presumptions that require colleagues to police and harass each other because they think there is a high likelihood that any particular other is dishonest. Argument and dialogue, so critical to the existence of the academic community, are impossible in an environment of distrust ... Finally, I am aware of no evidence that such presumptions are associated with a higher frequency of wrong doing. I believe that persons generally behave as they are expected to behave; most of them live up (or down) to the community's expectations (Levine, 1988, p. 349).

This chapter will explore the perception of IRBs as ethics police. It will trace the history of police power and provide some insights into the current system of human research protections, specifically, why it is frustrating for some researchers to work within the system, and why the system is relatively unresponsive to calls for it to become more effective, efficient and user-friendly. It will explore how public policy, accreditation and an external appeal process can limit IRB excesses. A macro or systems perspective shifts the focus from ensuring the ethical behavior of individuals to ensuring the ethical behavior of groups and organizations.

3.1.1 IRBs

IRBs are the means by which the United States protects the interests of research participants and ensures that research is conducted in an ethically acceptable manner. Each IRB addresses local interests and sensibilities through the wording of informed consent documents and procedures that minimize actual and/or perceived risks to the research participants (Baker et al., 2002).

Decision-making bodies such as IRBs are expected to be rational, fair and consistent. Neither the Common Rule (45 CFR 46) promulgated in 1991 and revised in 2018 nor the 1978 *Belmont Report* mention IRBs or how they are to apply research ethics to the proposals they review (Bankert et al., 2022, p. 5). Cornell University (2022) lists seven criteria that IRBs should follow when evaluating research proposals: Importance, Content and Design, Population and Sampling Methodology, Timing, Data Management and Dissemination, Resources and Overall Impact. I conclude that the Belmont Principles are an educational tool and not a requirement for reviewing research proposals.

This means each proposal will be decided on a case-by-case basis according to the specifics of the submitted protocol rather than directly applying a set of ethical principles. Some IRBs have become bureaucracies of virtue (Bosk, 2007), with the head of the IRB making the key decision as the first among equals. Other IRBs, as noted above, are viewed as ethics police (Klitzman, 2011, 2015).

According to Max Weber (1978), a legal rational bureaucracy should select the most efficient means to achieve an end. The characteristics of such a bureaucracy include a decision-making hierarchy with channels of appeal, a consistent system of abstract rules which are applied to particular cases by trained personnel and decisions which are formulated and recorded in writing in order to inform the management of the agency (Weber, 1947, pp. 329–332; Weber, 1978, pp. 957–958).

In addition to IRBs in the United States, other examples of national governments promoting and enforcing research ethics include the REBs in Canada, Research Ethics Committees (RECs) in the United Kingdom and Human Research Ethics Committees (HRECs) in Australia and New Zealand.

These entities are based at universities, hospitals and medical centers that employ researchers and provide them with administrative support and facilities. Several Eastern European countries have national as well as local ethics committees. Some African countries also have local RECs while others are centralized, requiring all health research to be approved by a single REC.

In the United States, the 1973 National Research Act (93-348, 212a) requires that entities conducting biomedical or behavioral research involving human subjects to establish an IRB to review and protect the rights of human subjects in research protocols. The Act granted broad but unspecified power to the Department of Health, Education and Welfare (now Health and Human Services) to interpret and enforce the statute. Under the Administrative Procedure Act, agencies are permitted to promulgate detailed rules and regulations through a rulemaking process involving public comment followed by the publication of final rules and regulations in the *Federal Register*. The courts have held that regulations must be a reasonable interpretation of the underlying statute (*Chevron v Natural Resources Defense Council*, 1984).

Human research protections, then, can be considered to be a form of police power whereby specified procedures for conducting federally funded research involving human participants are delegated to local authorities with discretionary, nonreviewable power of selective enforcement (Davis, 1969; Shweder, 2006). In essence, human research protection does not criminalize researchers' behavior but attempts to control the behavior of individual investigators and prevent undesirable and unethical research activities and practices.

The third edition of the *Institutional Review Board Management and Functions* (Bankert et al., 2022) reflects the 2018 revisions to the Federal Policy for the Protection of Human Subjects (45 CFR 46). It states that:

> IRB institutions have a shared responsibility for creating an institutional culture of ethical research, rather than a culture of mere compliance. Institution, policies, procedures and practices that emphasize ethical principles will encourage well-conceived and properly executed research and may help mitigate the view of IRBs as the "ethics police" (Bankert et al., 2022, p. 15).

In a similar vein, Steven Peckman (2006, pp. 17–18), the associate director for administration and planning at the UCLA Institute for Stem Cell Research and Medicine, focuses on shared responsibility. He wrote that when scientists, society and individual human subjects acknowledge their shared ethical responsibilities at the institutional and federal levels, a balance of interests is reached which creates a culture of trust. This facilitates the review and conduct of human research in an ethical and collegial environment. He noted that a breakdown at any level of compliance will weaken the protection of human subjects, erode the public's trust in scientific research and result in a demand for broader and strong regulation and oversights.

Furthermore, IRBs can work closely with researchers to ensure that the application of polices is fair to the investigators and to contribute to ethics research education within their institution and the public. They can become resource centers for information concerning ethical standards and federal requirements and communicate with federal officials and other IRBs about matters of common concern (Peckman, 2006, p. 18).

In most cases, differences over a research protocol are resolved through negotiations between the researcher and their IRB. Until the 2018 revisions to 45 CFR 46, investigators collaborating on multisite studies often had to negotiate with each investigator's IRB to gain approval for protocols, with only minor differences in the wording of informed consent or incentives to participate in the study.

Since only a few protocols are ultimately disapproved, most researchers view the IRB process as their private trouble. In general, people do not usually link their private work troubles to broader matters concerning social policy (Mills, 1959, p. 8). Most make the required changes, while a few withdraw their research proposal. In doing so, they accept the institutionalized ethical values of protecting the rights and welfare of human subject research participants. According to N.H. Steneck, these shared ethical values concerning the responsible conduct of research include: honesty in conveying information truthfully, accuracy in reporting findings and avoiding errors, efficiently using resources wisely and objectivity by letting the facts speak for themselves and avoiding improper bias (Steneck, 2007, pp. 2–3).

The Department of Health and Human Services (HHS) first issued rules and regulations governing human research protections (*45 CFR 46*) in 1981. In order to receive federal funds, institutions carrying out research involving human subjects must have an IRB. Five individuals are the minimum for a review panel, but most are much larger to ensure the needed expertise, especially for reviewing social behavioral and education research proposals. One must be a scientist, preferably with expertise in the area of the research, who can assess the scientific validity of the hypothesis and/or proposed methodology; one, a nonscientist whose professional experience includes no direct involvement in any scientific work; and one, an unaffiliated member who is often referred to as the community member. These two roles can be filled by a single IRB member. If the research involves a vulnerable population, e.g., children, cognitively impaired persons or prisoners, the review panel should include someone who is knowledgeable about and experienced in working with that population.

The regulations do not address term limits or length of service for IRB members or chairs. For that and other reasons, the IRB system is not easy to revise (Williams, 2005). For instance, although HHS has the authority to amend *45 CFR 46*, such changes would only apply to HHS funded research since other federal departments and agencies would have to agree to such changes. This was accomplished in 1991 with the establishment of the *Common Rule*, when 14 (now 20) federal departments and agencies adopted suggested changes into their own CFRs, e.g., Department of Education (*34 CFR 97*), Agriculture (7 CFR 1c) and Environmental Protection Agency (*40 CFR 1230*). In 2018, the Common Rule (*45 CFR 46*) was revised to better protect human subjects involved in research while easing the burden on investigators and making the IRB process more efficient and effective.

Until the 2018 revisions, one IRB did not have to accept a protocol for a multisite study approved by another IRB at a different university, hospital or research institution. For example, if researchers at three different universities are collaborating on a grant to study smoking prevention efforts in middle schools, one researcher's IRB may require active parental consent in the form of a signed card before their child can be approached directly with respect to the research. A second IRB may allow researchers to offer an incentive, such as throwing a pizza party for each eighth-grade class where 90 percent have returned a signed consent form. A third researcher's IRB may accept a "passive" parental consent whereby a child may participate as long as their parents did not return a form indicating their lack of consent (see Bachman & Schutt, 2017, p. 79).

Under the revised rules, when the research is utilizing the same research protocol, one participating site agrees to be the IRB of record. It will review the proposal and the other participating sites will cede oversight to the IRB of record.

3.2 Folkway, Mores and Laws

To better understand the perception of IRBs as "ethics police," this chapter now turns to discussing ways of regulating human behavior.

Social values evolve over time from folkways to mores to law (Sumner, 1907). The term folkways was coined by William Graham Sumner, a professor of sociology (the first in the United States) as well as politics at Yale College, and president of the American Sociological Association from 1908 to 1909. He coined the term to denote the habits and customs of a society. Folkways are the traditional accepted ways of doing things, often learned from childhood and are universally followed within a group or society. Examples include dressing appropriately for work or religious services, displaying suitable manners at public gatherings or using proper language. Folkways are part of a culture in that they emerge out of the repetition and routines of daily life.

As distinct from folkways, social mores, according to Sumner, are unformulated and undefined, reflecting the nonrational sentiments and beliefs of the society or group. Over time, certain social mores may become more definite and value laden by labeling actions as right or wrong. Forbidden actions may be subject to sanctions and penalties. Some become enshrined in religious codes of ethics, others enacted into laws, and still others formalized as discretionary regulations to protect the safety and welfare of a local community.

Local control, to give one example, involves cities, counties or states requiring bars to close at a specific hour, e.g., midnight or 4 a.m. Sumner concluded that expediency determined whether to place control in the hands of the local community or the state.

Philosopher Alasdair MacIntyre (1980) discussed the need to balance a regard for virtue and community with the need to protect individuals from each other and from government regulations. He considers regulation as the minimal means and law as the last resort to promote virtue. Ideally, regulations should enable individuals to behave better by reinforcing a moral community within a profession, institution or corporation. MacIntyre states that a new moral concern first emerges in incoherent and inchoate ways, resulting in a set of phases that will transform the concern into both individual and civic virtue.

In contrast, Max Weber (1978, p. 34) focused on the formal and legalistic aspects of social mores, which he termed social conventions. He thought that they were externally guaranteed by the probability that deviation from them within a social group will result in a general reaction of disapproval. But the more law like the social conventions, the greater the probability that a staff of people, including administrative officials, such as police and judges, will be expected to enforce them. According to Weber, bureaucracy slowly emerges in closed social groups like the clan, firm, school or church.

Some groups and societies were repressive and punishment oriented in the belief that labeling violators as deviant and making them suffer for their transgressions would serve as a deterrent to others, a belief that has been scrutinized by many artists and thinkers, e.g., Nathaniel Hawthorne in his *The Scarlet Letter*. In modern society, individuals who do not follow the social mores of such groups are usually disciplined in an attempt to change their behavior. Some examples of disciplinary actions are a teenager being grounded, a worker being suspended, a student being sent to detention or a congregant being shunned (Rothe, 1998).

Legislatively enacted laws can be considered as a set of special rules for the purpose of determining which behavior will be enforced and punished when the executive branch uses coercive power, e.g., the Federal Bureau of Investigation or National Guard. Moral rules in contrast identify acceptable social interactions and practices that community members are obliged to follow, which will be enforced through friendly persuasion or peer pressure.

3.2.1 *Types of Law*

Weber (1978, p. 654ff) identifies four types of law: formally rational, substantively rational, formally irrational and substantively irrational. Rational laws follow general criteria applicable to all cases; under irrational law, there is no guarantee that all similar cases are dealt with in the same way. Formal laws apply rules and procedures within any given legal system, while substantive laws apply external criteria outside a formal system. Under formally rational law, only unambiguous characteristics of the facts of the case are taken into account through the logical analysis of meaning and applying an abstract legal proposition found in a constitution, existing legislation or judicial decisions, e.g., case law, to guarantee uniformity and continuity in the legal system.

In substantively rational law, the decision is influenced by norms different from those obtained through logical generalization of abstract interpretations of meaning. These norms include ethical imperatives, utilitarian and other expediential rules, and political maxims. For example, under Roman Catholic canon law, the rules are organized around extralegal principles and the legal order itself is subservient to religious and political orders (Savelsberg, 2018, p. 494).

Laws are formally irrational when they are not controlled by intellect but instead decided by oracles; by public, religious or political show trials, in which the judicial authorities have already determined the guilt or innocence of the defendant; or by khadi justice, where cases are not decided on precedent resulting in verdicts in similar cases that vary widely. Laws are substantively irrational "to the extent that the decision is influenced by the concrete factors of the particular case as evaluated upon an ethical, emotional or political basis rather than by general norms" (Weber, 1978, p. 656).

An example of a substantively irrational law is the Three Strikes and You're Out rule for mandatory sentencing. It came from baseball, where the batter is out if the umpire calls a third strike. This extra-legal standard was the basis for a 1994 California law. The law requires a minimum sentence of 25 years to life for a defendant who has been convicted of two prior felonies from an enumerated list of violent and serious felonies (Vitiello, 2004, p. 1).

In early 1995, a District Court of Appeals in San Diego ruled that judges may not dismiss prior felony convictions in setting prison terms (Legislative Analyst's Office, 1995). The political agenda behind the "Three Strikes Law" was to allay the fears of many politicians and their constituents that they were soft on crime. They made the law difficult to amend by requiring a super-majority to do so (Vitiello, 2004, p. 4).

IRBs share a number of the features that characterize these different types of law, regulation and ethics. In making decisions, IRBs must develop and follow written procedures that comply with federal law and institutional policies. For example, the concrete factors in a particular research protocol would include the following: documentation of the equitable selection of research subjects, what risks to subjects are reasonable in relation to anticipated benefits, an informed consent process with sufficient information to enable a person to make a knowledgeable decision whether or not to voluntarily participate in the research, as well as proposed measures to protect the privacy and dignity of subjects, and safeguard any vulnerable subjects.

Interestingly, nowhere does the *Common Rule* (*45 CFR 46*) explicitly mention the *Belmont Report* or its three ethical principles of respect for persons, beneficence and justice. It states (45 CFR 46 §103(b)1) that each research institution must submit a statement of principles for protecting the rights and welfare of human subjects that may include an appropriate existing code (presumably The Nuremberg Code), declaration (presumably The Helsinki Declaration), statement of ethical principles (presumably *The Belmont Report*) or a statement formulated by the institution itself (Vanderpool, 2001, p. 10).

Rosenfeld (2020, p. 11) points out that the decision and minutes of the initial IRB review of a submission often contain minimal information to guide any subsequent continuing review of that research. This means that without easy access to prior decisions and their rationales, subsequent IRB panels may render inconsistent decisions. This could result in substantively irrational decisions based on each panel's interpretation and application of the regulations and ethical principles at the time of its review.

Peckman (2006, p. 17) called this "the Belmont Circle," which links interactions among IRBs' members and support staff, investigators, sponsors/funders and federal agencies in a circular horizontal fashion rather than as a hierarchy. All parties are obligated to uphold the letter and spirit of *The Belmont Report*. He added that:

> Using various ethical codes and regulations, they create an environment that ensures the protection of human subjects as well as the advancement of science. The collaboration must exist in a culture of trust, complete openness, and honesty. By upholding the highest ethical principles and standards, they build public support for the pursuit of greater knowledge in a safe research environment (Peckman, 2006, p. 18).

Peckman holds that the investigator, the IRB and the institutional official who is legally authorized to act on behalf of the institution, e.g., the Vice President for Research, are expected to play a role to ensure accountability. Fordham University, for instance, states that:

> In accordance with CFR 46.112, University officials may not approve of a research study if it has not been approved by the IRB nor may they overturn a final determination of disapproval. University officials may, however, disapprove of an IRB-approved study being conducted at or affiliated with Fordham. Officials may also impose additional restrictions or stipulations to an approved study but may not amend the IRB's terms of approval or take any actions that serve to lessen any measures deemed necessary for protection of human subjects in research (Fordham University, n.d.).

The IRB Chair or Director may review the researcher's statement that the proposed research is of minimal risk to the participants. Such proposals can be declared exempt research if they use commonly accepted educational practices conducted in a standard school setting, anonymous surveys, interviews, observation studies that are not "sensitive," or analyses of existing, deidentified or publicly available data.

In contrast, expedited reviews may be conducted if the proposal includes "sensitive" interviews or surveys, or analyses of identifiable data collected from voice, video, digital or image recordings made for research purposes by anthropologists, psychologists or sociologists who employ ethnomethodology. These must involve no more than minimal risk to subjects that are not greater than those ordinarily encountered in daily life (Michigan State University, n.d.).

A survey of 886 experienced biomedical and social and behavioral scientists by Keith-Spiegel et al. (2006, p. 73) found that social and behavioral researchers were more concerned about the competence of their IRB administrative staff to make the distinction between exempt and nonexempt research than biomedical researchers. The regulations are complicated and an in-depth understanding of the terms and definitions is necessary in order to properly apply them (OHRP-E, n.d.).

From a social science perspective, accountability means that a person, group or institution is responsible for a set of duties. They can be required to give an account of their activities, outcomes and consequences to an individual or organization that is in a position to issue rewards or punishment (Castiglione, 2012). Political scientist Guillermo O'Donnell (1998, p. 119) argued that in order for horizontal accountability to be effective in the absence of a hierarchy, one of the parties must be authorized and willing to oversee, control, address and, if necessary, sanction unlawful actions by one of the other parties. He would agree that the parties must be part of an interacting network committed to upholding the regulations governing the protection of human subjects. This suggests that the parties should agree on a way to have a system of checks and balances in order to rectify a possible imbalance that may have arisen within the culture of shared trust, including overreach by the IRB itself.

These checks and balances may be of higher concern to social behavioral scientists because they focus on interpersonal issues, matters of equity and organizational performance in their teaching and research. The social behavioral and education research environment may be more skeptical of authority than the medical research environment of medical schools, centers, hospitals and outpatient clinics.

3.3 Police Power

US Supreme Court Justice Stephen Field wrote that under the US Constitution, states have the right "to prescribe regulations to promote the health, peace, morals, education, and good order of the people" (Field, 1885, p. 31). In turn, counties, cities or townships are delegated police powers to pass laws or regulations governing and enforcing zoning, speed limits, retail liquor sales and public health.

Contrary to Sumner's theory, police power in France did not develop directly from folkways and social mores but, like Moses in *Exodus*, as a way for a central government to delegate control over everyday matters to local authorities. It was the first country in Europe to create a local police to enforce the policies of the monarch, in this case, Louis XIV (Bayley and Perito, 2011).

In 1666, Jean Baptiste Colbert, the Controller-General of Finances for Louis XIV, created the Council of Police of Paris and asked them to come up with a system for controlling the book trade with the goal of reducing the number of printers to only a sanctioned few (Novak, 2002). One of the 44 commissioners, Nicolas Delamare, a former high-level judicial officer of administrative law, began a treatise on the history of police and public administration. By "police," Delamare meant the ways of governing a city or "polis" (Korkman, 2007, p. 24). Delamare identified 11 areas of police regulation and administration, some of which are still governed by local ordinances including manners (and morals), health, provisions (food and drink), travel (roads and highways) and commerce and trade (Novak, 2002, p. 191). Unfortunately, Delamare died before he could complete the work, and one of the unfinished chapters was to explore police power with respect to science and the liberal arts (Foucault, 2007, p. 359).

In the United States, the enforcement of public rules and regulations that are delegated to local government and nongovernment entities to benefit the local community is known as police power (West's, 2005). In 1885, the US Supreme Court recognized that "it would be an extraordinary usurpation of the authority of a municipality (City of San Francisco), if a federal tribunal should undertake to supervise such regulations" (Barbier v. Connolly, 1885, p. 30) to prohibit public laundries from operating between ten o'clock at night until six o'clock in the morning to prevent fires. Furthermore, counties, cities or townships are delegated the ability to pass laws or regulations governing zoning, water supply sanitation and public health. Similarly, it would be inappropriate for a federal department or agency to directly supervise a research institution and its IRBs, or receive appeals of IRB decisions.

Several states permit the delegation of police power to nongovernmental entities such as private security companies (North Carolina), solid waste management authorities (New York) or nonprofit community development corporations (New Jersey).

By extension, research institutions and their IRBs have police power to protect the subjects of biomedical and behavioral research. However, while IRB procedures are specified in *45 CFR 46*, their decisions are not based on ordinances but rather on moral and ethical principles, i.e., substantively irrational law.

In general, courts are often called upon to determine whether adequate safeguards exist to guide the exercise and administration of delegated power (*NJ Firefighters Mutual Benefit Association vs N. Hudson Reg. Fire & Rescue*, 2001, pp. 52–53). Federal courts have held that such laws cannot be contrary to federal law (Prigg v. Pennsylvania, *41 U.S. 539,* 1842). To some extent, this is moral federalism under which the federal and state governments do not get involved with, or take responsibility for, local community matters such as inculcating virtue, keeping the peace and encouraging civic participation (Hendrickson, 2002). One example of moral federalism is the US Supreme Court decision allowing prosecution of obscenity under contemporary community rather than national standards (Miller v. California, *413 US 15*, 1973).

At the turn of the twentieth century, legal scholars carefully considered the nature of police power in the United States. John W. Burgess (1890, p. 215), a faculty member at the Columbia University Law School and the founder of *Political Science Quarterly,* wrote that police power is essentially administrative in nature, and that the community in its most local organization should participate, so far as possible, in the exercise of police power.

Ernst Freund (1904, pp. 3–7), a professor of political science and law at the University of Chicago, thought that police power allowed the state to exercise its compulsory power to prevent and anticipate an individual's failure to conform her or his actions due another person, business organization or social standard, by moving beyond common law and social mores (see Sumner above), but not making those actions statutory crimes. He held that every individual must submit to such restraints on his liberty in order to remove or reduce the likelihood of abuse by those who are unskillful, careless or unscrupulous. He noted that the police power is not a fixed quantity, but reflects the social, economic and political conditions in the community.

This means that the police power must be elastic and changeable and will vary from community to community.

He went on to explore police power with respect to science and the liberal arts, aspects not addressed by Delamare. Freund (1904, p. 223) wrote that the investigation and publication of truth for the promotion of human knowledge is the essence of science and must be beyond the interference of the police power.

However, every true fact is not always a contribution to science, so a set of ordinances and regulations will furnish the safest guide.

In the United States, with respect to medical, social and behavioral science research, that safest guide begins with the federal government, which must provide research institutions and their IRBs with adequate guidelines and regulations to ensure the proper administration of their delegated functions. The Common Rule (*45 CFR 46* §103(a) and (b)) requires every institution engaged in human subjects research to provide a satisfactory assurance that it will comply with the regulations and certify that the research has been reviewed and approved by an IRB designated in the assurance. However, the NBAC (2001, p. 1) found that "the federal protections were difficult to enforce and improve effectively across the government, in part, because no single authority or office oversees research protections across all federal agencies and departments."

In 2008, the Department of Health and Human Services (HHS) addressed this concern in creating the FWA. It is a legally binding agreement which standardized the assurance process and centralized oversight in the HHS OHRP (2008). OHRP required that in order to receive federal funding for research, each research institution must first create or identify an institutional or external IRB and then register it with OHRP. Once registered, the institution applies for an FWA from OHRP so that it may receive federal support from any government agency or department for research involving human subjects. Each Institution must renew its FWA every 5 years, even if no changes have occurred, in order to maintain an active FWA. After a research institution submits all of the documentation OHRP requires, it is committed to continue to comply with the *Common Rule* (45 CFR 46).

Despite the Common Rule, no single federal authority directly oversees research protections across all federal agencies and departments. The regulations, which are complicated, are interpreted and applied by each IRB. This is a classic example of delegated police powers to local research institutions and their IRBs to oversee the protection of research with human subjects. The FWA five year renewal requirement, even if no changes have occurred, is a soft check on IRBs.

3.3.1 Bureaucracies of Virtue

Sumner's shift from folkways to mores to law requires the development of an organization of specialists to manage and ensure that a formal set of rules and regulations are impersonally carried out. This is, in Max Weber's terms, a bureaucracy. IRBs follow a set of ethically driven criteria to impersonally review a research proposal. Legal scholars Jacob and Riles (2007, p. 181) coined the term "bureaucracies of virtue" to describe the bureaucratization of research ethics in the United States, which they saw as developing out of efforts to establish and closely document its principles and procedures.

According to Lincoln and Tierney (2004, pp. 219, 223), IRBs make qualitative and participatory action research undergo numerous revisions in an attempt to make them appear more conventional. They suggest that some IRB members expect the proposals to resemble what they consider to be sound research, that is, to be like clinical and biomedical proposals.

Sociologist Charles Bosk (2007, pp. 194, 197–198) noted that those IRB members, who are accustomed to reviewing protocols for randomized clinical trials, may perceive qualitative social science and ethnomethodology research proposals as a grab bag of questions from which the investigator may choose to study after early observations in the field, and therefore may require revising the protocol and informed consent documents. The problem, according to Bosk (2007, pp. 198, 201–202), can be boiled down to what Robert Merton (1957, pp. 199–201) termed goal displacement, where people follow bureaucratic rules and regulations for their own sake rather than working toward the larger organizational goals or mission. Organization members prioritize and even sanctify the means or operating rules and procedures. They focus on the wording of consent procedures and the proximal risks and benefits to the individual subjects, which are to be judged against local community standards. For Bosk, their goal displacement is akin to Weber's concept of substantive rationality, which centers on the ultimate goals of an organization or society.

Meanwhile, IRB staffs bureaucratized. They formed their own professional association and developed accreditation for their training and programs (Dingwall, 2012, pp. 13–14). The Association for the Accreditation of Human Research Protection Programs (AAHRPP) was founded by seven nonprofit organizations that represent the leadership of universities, medical schools and teaching hospitals; biomedical, behavioral and social scientists; IRB professionals; and patient and disease advocacy organizations. Its accreditation program was officially launched in 2002 and the first accreditations were awarded in 2003.

Technically, IRBs can be considered quasi-nongovernment organizations (quangos), an entity that has some legal relation or association, however tenuous, to the federal government (Kosar, 2011). They are "organizations that utilize private sector methods to achieve public aims in the most efficient manner possible. They are hybrids and quasi in every respect: quasi-independent, quasi-public, quasi-private, quasi-legitimate and quasi-accountable" (Flinders, 1999, pp. 3–4).

IRBs are empowered with very broad discretion to exercise their administrative authority within the bounds of the Common Rule (Shelton, 1999). The several thousand IRBs scattered across the United States make decisions based on ethical principles that are not always consistent or evenly applied. As a result, their decisions are, in Weber's terms, substantively rational (*Wertrational*). They appear to be oriented to the protection of human subjects at the expense of advancing scientific knowledge that could benefit society.

When combined with excessive paperwork and expanding obligations to review protocols that pose little risk to subjects, the result is mission creep that could compromise the central goals that motivated the long formation of IRBs in the first place (Gunsalus et al., 2006).

Furthermore, forming quangos and granting them police power shifts the responsibility of dealing with sensitive issues from the national political agenda and party politics, to nongovernmental entities (Flinders, 1999). The main exceptions are federal funding for research involving fetal tissue transplants, *in vitro* fertilization and human embryonic stems cells (Boonstra, 2001).

3.3.2 A Collegial IRB

According to Weber (1978, pp. 36, 325), an ethical standard contains a certain type of value which can become a valid norm governing social actions. Such ethical beliefs are generally upheld by social or legal sanctions or by police. Only an abstract standard of conduct subjectively conceived as derived from ultimate axioms or principles, Weber suggested, could be regarded as an exclusively ethical norm and would significantly determine one's conduct. In contrast to the legal order, social norms and conventions lack specialized personnel who enforce the standard, e.g., priests, judges or police.

An ethical and collegial environment facilitates the review and conduct of human research (Peckman, 2006, p. 17). Sociologist Malcom Waters (1989, pp. 946–947, 969), in his survey of the literature on collegiality as a type of organization, noted that Weber (1978, pp. 272–278, 997) focused on monocratic bureaucracy with a leader and staff that is more efficient and effective than collegial bureaucracy. Waters considered both to be rational organizational forms that utilize technical expertise to realize specific goals.

Weber gave 13 examples of collegial bureaucracy, some of which serve to limit the powers of a monocratic chief. This may occur when a central state transfers decision-making to subordinate or local authorities because the decision requires a thoroughness that is often missing when making a decision. In some instances, the good decision-maker needs to know and explore all possibilities in order to decide when the maximum benefit is satisficing, that is, when it is pursuing the minimum satisfactory condition or outcome (see Simon, 1956, p. 136). An administrative action may be legitimated by the cooperation of a plurality of people unanimously or by majority vote. IRBs have such devolved decision-making powers.

Waters (1989, p. 965) identified several characteristics of an ideal-typical collegiality that can be applied to IRBs. Formal autonomy would enable researchers and IRBs, without bureaucratic interference, to meet transcendental ethical standards, in part through self-policing. Collective decision-making by faculty colleagues would promote trust among the institution's researchers and minimize their career self-interests for the collective good of scientific research.

The Collaborative Institutional Training Initiative (CITI Program) at the University of Miami, Coral Gables, FL, was founded in 2000 with a focus on biomedical research, but in 2004 added social, behavioral and education research. It covers major topics on protecting human subjects and uses case studies as examples. Robert Amdur, MD (2003), published the first edition of *Institutional Review Board: Member Handbook*, which provided practical information for IRB members to prepare for and participate in full IRB committee meetings.

The *Handbook* contains an IRB Reviewer Template which links specific criteria for IRB approval with the Belmont Principles of beneficence, respect for persons and justice. This helps IRB members apply the principles to the protocol being reviewed. Beneficence is assessed by investigator qualifications, conflict of interest, subject recruitment, payment or reimbursement, risk/benefit analysis, potential benefit to the subjects and data oversight. Respect for persons is assessed by the vulnerability of subjects, written or surrogate informed consent, costs, confidentiality including data monitoring and stopping rules, as well as consent documents that describe the essential protocol elements so that they can be understood by the expected subject population. Justice is assessed by whether subject selection is likely to be equitable. The final IRB decision should inform the researcher where the protocol failed to meet specific criteria and which principles would need to be addressed in a revision.

3.4 Limiting IRB Excesses

Codes of research ethics are responses to major scandals in biomedicine and social and behavioral sciences. If successfully adopted and implemented, they seek to reestablish responsibility, trust and institutional legitimacy through new social and political arrangements (Metcalf, 2014, p. 1). Key examples this book has noted include the 1947 Nuremberg Code, the 1964 WMA's Helsinki Declaration and, in the United States, the passage of the 1973 National Research Act, and subsequently, the promulgation of the *Belmont Report*. While research ethics can be successfully implemented, they can also be unsuccessfully implemented, as this chapter and Chap. 2 have demonstrated. In the case of IRBs, the challenge is how to limit their excesses.

After attending the Summit of Psychological Sciences with the theme "IRBs: All Checks and No Balances," Jeffrey Cohen (1999, p. 6), the newly appointed Association Director for Education in the OPRR, identified a need to improve the review process at the local level, regularize IRB procedures that were resulting in a lack of consistency and a wide variation in the interpretation of the regulations within a given IRB and educate IRB members and researchers on ethical issues, the related regulations and best practices and the appeal process. These aims would eventually be met through public policy and accreditation and certification, but attempts to establish an appeal process would fail.

3.4.1 Public Policy

In July 1972, Jean Heller published an article exposing the unethical methods in an ongoing US Public Health study of untreated syphilis among Black male sharecroppers in Macon County, AL (Chap. 4). In February 1973, Sen. Hubert Humphrey introduced the National Human Experimentation Standards Board Act, a bill to create an independent board to establish guidelines for experiments involving human beings funded by the Federal government. The Board would review all planned medical experiments to determine if the guidelines established are being complied with and to obtain an injunction to prevent such experimentation when the experiment is found not to comply.

Had this been enacted, it would have centralized the review of all biomedical research proposals into a single federal agency. Senator Edward Kennedy then sponsored the National Research Act, which established the National Commission for the Protection of Human Subjects of Biomedical and Behavioral Research. The Council produced the *Belmont Report.*

The end result was to place federal oversight, not in a single national regulatory board, but in those federal agencies funding research involving human subjects (ACHRE, 1995, pp. 180–181). In turn, HEW (1979) published proposed regulations which would delegate authority and oversight to research institutions and their IRBs and shifted operating costs to the research institutions. Granting research institutions police power and shifting the operating costs for research regulation, review and enforcement saved the federal government time and money as well as not getting enmeshed in local community beliefs, interests and sensibilities concerning research ethics.

As discussed in Chap. 2, some social scientists were skeptical that this grant of police power to research institutions and their IRBs was in their best interests. Among them was MIT political science professor Ithiel de Sola Pool. After he wrote an op-ed piece for the *New York Times* in December 1979, Pool received a letter from Antonin Scalia, then a law professor at the University of Chicago, who would be appointed to the US Supreme Court in 1986. Scalia wrote that as an IRB member himself, he was "disturbed by the authority I find myself and my colleagues wielding over the most innocuous sorts of intellectual inquiry" (Schrag, 2010, p. 104). Although the interests of the social and behavioral sciences were championed by well-known and respected scholars and researchers, at the time, most social science researchers had little if any interactions with IRBs.

In November 1980, Ronald Reagan, who opposed increased regulations, was elected President. This short-circuited attempts to revise the 45 CFR 46. The January

1981 revised regulations contained several compromises (Schrag, 2009, p. 17ff; Moreno, 2005). It no longer required but strongly recommended that any institution receiving PHS funds review all human subjects research to be carried out by their researchers, regardless of funding source. It expanded the categories of exempt research involving little or no risk of harm to participants to include some interviews and survey research (unless subjects could be identified and a breach of confidentiality might invoke legal liability for the respondent), and purely observational research in most public contexts.

3.4.2 Accreditation and Certification

It would take another ten years, from 1981 to 1991, to revise 45 CFR 46. It became the Common Rule when 15 federal departments and agencies agreed to follow the Department of Health and Human Services (HHS) research regulations. Meanwhile the question was how to enforce the HHS rules and ensure that research institutions and their IRBs were in compliance.

A February 5, 1993, memorandum from the director of the Office of Protection from Research Risks (OPRR) stated that if an institution was found not to be in compliance with the Department of Health and Human Services (DHSS) regulations or PHS policy, then OPRR can impose a range of sanctions (McCarthy, 1995). The sanctions ranged from a letter of reprimand to suspension of some or all research projects to declaring the investigator ineligible for HHS supported research.

In 1998, the Office of the Inspector General of Health and Human Services (OIG) issued a series of reports on IRBs. The first, *Institutional Review Boards: Their Role in Reviewing Approved Research* (OIG, 1998a, p. 12) noted that the substantive continuing review of ongoing research projects is regarded with suspicion at best, and was counterproductive at worst. Many of the IRB officials interviewed for the report and a review of the literature strongly suggested that any movement toward IRBs becoming "watchdogs" or "policing" could undermine their credibility.

The second report, *Institutional Review Boards: A Time for Reform* (OIG, 1998b) recommended increasing IRB awareness of on-site research practices involving human subjects. While acknowledging that this might be interpreted as surveillance and policing that could compromise the research enterprise, the report argued that trust alone does not provide sufficient continuing protection. It concluded that additional verification of IRB activities is allowable under current federal regulations and is consistent with the intent of the National Commission that laid the groundwork for those regulations.

In response to the OIG report, the Association of American Medical Colleges (AAMC, 1998) contended that the report presumed a policing or auditing role that was inconsistent with the mission articulated for IRBs in the *Belmont Report*. The AAMC noted that the current system had worked remarkably well and was not on the verge of collapse. It argued that the alarmist tone in some sections of the OIG report should be revised to make the level of concern proportional to the magnitude of the problems identified and that the text suggesting an auditing or policing role for IRBs should be eliminated.

The first report noted that the Commission had recommended that federal law permit HEW to establish a single office that would accredit IRBs. The accreditation would include documenting an IRB's membership, staff, meeting facilities, review and monitoring procedures, provisions for recordkeeping and their compliance activities. The accrediting office could conduct site visits and audits of IRB records, in order to examine the performance of the boards and their fulfillment of institutional assurance and regulatory requirements. But 45 CFR 46 lacked any mention of accreditation, audits or site visits, and, by omission, gave OPRR great discretion in developing compliance policies and procedures.

OPRR responded to the OIG reports, complaints from patient groups and congressional criticism that federal protections for human research subjects are inadequate or poorly enforced, as well as criticisms of the slow pace of some of its investigations (Weiss, 1999). From 1990 to mid-1995, OPRR imposed some type of restriction on an institution's authority to conduct human subject research 17 times (GAO, 1996). In the spring of 1999, OPRR shut down or suspended research activities at the Veterans Administration Greater Los Angeles Healthcare System (Puglisi, 1999), Duke University Medical Center (Weiss, 1999), University of Illinois, Chicago, and Virginia Commonwealth University. In September 1999, the Food and Drug Administration suspended human gene therapy experiments at the University of Pennsylvania following the death of 18-year-old Jesse Gelsinger in a clinical trial (Institute of Medicine, 2001, p. 31).

A few months later, OPRR was replaced by the OHRP. In 2006, it suspended all federally funded research projects at Bluefield State College, a small historically black commuter college in southeastern West Virginia, because the college had approved three faculty research projects without having a legitimate IRB (Guess, 2007). It suspended a research study involving almost 200 children on the NIH campus in Bethesda because it presented a risk to the children (Weiss, 2009).

As the debate over how best to regulate research continued, the Institute of Medicine (IOM, 2001, pp. 45–47) weighed in, noting that accreditation can be an alternative to government oversight. Universities and colleges as well as schools of medicine, nursing and social work have accreditation systems in place. Some advantages to this alternative are that the government is not directly involved in establishing the criteria for and awarding of accreditation and that accreditation is paid for by user fees and not taxes. An independent accreditation organization has more leeway to modify and improve its standards than federal agencies carrying out mandatory programs. Disadvantages are that the accreditation system is not accountable to the public and that the process may be self-serving or unduly influenced by the entities being accredited.

The Institute of Medicine (IOM, 2001, pp. 47, 55, 58) contended that accreditation can require educational training for IRB members, staff and researchers that could change norms and behaviors, thereby improving the overall climate of research ethics at the institution (Institute of Medicine, 2001, pp. 47, 55, 58). If accredited institutions and their IRBs are deemed to be in compliance with respect to structure, policies and procedures, federal agencies can then focus on investigating violations and issuing sanctions.

In 1999, Public Responsibility in Medicine and Research (PRIM&R) endorsed the concepts of accreditation of institutions and certification of administrators/staff conducting human subjects research. A working group was formed and its preliminary draft presented to the Institute of Medicine (IOM) in December 2000. The IOM recommended that a nongovernment organization develop the accreditation process and should decide on either a single set of standards for all research institutions or on different standards for different kinds of research institutions (IOM, 2001, p. 15). This resulted in establishing the AAHRPP in 2001.

At the same time, the Association of American Medical Colleges (AAMC) became concerned about the growing adverse publicity about the integrity of research conducted at academic medical centers. The AAMC and the American Medical Association (AMA) sponsor the Liaison Committee on Medical Education (LCME) which accredits all M.D.-granting institutions in the United States and Canada. After consulting with PRIM&R, the AAMC agreed to be the signatory and holder of the original loan to establish AAHRPP as well as spending 18 months lining up support from six other professional organizations including the Association of Public and Land-grant Universities (APLU), the Consortium of Social Science Associations (COSSA) and National Health Council (Mather & Hartnett, 2008).

Meanwhile, the debate over how best to regulate research continued. The Institute of Medicine (IOM, 2001, pp. 45–47) weighed in, noting that accreditation can be an alternative to government oversight. Universities and colleges as well as schools of medicine, nursing and social work have accreditation systems in place. Some advantages to this alternative are that the government is not directly involved in establishing the criteria for and awarding of accreditation and that accreditation is paid for by user fees and not taxes. An independent accreditation organization has more leeway to modify and improve its standards than federal agencies carrying out mandatory programs.

The AAHRPP (2020) accreditation established performance standards in three domains: Organization, IRB or Ethics Committee and Researcher and Research Staff. The standards require compliance with all applicable laws, regulations, codes and guidance, and clearly reflect 45 CFR 46. Researchers and staff are expected to adhere to ethical principles and standards appropriate for their discipline. The accreditation is voluntary, although its recognition by OHRP and the accreditation of major universities and research centers has encouraged others to seek accreditation. AAHRPP had accredited over 600 entities worldwide, including all major independent IRBs in the United States. More than 70 percent of US medical colleges and 85 percent of the top US NIH-funded academic medical centers are either accredited or have begun the accreditation process.

Klitzman (2015, pp. 344–346) found that while accreditation forces IRBs to self-evaluate their procedures and policies, which can be helpful in identifying gaps, it often focuses on paperwork. He noted that some wanted the accreditation agency to directly confront the large differences in the content of committee decisions. The real problem, according to one IRB chair he interviewed, is that many IRBs do not have a good understanding of the regulations or how to apply them. Another IRB chair thought that what was needed was the equivalent of a Law or Court Reporter that contains judicial opinions from previous court decisions of similar cases.

Like federal Court Reporters, an IRB Case Reporter would consist of selected IRB decisions from medical schools and the 131 Carnegie R1 Doctoral Universities with very high research activity. A case report would include the IRB's interpretation of *45 CFR 46* requirements and application of ethical principles to the specific protocol under review. An IRB Case Reporter could serve as a reference for IRBs when making a decision and for researchers questioning or appealing their IRB's decision. It would provide precedent for deciding subsequent appealed cases involving identical or similar facts, or similar ethical issues. Currently this may be difficult since IRBs are only required to retain IRB records and documents for at least three years.

Were IRBs to adopt the Law or Court Report model, the move would effectively incorporate Cohen's (1999, p. 6) suggestion that identifying best practices could reduce the variability in IRB reviews. IRB staff and members would become more familiar with the regulations and how to interpret and apply them. A small measure of Weber's formally rational law could be introduced into the IRB decision making process. This would improve consistency and fairness in IRB decisions. Like accreditation and certification, this could be accomplished without government authorization or support.

3.4.3 Appeal Process

Another tool for potentially limiting the excesses of IRBs is an appeal process for researchers. Yet, as noted above, attempts to secure that process failed. The absence of an external appeal process, as Klitzman (2011, p. 6) has argued, gives IRBs a great deal of de facto power. Ignoring that absence can only make tensions between IRBs and principal investigators (PIs) worse. However, acknowledging this perceived power can help IRBs better facilitate interactions with PIs and thus, in the end, best help protect human subjects.

An example of a formal procedure to question an IRB's negative decision can be found in the University of Minnesota Investigator Manual (2002, pp. 67–68). The manual explicitly instructs a researcher who disagrees with their IRB's decision to request the IRB to reconsider a decision by submitting a written response within five business days. The researcher must provide a rationale for the request, including any additional supporting documents. Grounds for a request are limited to the following reasons: new information was not reasonably available during the IRB review/investigation, there was material failure by the IRB to follow IRB policies and procedures, the IRB-issued sanction exceeds the severity of the noncompliance violations, and the IRB action is disproportionate to the risks to the research subjects' safety and welfare.

Researchers may also ask for reconsideration where the IRB has suspended or terminated the human research. It should be noted that a request to reconsider is directed to the deciding IRB, as opposed to an appeal, which goes to a different IRB within or outside the research institution.

The appeals process was addressed by the Department of Health and Human Services (HHS) in its ANPRM (ANPRM, 2011) on Human Subjects Research Protections: Enhancing Protections for Research Subjects and Reducing Burden, Delay and Ambiguity for Investigators. Readers will recall that the publication requested comments and recommendations on a series of complex matters relating to the approval of research proposals.

Question 28 began by stating that the Common Rule does not currently require that the researcher always be allowed some form of appeal of a decision. It noted that some institutions have voluntarily chosen to provide appeal mechanisms by, for example, allowing the researcher to present the project to a different IRB or by having it reviewed by a special appeal IRB panel that is composed of members chosen from among the membership of the institution's other IRBs. It then specifically asked:

> Should the Common Rule include a requirement that every institution must provide an appropriate appeal mechanism? If so, what should be considered acceptable appeal mechanisms? Should such appeal mechanisms, or different ones, be available for appeals asserting that the investigation is not research, or that the research does not require IRB approval? (ANPRM, 2011, p. 44521)

In its response to Question 28, the American Association of University Professors (AAUP, n.d., p. 5) wrote that an appeals process would not only protect researchers against arbitrary decisions by IRBs but would increase the credibility of IRBs among researchers. Likewise, the NRC (2014, p. 145) recommended that research institutions should develop a system for the appeal of IRB decisions. An appeals committee, it suggested, could operate either within the institution or in conjunction with an outside agency. If the appeals committee should find an error in the IRB's understanding or interpretation of federal or institutional policy, it would return the protocol to the IRB for a re-review guided by the correct interpretation of the regulation or policy. If the appeals committee has the authority to reverse or alter the decision of the IRB, it must be established and perform according to the rules set forth in the Common Rule.

The need for an independent appeal process is most evident in multisite research. For example, two researchers, one at Cornell University and the other at Johns Hopkins University, proposed a multisite study (Ceci & Bruck, 2009, p. 28). The researches proposed to have 6- to 10-year-old children view a 4-min videotape in which a fireman told a child actor not to play with the fireman's hat. After suggestive questioning by a policeman, the child actor incorrectly claimed that the fireman had hit him. The researchers proposed to ask the children who viewed the video why the child actor made the incorrect statement.

One IRB refused to approve the proposal because it was deemed unethical to show children public servants in a negative light. Upon appeal, the IRB held firm in its rejection despite the fact that (a) the National Science Foundation (NSF) and the NIH had reviewed this proposal without noting any ethical concerns and the NSF had approved it for funding. Ceci and Bruck (2009, p. 29) argued that an independent appeal procedure would permit researchers to challenge decisions that "reflect the scientific ineptitude or the social or political values of the reviewers."

When it comes to an appeal process for investigators challenging a decision on research involving human subjects, the United States is an outlier. The World Health Organization (WHO, 2011) recommended that institutions provide written procedures for researchers to request reconsideration of REC decisions, either by the REC itself or by other entities. If appeals to entities outside the REC are authorized, written procedures address the process for appeals, what materials must be submitted and to whom, and who will be the ultimate decision-maker.

In contrast to the US's Common Rule, the Canadian TCPS (Tri-Council, 2018, pp. 85–86), for example, contains a section addressing the appeal of REB decisions. It is joint policy of Canada's three federal research agencies—the CIHR, the Natural Sciences and Engineering Research Council of Canada (NSERC) and the Social Sciences and Humanities Research Council (SSHRC).

In cases when researchers and REBs cannot reach agreement through reconsideration, and the REB has issued a final negative decision, the researcher can utilize the institution's established appeals process. The appeal committee reflects a range of expertise and knowledge similar to that of the REB. It can be an ad hoc or permanent committee. Members of the original decision-making REB may not serve on that appeal committee. After a review of the researcher's grounds for the appeal, the process and any elements of the REB decision that are not supported by the Tri-Council Policy, the appeal committee has the authority to approve, reject or request modification of the research proposal. Its decision is final. At that point, the only remaining recourse for a researcher is judicial review by Canadian courts.

An example of a formal appeals process is that of The University of Waikato (2008), a public university in Hamilton, New Zealand. When the HREC receives a complaint about research activity, it first considers the seriousness of the issue. If the complaint is sufficiently serious, it may refer the matter to the university's Vice-Chancellor who would arrange for it to be dealt with as an infraction of the student discipline regulations, a breach of the staff code of conduct. Otherwise, the HREC itself may take informal action, at its discretion, to deal with the complaint or dispute. A researcher can appeal any decision of the HREC to the Academic Board, a committee of the Council which governs the University. The decision of the Academic Board (or delegated authority) on an appeal is final. As these examples show, there are numerous models for instating a judicious, formal set of mechanisms for researchers to question negative decisions on their work. Furthermore, these models are explicitly recommended by the WHO. The United States remains uniquely deficient in that respect.

3.4.4 The Revised Common Rule 2018

The Department of Health and Human Services (HHS) first issued rules and regulations governing human research protections (*45 CFR 46*) in 1981 which became the Common Rule in 1991. Steps to revise the Common Rule began in 2011 and were implemented in 2018. An ANPRM (ANPRM, 2011) seeking comments on potential revisions to the Common Rule was issued in July 2011. As required by law, the government sought public input on an array of issues related to the ethics, safety and oversight of human research.

Four years later, an NPRM (2015) seeking comments on proposals to comprehensively revise the Common Rule was issued. The general public accounted for 906 (41.4 percent) of the 2186 responses, followed by researchers with 401 (18.3 percent), patients with 245 (11.2 percent) and university/medical Centers/IRBs with 204 (9.3 percent). Responses were also received from professional associations, advocacy groups, industry, health departments and tribal nations (COGR, 2016).

Several significant changes to the Common Rule proposed in the NPRM addressed the concerns of social and behavioral researchers. The NPRM (2015, p. 54054) identified categories of activities that should not be deemed research because they were inherently low risk. These included oral history, biography, legal research and historical scholarship which involve the collection and use of information that focuses directly on the specific individuals about whom the information is collected.

The NPRM (2015, p. 54048) expanded the categories of exempt research, which would allow studies to be considered exempt without requiring any administrative or IRB review. The new categories included certain research involving benign interventions with adult subjects, educational tests, surveys, interviews or observations of public behavior when sensitive information may be collected, provided that data security and information privacy protections policies are followed. In cases of secondary research use of identifiable private information originally collected as part of a nonresearch activity, when notice of possible use has been given, then identifiers must be removed. Secondary research data should also be stripped of personal and geographic identifying information.

It eliminated the continuing review requirement for studies that undergo expedited review and for studies that have completed study interventions and are merely analyzing data or involve only observational follow-up in conjunction with standard clinical care. It also mandated that US institutions engaged in cooperative research rely on a single IRB for that portion of the research that takes place within the United States.

The Revised Common Rule became effective in July 2018, with the implementation of several sections delayed until January 2019. Notably missing was an appeal process beyond a hearing by different members of the IRB at the researcher's institution. The NPRM failed to bring the United States in line with the WHO and Canada regarding an independent appeal process. Schrag (2019) noted that an appeal process could have been another mechanism to force IRBs to base their decisions on evidence, by giving researchers the chance to challenge gut reactions.

3.5 Conclusion

Although often considered a pejorative term, police power is an effective and efficient way for central authorities to deal with local issues such as zoning, schools, sanitation and health. As this chapter has discussed, the human research protection system contains a legitimate police power through which it accommodates community standards, ethical values and normative behavior without criminalizing actions. As such, it is more likely to embody what Weber classified as substantively irrational law, which prioritizes ethics and general principles over formally rational law, which focuses on legislation and case law precedent. Because US IRB decisions are based on applying ethical principles from the *Belmont Report* to a research protocol and then weighing a range of positive and negative consequences which individual human subjects and communities may experience, IRBs have considerable discretion within the bounds of 45 CFR 46 (USAID, 2006).

In the United States, a local IRB has the ability, within federal guidelines, to make decisions based on its chosen ethical principles and deal with similar protocols differently. This can be considered an instance of moral federalism. And according to Weber's terms, it can be considered a substantively irrational legal system which results in a lack of uniformity or consistency in decisions within and across research institutions. While IRBs that receive federal funds must have an FWA from the HHS OHRP, they are not routinely held accountable for their decisions through reviews or an appeal.

The US human protection research approach reflects the American obsession with rugged individualism and favors local over state and national interests. The *Belmont Report*'s principle of respect for persons is operationalized as informed consent to freely choose to participate in the research.

This implies an autonomous and self-directed, rather than other-directed individual who, given relevant information, can decide to volunteer as a subject in a research project. Sociologist David Reisman (2001, p. 24) proposed three types of directedness that correspond closely to Weber's types of social action—traditional, *Wertrational* or value oriented, and *Zweckrational* or goal/purpose oriented (Heberle, 1956, p. 34). A tradition directed person depends on and follows external rules in order to behave in an approved way and not be shamed; an inner-directed value-oriented person follows her or his moral compass in the pursuit of goals which they perceive as valuable because their inner voice tells them they are, and an other-directed person chooses a given way of acting because she or he is anxious to receive the approval of others in order work together to achieve common goals.

American research ethicists appear to hold individual virtue above civic virtue. They also favor direct benefits to the research subjects over nonsubjects who have similar conditions or statuses and may benefit from the research, and they discount altruistic motivations for participating in research. The failure of the American human research protection system to require an independent appeal process makes it an outlier compared to the recommendations of the World Health Organization (2011) and practices of other developed countries. Explicitly requiring an independent review process would create a necessary balance to protect the integrity of the US human protections system and increase the credibility of IRBs among researchers and the scientific community.

Acknowledgments I wish to thank Manfred Stommel for his review and suggestions on this chapter and John Kennedy for his insights on social science ethics and IRBs. I learned about Weber and Sumner in my graduate classes at the University of Chicago with Peter M. Blau, Morris Janowitz and Peter H. Rossi.

References

AAHRPP. (2020). Accreditation of Human Research Protection Programs. (2020). *AAHRPP accredits three more research organizations: Harvard University, Tampa General Hospital and Castle IRB.* Retrieved November 1, 2021, from https://admin.aahrpp.org/Website%20Documents/4th%20Q%202020%20accreditations%20release%20FINAL%20-AAHRPP%20accredits%20three%20more%20research%20organizations.pdf

AAMC. (1998, May 4). Association of American Medical Colleges. Letter to the inspector general of DHHS, May 4, 1998. In Office of Inspector General (1998b), *Institutional Review Boards: A time for reform.* Appendix D 31–35. https://oig.hhs.gov/oei/reports/oei-01-97-00193.pdf

AAUP. (n.d.). American Association of University Professors. *Comments in reply to "Human subjects research protections: Enhancing protections for research subjects and reducing burden, delay, and ambiguity for investigators". Letter to Dr. Jerry Menikoff, Director Office of Human Research Protections.* Retrieved February 9, 2020, from http://dataprivacylab.org/projects/irb/aaup.pdf

ACHRE. (1995). Advisory Committee on Human Radiation Experiments: Final Report, Washington DC: Superintendent of Documents, U.S. Government Printing Office. October 1995.

Amdur, R. J. (2003). *Institutional Review Board: Member handbook.* Jones and Bartlett.

ANPRM. (2011). *Advance Notice of Proposed Rulemaking on human subjects research protections: Enhancing protections for research subjects and reducing burden, delay, and ambiguity for investigators 76 Fed. Reg. 44521*(July 2016).

Bachman, R. D., & Schutt, R. K. (2017). *The practice of research in criminology and criminal justice* (6th ed.). Sage Publications, Inc..

Baker, M., McDaniel, D., & Lansink, J. (2002). IRB accreditation and human subject protection. *Applied Clinical Trials, 11*(1), 32–38. Retrieved February 10, 2020, from http://www.appliedclinicaltrialsonline.com/irb-accreditation-and-human-subject-protection

Bankert, E. A., Gordon, B. G., Hurley, E. A., & Shriver, S. P. (2022). *The Institutional Review Board management and functions* (3rd ed.). Jones and Bartlett Learning.

Bayley, D., Perito, R. (2011). Police corruption: What past scandals teach about current challenge. *Special Report.* 294: Washington DC. United States Institute of Peace.

Belmont Report. (1978). *The Belmont Report: Ethical principles and guidelines for the protection of human subjects of research.* DHEW Publication No. (OS) 78-0013. U.S. Government Printing Office, Washington, D.C. Retrieved February 10, 2020, from https://www.hhs.gov/ohrp/regulations-and-policy/belmont-report/read-the-belmont-report/index.html

Boonstra, H. D. (2001). Human embryo and fetal research: Medical support and political controversy. *The Guttmacher Report on Public Policy, 4*, 1. Retrieved February 10, 2020, from http://www.guttmacher.org/pubs/tgr/04/1/gr040103.html

Bosk, C. L. (2007). The new bureaucracies of virtue or when form fails to follow function. *PoLAR: Political and Legal Anthropology Review, 30*(2), 192–209.

Burgess, J. W. (1890). *Political science and comparative constitutional law Vol I: Sovereignty and liberty government*. Ginn and Company.

Castiglione, D. (2012). Accountability and social science. *Britannica*. Retrieved October 27, 2021, from https://www.britannica.com/topic/accountability

Ceci, S. J., & Bruck, M. (2009). Do IRBs pass the minimal harm test? *Perspectives on Psychological Science, 4*(1), 28–29. https://doi.org/10.1111/j.1745-6924.2009.01084

Chevron. (1984). *Chevron U.S.A., Inc. v. Natural Resources Defense Council, Inc.* 467 U.S. 837.

COGR. (2016). Council on Governmental Relations. *Analysis of common rule comments*. Retrieved October 28, 2021, from https://www.cogr.edu/analysis-common-rule-comments

Cohen, J. (1999). The federal perspective on IRBs. *APS Observer, 12*(9), 6–19.

Davis, K. (1969). A new approach to delegation. *The University of Chicago Law Review, 36*(4), 713–733. https://doi.org/10.2307/1598971

DHEW. (1979, August 14). Department of Health Education and Welfare. Proposed regulations: Amending basic HEW policy for protection of human research subjects. *44 Fed. Reg. 47693.*

Dingwall, R. (2012). How did we ever get into this mess? The rise of ethical regulation in the social sciences. In K. Love (Ed.), *Ethics in social research: Studies in qualitative methodology* (pp. 3–26). Emerald Group Publishing Limited.

Field, S. (1885). *Barbier v Connolly, 113 US Reports 27.*

Flinders, M. V. (1999). Setting the scene: Quangos in context. In M. V. Flinders & M. J. Smith (Eds.), *Quangos, accountability and reform: The politics of quasi-government* (pp. 3–16). St Martin's Press.

Fordham University. (n.d.). *Policy on human subjects research*. Retrieved October 31, 2021, from https://www.fordham.edu/info/24326/institutional_review_board/6727/policy_on_human_subjects_research

Foucault, M. (2007). *Security, territory, population: Lectures at the College de France 1977-1978*. Palgrave Macmillan.

Freund, E. (1904). *The police power: Public policy and constitutional rights*. Callaghan & Company, University of Chicago Press. Retrieved February 15, 2020, from https://books.google.com/books?id=2CksAAAAMAAJ&q=callghan#v=snippet&q=callghan&f=false

GAO. (1996). General Accounting Office. *Scientific research. Continued vigilance critical to protecting human subjects*. Retrieved February 11, 2020, from https://www.gao.gov/archive/1996/he96102t.pdf

Gunsalus, C. K., Bruner, E. M., Burbles, N. C., Dash, L., Finkin, M., Goldberg, J. P., Greenough, W. T., Miller, G. A., & Pratt, M. G. (2006). Mission creep in the IRB world. *Science, 312*(5779), 1441. https://doi.org/10.1126/science.1121479

Heberle, R. (1956). Note on Riesman's the lonely crowd. *American Journal of Sociology, 62*(1), 34–36.

Hendrickson, K. A. (2002). The survival of moral federalism. *Public Interest, 148*, 96–111.

IOM (Institute of Medicine). (2001). *Preserving public trust: Accreditation and human research participant protection program*. The National Academies Press. https://doi.org/10.17226/10085

Jacob, M. A., & Riles, A. (2007). The new bureaucracies of virtue: Introduction. *Political and Legal Anthropology Review, 30*(2), 181–191. https://doi.org/10.1525/pol.2007.30.2.181

Keith-Spiegel, P., Koocher, G. P., & Tabachick, B. (2006). What scientists want from their research ethics committee. *Journal of Empirical Research on Human Research Ethics, 1*(1), 67–82. https://doi.org/10.1525/jer.2006.1.1.67

Klitzman, R. (2011). The ethics police? IRBs' views concerning their power. *PLoS ONE, 6*(12), e28773. https://doi.org/10.1371/journal.pone.0028773

Klitzman, R. (2015). *The ethics police? The struggle to make human research safe*. Oxford University Press.

Korkman, P. (2007). Conscience and police in the *Bibliotheque raisonnee des savans de l'Europe. International Review of Eighteenth-Century Studies, 1*, 19–35. Retrieved February 11, 2020, from http://www.helsinki.fi/historia/1700/IRECS/proofs/IRECS_korkman.pdf

Kosar, K. R. (2011). The quasi-government: Hybrid organizations with both government and private sector legal characteristics. *Congressional Research Service Report for Congress*. Retrieved February 14, 2020, from http://www.fas.org/sgp/crs/misc/RL30533.pdf

Legislative Analyst's Office. (1995). *The three strikes and you're out law*. Retrieved March 3, 2020, from https://lao.ca.gov/analysis_1995/3strikes.html

Levine, R. J. (1988). *Ethics and regulation of clinical research* (2nd ed.). Yale University Press.

Lincoln, Y. S., & Tierney, W. G. (2004). Qualitative research and Institutional Review Boards. *Qualitative Inquiry, 10*(2), 219–234. https://doi.org/10.1177/1077800403262361

MacIntyre, A. (1980). Regulation: A substitute for morality. *The Hastings Center Report, 10*, 31–33. https://doi.org/10.2307/3560503

Mather, J. H., & Hartnett, T. (2008, February 20). HSP and accreditation: Growing pains and successes mark first seven years. *Medical Research Law & Policy Report, 7*(4).

McCarthy, C. R. (1995). When OPRR comes calling: Enforcing federal research regulations. *Kennedy Institute of Ethics Journal, 5*(1), 51–55. https://doi.org/10.1353/ken.0.0049

Merton, R. K. (1957). *Social theory and social structure* (revised and enlarged ed.). The Free Press.

Metcalf, J. (2014). Ethics codes: History, context, and challenges. *Council for Big Data, Ethics, and Society*. Retrieved November 1, 2021, from https://bdes.datasociety.net/council-output/ethics-codes-history-context-and-challenges/

Michigan State University. (n.d.). Expedited Categories, Human Research Protection Program. Available at Expedited Categories | Human Research Protection Program | Michigan State University (msu.edu). Retrieved December 5, 2022

Mills, C. W. (1959). *The sociological imagination*. Oxford University Press.

Moreno, J. D. (2005). The end of the great bioethics compromise. *Hastings Center Report, 35*, 14–15. https://doi.org/10.1353/hcr.2005.0011

National Bioethics Advisory Commission. (2001). *Ethical and policy issues in research involving human participants* (Vol. I). Bethesda, MD.

National Research Council. (2014). *Proposed revisions to the common rule for the protection of human subjects in the behavioral and social sciences*. The National Academies Press. https://doi.org/10.17226/18614

NJ Firefighters Mutual Benefit Association vs N. Hudson Reg. Fire & Rescue, New Jersey Superior Court. (2001, May 15). Retrieved February 11, 2020, from https://www.courtlistener.com/opinion/2050731/fmba-v-n-hudson-reg-fire-rescue/

Novak, W. J. (2002). Governance, police and American liberal mythology. In L. O. Gostin (Ed.), *Public health law and ethics: A reader* (pp. 186–192). University of California Press.

NPRM. (2015). *Notice of Proposed Rulemaking*. Federal Policy for the Protection of Human Subjects. Retrieved January 24, 2023, from https://www.govinfo.gov/content/pkg/FR-2015-09-08/pdf/2015-21756.pdf

O'Donnell, G. A. (1998). Horizontal accountability in new democracies. *Journal of Democracy, 9*(3), 112–126. https://doi.org/10.1353/jod.1998.0051

Office for Human Research Protections. (2008). Engagement of institutions in human subjects research, 73 *Fed. Reg*. 63150. (10/23/2008)

OHRP-E. (n.d.). Lesson 4: Independent review of research. *HHS.gov*. Retrieved November 23, 2021, from https://www.hhs.gov/ohrp/education-and-outreach/online-education/human-research-protection-training/lesson-4-irb-review-of-research/index.html

OIG. (1998a). Office of the Inspector General. *Institutional Review Boards: Their role in reviewing approved research*. Retrieved February 20, 2020, from https://oig.hhs.gov/oei/reports/oei-01-97-00190.pdf

OIG. (1998b). Office of the Inspector General Institutional Review Boards: A time for reform. Retrieved February 20, 2020, from https://oig.hhs.gov/oei/reports/oei-01-97-00193.pdf.

Peckman, S. (2006). A shared responsibility for protecting human subjects. In E. A. Bankert & R. J. Amdur (Eds.), *Institutional Review Board: Management and function* (2nd ed., pp. 16–20). Jones & Bartlett Learning.

Puglisi, J. T. (1999, April 21). *Suspension of medical research at the west Los Angeles and Sepulveda VA medical facilities: Testimony before the house committee on veterans' affairs, subcommittee on oversight and investigations and subcommittee on health.* http://www.hhs.gov/asl/testify/t990421d.html

Reisman, D. (2001). *The lonely crowd.* Yale University Press.

Rosenfeld, S. J. (2020). Managing what you can't measure—Institutional Review Board decision support software. *Ochsner Journal, 20*(1), 10–14. https://doi.org/10.31486/toj.19.0074

Rothe, J. (1998). *Redefining education and traffic safety with a socio-cultural set of lenses.* http://citeseerx.ist.psu.edu/viewdoc/download?doi=10.1.1.34.3141&rep=rep1&type=pdf

Savelsberg, J. J. (2018). Max Weber's formal and substantive rationality: Tensions in international criminal law. In W. Gephart (Ed.), *Law as culture: Max Weber's comparative sociology of law* (pp. 493–510). Vittorio Klostermann.

Schrag, Z. M. (2009). How talking became human subjects research: The federal regulation of the social sciences, 1965-1991. *Journal of Policy History, 21*(1), 3–37. https://doi.org/10.1017/S0898030609090010

Schrag, Z. M. (2010). *Ethical imperialism: Institutional Review Boards and the social sciences.* Johns Hopkins University Press.

Schrag, Z. M. (2019). Vexed again: Social scientists and the revision of the common rule, 2011-2018. *Journal of Law, Medicine & Ethics, 47*, 254–263. https://doi.org/10.1177/1073110519857281

Shelton, J. D. (1999). How to interpret the federal policy for the protection of human subjects or "common rule" (Part A). *IRB: Ethics and Human Research, 21*(6), 6–9. https://doi.org/10.2307/3564451

Shweder, R. A. (2006). Protecting human subjects and preserving academic freedom: Prospects at the University of Chicago. *American Ethnologist, 33*(4), 507–518.

Simon, H. A. (1956). Rational choice and the structure of the environment. *Psychological Review, 63*(2), 129–138.

Steneck, N. H. (2007). *ORI introduction to the responsible conduct of research* (updated ed.). Government Printing Office. ISBN 978-0-16-079043-0.

Sumner, W. G. (1907). *Folkways: A study of the sociological importance of usages, manners, customs, mores and morals.* Ginn & Company. Paperback. Retrieved February 16, 2023, from https://www.amazon.com/Folkways-Study-Manners-Customs-Morals/dp/1602067589

The World Health Organization (WHO:2011). *Guidance for Ethics Review of Health-Related Research with Human Participants* (2011: Annex 3) check the two WHO references and how in text.

Tri-Council. (2018). *Tri-Council Policy Statement Ethical Conduct for Research Involving Humans– TCPS 2.* Retrieved November 2, 2021, from https://ethics.gc.ca/eng/policy-politique_tcps2-eptc2_2018.html

University of Waikato. (2008). Ethical conduct in human research and related activities regulations. Retrieved February 23, 2020, from https://calendar.waikato.ac.nz/assessment/ethicalConduct.html

USAID (United States Agency for International Development). (2006, December 26). *Protection of human subjects in research supported by USAID: A mandatory reference for ADS Chapter 200.* File Name: 200mbe_122606_cd16. https://www.usaid.gov/sites/default/files/documents/1864/200mbe.pdf

Vanderpool, H. Y. (2001). Unfulfilled promise: How the Belmont Report can amend the Code of Federal Regulations title 45 part 46—Protection of human subjects. *Ethical and policy issues in research involving human participants* (Vol. II, pp. 1–20). Bethesda, MD.

Vitiello, M. (2004). Reforming three strikes' excesses. *Washington University Law Quarterly, 82*(1). https://openscholarship.wustl.edu/law_lawreview/vol82/iss1/1

Waters, M. (1989). Collegiality, bureaucratization, and professionalization: A Weberian analysis. *American Journal of Sociology, 94*(5), 945–972.

Weber, M. (1947). *The theory of society and economic organization*. Translated by A.M. Henderson and T. Parsons, New York: The Free Press.

Weber, M. (1978). *Economy and society: An outline of interpretive sociology*. University of California Press.

Weiss, R. (1999, May 12). U.S. halts human research at Duke. *Washington Post*, A1

Weiss, R. (2009). Child Research Study Halted. *The Washington Post*. November 7, 2000. Retrieved April 15, 2022, from https://www.washingtonpost.com/archive/politics/2000/11/07/child-research-study-halted/cfb234df-8f95-4686-b956-4fe95e08ad9a/

West's. (2005). Police Power *Encyclopedia of American Law*. eds. Vol. 8. 2nd ed. Edited by S. Phelps and J. Lehman, Detroit, MI: Gale. P 10.

Williams, E. D. (2005, June 2). Federal protection for human research subjects: An analysis of the *Common Rule* and its interactions with FDA regulations and the HIPAA privacy rule. *CRS Report for Congress*. Retrieved February 11, 2020, from http://www.fas.org/sgp/crs/misc/RL32909.pdf

World Health Organization. (2011). Standards and operational guidance for ethics review of health-related research with human participants. *World Health Organization*. Retrieved February 17, 2020, from https://www.ncbi.nlm.nih.gov/books/NBK310669/

Part II
Case Studies

Chapter 4
The US Public Health Tuskegee Syphilis Study: A Sociological Perspective

> I often tell my students that syphilis is the only disease which they require to study thoroughly.
>
> Know syphilis in all its manifestations and relations, and all other things clinical will be added unto you.—William Osler (1897)

4.1 Introduction

The US Public Health Tuskegee Syphilis Study, officially titled the "Tuskegee Study of Untreated Syphilis in the Negro Male," observed the course of the untreated disease in over 300 African American men who had third stage syphilis. It began in 1934 and ended in 1972 with Jean Heller's 1972 exposé in the *Washington Star* that highlighted its racist dimensions and ethical failings. Reasons for its longevity include structural racism, as the exposé made plain, along with bureaucratic inertia and the personal motivation of the physician-researchers to study and control syphilis (Lombardo & Dorr, 2006, p. 291).

This chapter will cover the history of syphilis as a communicable disease with race-related differences in its signs, symptoms and course. The study began as a survey of the prevalence of syphilis among the African Americans in the South. The USPHS took over the project in 1932 and designed a passive observation of the course of syphilis in 399 men with and 201 without syphilis. No one in the study would receive treatment for syphilis, even after penicillin became available. The study continued for 40 years, despite criticisms, until the 1972 exposé. This led to a successful class action law suit, a presidential apology and a Legacy Project to help investigators conduct ethically responsible research on the impacts of the Study.

Sociological insights can help us better understand the rise and decline of syphilis as a social problem, the roles of state and local governments, universities and philanthropies, as well as under what conditions individuals will break rules and become whistleblowers. Furthermore, what we now call clinical or applied

H. Perlstadt, *Assessing Social Science Research Ethics and Integrity*, Clinical Sociology: Research and Practice, https://doi.org/10.1007/978-3-031-34538-8_4

sociologists were directly or indirectly involved in the early days of the Study as administrators, program staff, consultants, evaluators and researchers.

It is possible that "the Tuskegee Study revealed more about the pathology of racism than it did about the pathology of syphilis" (Brandt, 1978, p. 27). It was designed not as an experiment but to scientifically observe the natural history of syphilis in a group of untreated African American men living in Macon County, Alabama, in the 1930s. Almost a century later, it is still evident that the USPHS Tuskegee study has had harmful effects on African American confidence in the American health care system.

For example, some African Americans refused to acknowledge the prevalence of the AIDS epidemic in their communities, were reluctant to become bone marrow donors, or hesitated to be vaccinated against the COVID-19 virus because they believed that the men in the Tuskegee study were actually injected with syphilis. It is true that some White physicians, especially in the South, frequently used African American patients as guinea pigs, but this was not the case in the Tuskegee Study (Gamble, 1997, pp. 11774–775). Myths and falsehoods concerning the Study were promulgated by African American leaders, including Harlon Dalton, a Yale Law School professor, and Dr. Eleanor Walker, a Detroit radiation oncologist, as well as other prominent individuals like Tom Brokaw on "NBC Nightly News."

The major ethical questions that the study raises have tended to focus on its lack of informed consent, its excessive or inappropriate inducements and its prohibiting participants from leaving the study. One rarely discussed ethical question in a passive observation study like Tuskegee was whether and when to begin treating the patients and any controls. Today, IRBs are required to review and approve all nonexempt research projects at intervals appropriate to the degree of risk, but not less than once a year (*43 CFR 56.109(e)*). Continuing review is required as long as the research remains active for long term follow-up of research subjects (University of Iowa, n.d.). In the case of the Tuskegee study, continuing reviews would have raised questions when penicillin became the widely available and preferred treatment for syphilis but was not thereafter offered to the participants.

4.1.1 Syphilis

Syphilis is a bacterial infection which starts out as a painless sore usually following sexual contact. The bacteria can remain inactive for decades before becoming active again. It develops in three stages but the stages may overlap and the symptoms don't always occur in the same order. The secondary or latent stage exhibits no symptoms and can last for years. Between 15 and 30 percent of people with untreated syphilis move on to the third stage.

Complications include damage to the brain, nerves, eyes, heart, blood vessels, liver, bones and/or joints (Mayo Clinic, 2020).

The history of modern medical research into syphilis begins with Caesar Boeck, who in 1880 founded what would become the *Journal of the Norwegian Medical*

Association. He became chief of the dermatologic clinic of the Rikshospitalet in 1889 (JAMA, 1970, p. 1538). He began the Oslo study of the natural history of untreated syphilis which lasted almost 20 years (1891–1910). He believed that the then-common mercury treatment for syphilis tended to interfere with the patient's own defense mechanisms, and practically forbade its use in his wards. Most of his approximately 2000 patients were residents of the poor district of Oslo (Harrison, 1956, p. 71). Approximately 40 percent of the patients were treated with potassium iodide and 3.6 percent with mercury in some form. Patients were kept in the hospital as long as they showed any signs of syphilis. Males with primary and secondary syphilis stayed fewer days than females.

Boeck died in 1917. In 1929, his research successor, E. Bruusgaard, published a report on patients 15 to 20 years after their infections. He found that 10 percent of untreated syphilitics would develop neurosyphilis, 13 percent cardiovascular syphilis and 12 percent benign late syphilis. Almost two-thirds (64%) appeared to be symptom free. Although he obtained information from only 22 percent of the original patients, his report became the standard for prognostics statements for the next 25 years (Clark & Danbolt, 1955, pp. 311, 341; Harrison, 1956, p. 71; Gray, 1998).

Meanwhile, around 1905, Fritz Schaudinn and Erich Hoffmann discovered the causative agent of syphilis, *Spirochaeta pallida*, and August Wassermann developed the first serologic test for syphilis. Paul Ehrlich received the Nobel Prize in Physiology and Medicine in 1908 for his discovery of arsphenamine (Salvarsan), the first effective treatment for syphilis. He called it a "magic bullet" because it would target a highly specific site and treat only that site.

4.1.2 Syphilis Becomes a Public Health Problem

These scientific breakthroughs meant that syphilis could be identified and treated. The problem was that in the United States at the time, sexual vice and venereal disease (VD) were not discussed publicly. VD is a sexually transmitted disease (STD) through sexual intercourse or genital contact with an infected partner. Syphilis and Gonorrhea are two common VDs. The terminological distinctions of sociologist C. Wright Mills (1959, pp. 8–9) are useful here: on the one hand, there are private matters, and on the other hand, there are public issues. Sexual vice and venereal disease were simultaneously private matters that threatened an individual's health and social reputation, as well as public issues that threatened the health and wellbeing of others, including servicemen and women in the US military. To meet this challenge, the American Social Hygiene Association (ASHA) was established in 1914 to promote social health, to advocate for the highest standards of private and public morality, and, pertinent to this chapter, to conduct inquiries into the condition of prostitution and venereal disease in American towns and cities (Parascandola, 2008, pp. 26, 44–45).

At the end of the eighteenth century, Boston, New York, Philadelphia and Charleston considered venereal disease a public health problem. The almshouse in

Philadelphia reported that about 10 percent of its beneficiaries were infected with VD, including Mariners, prostitutes and some infants. State level statistics had their shortcomings. In 1911, California became the first state to require physicians to report VD cases. More generally, during this period physicians reported the number of cases seen, but not the names to protect patient confidentiality (Parascandola, 2008, pp. 44–45).

When the United States began its military buildup for World War I in the spring of 1917, the ASHA, along with the American Red Cross, Young Men's Christian Association (YMCA) and the General Federation of Women's Clubs opposed the presence of prostitution venues near the newly built training camps. The ASHA proposed to repress prostitution near the training camps, replacing them with wholesome recreation activities and educating the recruits about the nature and prevention of venereal diseases (Clarke, 1955, p. 422). The Secretaries of War and the Navy welcomed this offer.

Shortly after the American Expeditionary Force (AEF) landed in France in late June 1917, they discovered state-run brothels (Blackman, 2014, p. 95). General John Pershing, the AEF commander, declared regulated houses of prostitution off limits. To fill the gap, the YMCA operated 26 Rest and Recreation leave centers in rural France.

The government paid for food and lodging and the YMCA covered expenses for recreation and entertainment. The YMCA filled the seven days with organized sports and dances, sightseeing and movies. One aim was to keep the soldiers from contracting venereal diseases (Brandt, 1987, pp. 102–104, 109).

Venereal diseases exacted a high toll during the war, with about seven million days of active duty lost because of them. It was second only to influenza. Army records revealed very high rates of venereal disease among "colored troops." Brandt (1987, pp. 115–116) suggested that these high rates may reflect the tendency of Army physicians to diagnose African American soldiers as having sexually transmitted conditions.

By the 1930s, syphilis was most prevalent in the African American population. All treatment programs were lengthy, painful and potentially toxic, with a very poor completion rate and many obtained no relevant treatment (Benedek & Erlen, 1999, pp. 18–19).

4.1.3 Race-Related Differences in Disease

After World War I, Ernest Zimmermann (1921, pp. 83, 87) explored race-related differences in the manifestations of primary, secondary and tertiary syphilis. He reviewed the international literature and analyzed data from the syphilis department of the Johns Hopkins Dispensary, a charitable clinic in Baltimore. He found some striking differences between White and African American males with tertiary manifestations of syphilis. Neurosyphilis was more than twice as frequent among the White males (57.6% of 155 vs 28.6% of 71) but bone lesions were the most frequent complications among African American males (27.8% of 69 vs 14.4% of 39), as was aortitis, the inflammation of the aortic wall (20.9% of 52 vs. 11.8% of 32). He noted one limitation was that many of the African Americans studied "possess an admixture of white blood, and that this may modify results to a certain extent" (Zimmermann, 1921, p. 78).

4.2 Background and Context of Syphilis Study

It is important to place the USPHS Tuskegee Syphilis Study in the context of the segregated social caste system that existed in Macon County, Alabama after the Civil War. In 1880, African Americans composed a majority of the county population; one of this population's leader made a deal with a White candidate for the Alabama Senate establishing that if the candidate carried the county, he would work with the state to establish the Tuskegee Normal School for Colored Teachers, which would eventually become the Tuskegee Institute and, today, Tuskegee University. The school began in 1881 when Booker T. Washington, a 25 year old who was born into slavery, became its first principle. He would later serve as an advisor to US presidents William McKinley (1897–assassinated 1901), Theodore Roosevelt (1901 to 1909) and William Howard Taft (1909–1913) (Tuskegee University, n.d.).

4.2.1 Julius Rosenwald's Legacy for the African American Community

In 1910, Julius Rosenwald, the son of German Jewish immigrants, read Booker T. Washington's autobiography *Up from Slavery*. Previously, Rosenwald worked in his family's business manufacturing men's suits. In 1895, he invested in one of its clients, Sears, Roebuck and Company, of which he would become president. When Sears began selling its stock publicly in 1906, Rosenwald became extremely wealthy (Harter, n.d.). A few years later, he was introduced to Washington who, in December 1911, asked him to serve on the Board of Directors of the Tuskegee Institute (Ascoli, 2006, p. 89). Rosenwald also served on the Boards of the ASHA, the University of Chicago and the Rockefeller Foundation (Chicago Commission, 1922, pp. 652–653).

In 1912, Rosenwald gave $2500 to the Tuskegee Institute. Washington wanted to use a small amount for grants to enable African American communities near Tuskegee to build rural elementary schools. However, the communities were required by Rosenwald to contribute matching funds, thereby having a stake in the project. The first "Rosenwald School" was dedicated in Alabama in 1913. For the next 20 years, Rosenwald would provide funds that enabled African American communities in 15 southern states to build over 5300 schools for their children.

Through a combination of active leadership in the North Carolina Department of Public Instruction and enthusiastic fundraising by African Americans at the grass-roots level, over 800 Rosenwald buildings were erected in the state (Hanchett, 1988, pp. 387, 395–396; Hawkins, 2020).

In 1917, Rosenwald and his family established the Rosenwald Foundation (n.d.), also known as the Rosenwald Fund, for "the well-being of mankind." He gave over two million dollars to African American University Centers at Tuskegee, Howard, Fisk, Atlanta and Dillard Universities as well as approximately 1000 scholarships or fellowships to African American students. Over the years, the Foundation stimulated social change by granting money to pilot programs that involved public-private partnerships. The expectation was that the state or some other government agency would then take over their funding and administer them (Ascoli, 2006, pp. 314–315).

From 1917 until 1928, the Foundation remained largely under the personal control of Rosenwald. He donated a portion of his Sears stock to the Foundation, provided that it would spend all its funds and cease operations within 25 years of his death, which occurred in 1932 (Hawkins, 2020). The Foundation was reorganized in 1928 with a newly created Board of Directors and full-time staff headquartered in Chicago (Harter, n.d.).

Rosenwald would leave a lasting legacy on the African American community in both Chicago and throughout the United States, including in the American South and in Macon County, home of the Tuskegee Institute. Following the 1919 race riots in Chicago, Rosenwald was appointed to the Chicago Commission on Race Relations to identify the causes of the violence and propose solutions. The Commission's 1922 report was primarily written by Charles S. Johnson. Johnson had recently earned his PhD in sociology from the University of Chicago under Robert E. Park. Johnson would adapt Park's work on urban sociology and race relations to rural Macon County. Park met Booker T. Washington through the Congo Reform Association. From 1905 to 1914, Park worked at Tuskegee doing field research and serving as director of public relations (ASA1, n.d.).

Park suggested that Johnson be appointed Associate Executive Secretary and Research Director of the Commission. Throughout his career, Johnson was a full-time reformer (Dunne, 1998, p. 3). Along the way he founded and edited *Opportunity*, the *Journal of the National Urban League*, and headed the new Institute for Social Sciences at Fisk University, a private historically African American university in Nashville, TN. In 1946, he became Fisk's first African American president and was a member of the US delegation to UNESCO in Paris.

4.2.2 Macon County in the 1930s

A description of Macon County at the start of the Tuskegee Syphilis Study can be found in Johnson's (1934) book *Shadow of the Plantation*, as well as Olansky et al.'s (1954) article in *Public Health Reports* on Environmental Factors in the Tuskegee Study. The article was inspired by the work of Warner, Hill, et al. (1951) on the relationship between syphilis prevalence and community structure in Savannah, GA. W. Lloyd Warner was Chairman of the Department of Sociology and Anthropology at the University of Chicago and a Special Consultant to USPHS. He applied social science research methods to the complex problems of contemporary society.

In 1931, Johnson conducted a community study for the Rosenwald Foundation of 612 families consisting of 2432 persons living in eight settlements in Macon County. Macon County is about 40 miles east of Montgomery, the state capital. His study adapted the University of Chicago's empirical research on urban communities to an African American farming population that was located about 10 miles down a highway from Tuskegee, and then several miles along unpaved roads into the countryside. These communities reflected the physical layout of former plantations. Housing consisted of cabins on the edge of cotton fields. The local church or store was located at the country crossroads, but with no nearby dwellings.

Men and women walked along the roads on their way to work, children played in them and old folks chatted under nearby trees. Most of the African American farmers worked an average of 46 acres compared to 103 acres for Whites (Johnson, 1934, pp. 10–14). The men selected for the Tuskegee syphilis study came from a low income, low education group who lived in or near Macon County (Reverby, 2009, pp. 270–271 n17; Olansky et al., 1954, pp. 962–963). It is possible that of the 600 in the study, some could have come from one of the eight settlements Johnson studied.

At the start of the study, African Americans in the area had a few options for receiving health care, but they were limited. Macon County had nine White physicians and one African American physician in private practice.

Their offices were not located in southern and southwestern Macon County, where most of the African Americans lived. The John A. Andrew Memorial Hospital began as the student infirmary for Tuskegee Institute in 1912 and offered care for African Americans in the community who could afford it. The Veterans Administration Hospital located just outside Tuskegee had 2300 beds for African Americans who had fought in World War I, and its staff was entirely African American. It did not provide medical care to nonveterans. The Macon County Health Department was created in 1928 and was able to expand maternal and child health programs and venereal disease control with funding from the USPHS, the Rosenwald Foundation and the Alabama State Health Department (Olansky et al., 1954, pp. 693–694).

4.2.3 Prevalence Surveys

At the national level, from May 1926 to February 1929, the USPHS conducted a series of surveys on the prevalence of venereal disease in representative communities across the United States (Usilton, 1930).

Surveys were sent to physicians, clinics, hospitals and charity institutions in each community in several states, counties, small towns and major cities across the United States, covering an estimated 20 percent of the total US population. Overall, only a small proportion of physicians treated venereal disease cases. Data on race was obtained from surveys in Tennessee, Mississippi, Virginia and the city of St. Louis, including its five neighboring counties. While the number of cases were higher for White males than African American males (8520 vs 4824), and White females than African American females (4483 vs 3767), the rates per 1000 population were higher for African American than White males (8.04% vs 5.10%) and African American than White females (6.36% vs. 2.79%) (Usilton, 1930, p. 556).

According to Clark (1932) and Olansky et al. (1954), the problem was that existing case studies did little to identify the relative efficacy of treating tertiary syphilis. Surveys in the rural areas of the South revealed a high incidence of syphilis among the African American population and that many cases remained untreated. This provided the rationale that a long-term study of untreated syphilis might lead to a more knowledge-based syphilis control program.

The solution was a longitudinal study following a large number of patients for a long period of time (Clark et al., 1932, p. 135). Some longitudinal studies are observational in nature and include no treatment. Since no single clinic would have enough cases to achieve this goal, the USPHS sponsored the Cooperative Clinics Group (CCG) in 1929. The CCG consisted of research-oriented venereal disease clinics at Western Reserve University, Johns Hopkins University, the Universities of Michigan and Pennsylvania and the Mayo Clinic. Dr. Taliaferro Clark, the head of the USPHS Disease Section, was also a member of the CCG (Benedek & Erlen, 1999, p. 7; Crenner, 2012, p. 265).

In September 1929, the PHS asked the Rosenwald Foundation to fund a joint project dealing with the prevalence of syphilis among the African American population in Mississippi. The previous year, Michael M. Davis became the director of medical services at the Rosenwald Foundation. Davis had studied economics and sociology, earning his PhD in 1906 at Columbia University under Franklin H. Giddings. Giddings transformed American sociology into a research science utilizing statistical and analytic methodology (ASA2, n.d.). Afterward, Davis practiced what he learned in social settlements before becoming the director of the Boston Dispensary in 1910 and had worked with syphilis clinics in Boston. Beginning in 1920, he conducted a seven-year research project studying ambulatory care in New York City for the Rockefeller Foundation (Jones, 1993, p. 58; Davis, 1960).

Dr. Oliver C. Wenger, the Director of the USPHS Venereal Disease Clinic in Arkansas, was brought in to supervise the Mississippi surveys (Gray, 1998, p. 46). He advocated for public health programs for the poor (Poirier, 1995, p. 139). He proceeded to add a syphilis treatment demonstration component to these programs. As the Mississippi treatment demonstration neared completion, Wenger wrote to Dr. Thomas Parran, Jr., who had served as Chief of USPHS's Division of Venereal Diseases, that a meeting of southern health officers should be called to discuss the possibility of starting new testing and treatment programs. Parran had shifted the Division's orientation from sex education and prophylaxis to health surveys, scientific research and treatment demonstrations (Jones, 1993, pp. 57–58).

Later, at the request of Governor Franklin D. Roosevelt, Parran was loaned to New York State in April 1930 to serve as State Health Commissioner. When Roosevelt became president, he appointed Parran to the Committee on Economic

Security, which drafted the 1935 Social Security Act. The Act authorized $8 million for public health departments and $2 million for scientific research on diseases. In 1936, Roosevelt appointed Parran as US Surgeon General, a position he held until 1948 (Snyder, 1995, pp. 630–631).

Drawing heavily on Wenger's reports, Parran and Clark sent a proposal to the Rosenwald Foundation in early in October 1929 requesting funding to expand the program. The Foundation's then-director, Davis, made sure the program met the Foundation's long-term goals. It would provide training for both White and African American private physicians, promote the utilization of African American clinicians and nurses in county health departments and extend existing clinical services or establish new ones where needed (Jones, 1993, p. 59).

In November 1929, the Rosenwald Foundation voted to support the expansion of the pilot study. With this funding and the cooperation of local health departments, between 1929 and 1931, the PHS surveyed African Americans for syphilis in six rural southern counties: Albemarle County, VA, Glynn County, GA, Macon County, AL, Pitt County, NC, Scott County, MS, and Tipton County, TN (Thomas & Quinn, 1991, p. 1491; Gray, 1998, pp. 41–42; Benedek & Erlen, 1999, p. 19). Approximately 40,000 persons were tested for syphilis, and 25 percent were found to be infected. Macon County had the highest prevalence, with 36 percent infected. Of the 1400 cases recorded during the survey, only 33 had ever had previous antisyphilitic therapy and the average for these 33 was less than 5 arsenical injections.

Nearly a year later in October 1930, Davis met with Clark, who by that point had become Chief of the USPHS Venereal Disease Division. Together, they laid the groundwork for an outside review of the syphilis control demonstrations by a team of syphilologists and sociologists. After some negotiations, the USPHS, along with state and local officials, agreed that the Committee on Administrative Health Practice of the American Public Health Association (APHA) would serve as the review agency.

Clark favored an intensive sociological study on all of Macon County and its county level health promotion activities. This would bring an accepted community survey methodology that would yield reliable findings on the prevalence of syphilis in a large population according to race, age, gender and occupation. This would be followed by medical examinations to identify individuals with tertiary syphilis. After a lengthy search, Davis suggested Professor Charles Johnson, chair of the Department of Sociology at Fisk University. Johnson and his graduate student assistants began the study in 1931 and published their findings in 1934.

In April 1931, Davis convened a blue-ribbon panel at the Hotel Pennsylvania in New York City to discuss the proposed review. Joining Davis were Dr. William F. Snow from Stanford University, who was secretary of the California State Board of Health and a leader in the ASHA, Parran, who had returned to the USPHS, and two members of the Committee on Administrative Health Practice of the American Public Health Association. Johnson and Clark were principal speakers. Following Johnson's summary of his findings, they agreed that the evaluation should not be conducted until the demonstrations were completed (Jones, 1993, pp. 84–85).

The evaluation concluded that mass treatment could be successfully implemented among rural African Americans (Brandt, 1978, p. 22). Everyone involved realized they had documented a problem of enormous dimensions and solving it would take both public money and public resolve (Gray, 1998, p. 42). The questions established were where to site the treatment program, which type of research design would be chosen and who would pay for the study. Parran thought that "If one wished to study the natural history of syphilis in the Negro race uninfluenced by treatment, this county (Macon) would be an ideal location for such a study" (Bender, 2017). But by the spring of 1932, the Rosenwald Foundation realized that the government was not doing enough to take over the project, and, given the decline of the Foundation's stock market assets, the board of directors voted to end its support for the syphilis treatment program (Ascoli, 2006, p. 314).

4.2.4 Developing the Study

Without a formal application and detailed protocol as would be required today, the best we can do in an effort to interpret the USPHS Tuskegee Syphilis Study is examine a series of letters that reveal the thinking informing it, as well as how it gained initial financial and institutional support after the Rosenwald Foundation indicated it would be ending its funding (See Reverby, 2000, pp. 73–87). On August 29, 1932, Taliaferro Clark (1932), Chief of the USPHS Venereal Disease Division and author of the *Rosenwald Study Report*, decided that conditions in Macon County merited renewed attention. Clark believed the high prevalence of syphilis offered an "unusual opportunity" for observation (Brandt, 1987, p. 22). According to Brandt, Claude Bernard, one of the founders of experimental medicine, distinguished between two types of research: an experimental intervention to prevent, ameliorate or cure a disease, and a passive observation of the course of a disease. An experimental or clinical intervention compares an experimental group with a control group to identify the causes of different outcomes. A passive observation study requires that no one in the study receives treatment.

An observational study could document the spontaneous evolution of syphilis in study subjects, which could then be compared to the nineteenth-century Oslo study. Syphilologists debated whether complications of third or late-stage syphilis were more prevalent in African American males. Some argued that African Americans had a racially determined resistance to neurosyphilis infection, basing their argument on the racist belief that African Americans had a more rudimentary development of the brain and nervous systems. Dr. William A. Hinton, an African American syphilologist who devised the Hinton test for syphilis, suggested that African Americans had higher rates of cardiovascular syphilis because they were more likely to be engaged in hard physical labor (Crenner, 2012, pp. 248, 259).

Clark also wrote to Dr. J. N. Baker, the Alabama State Health Officer, asking him if he was interested in possible research work on syphilitic African Americans in Macon County that would be funded by the PHS with the cooperation of the

Tuskegee Institute's Andrews Memorial Hospital. Clark described the research as "an unparalleled opportunity of studying the effect of untreated syphilis on the human economy" (Reverby, 2009, p. 38).

A few weeks later, Clark and Wenger met with Baker, who wanted to treat everyone who was examined and found to be syphilitic. At that time, Clark was planning a short-term study, so they agreed that the syphilitics would receive eight doses of neoarsphenamine, a derivative of arsenic and some additional treatment with mercury pills, unless treatment with either drug was contraindicated on medical grounds. Clark then assigned Dr. Raymond Vonderlehr to Tuskegee in September 1932 to oversee the study. Vonderlehr had joined the USPHS in 1925 and then went on to study syphilis in clinics in Europe. He had an extensive background in syphilology and cardiovascular syphilis. In 1931, he was assigned to the USPHS's division of venereal disease. He was joined by Wenger, who had supervised the 1929 Surveys in Mississippi that led to the Rosenwald surveys (Gray, 1998, pp. 45–46).

Toward the end of September, Baker wrote a letter back to Clark that the Macon County Board of Health was enthusiastic about the previous project (the syphilis control demonstration) and was willing to support the suggested undertaking. But they insisted that treatment be provided to the participants. They liked the idea that interns from Tuskegee Institute would provide the treatment under the supervision of the County Health Officer. Since the Board could speak for organized medicine in the county, their endorsement meant that Clark could proceed (Selected Letters, 2000, pp. 74–75).

Meanwhile, Eugene H. Dibble, Jr., an African American physician and medical director of the Tuskegee Institute, wrote to Dr. Robert R. Morton, who had succeeded Booker T. Washington as head of the Tuskegee Institute. He told Morton that the USPHS was "very anxious to extend its research further into this problem, so that they can find out just what effect syphilis is having on people who have been untreated over a period of years" (Dibble, 2000, p. 75). He noted that the cost of treatment of syphilis was very high and a study on the effects of the disease on the cardiovascular and nervous systems would have worldwide significance. He added that both Surgeon General Hugh Cumming and Clark wanted to use the facilities of the Andrews Hospital on the Tuskegee Institute campus but that they would furnish the necessary supplies and equipment. Dr. Clark indicated that Tuskegee Institute and Andrews Hospital would get credit for this research.

In turn, Dibble recommended that the USPHS hire Eunice Rivers, an African American supervisor of night nurses. Appointing African American medical practitioners, readers will recall, was in keeping with the goals of Surgeon General Parran's 1929 proposal for studying syphilis in African Americans. Rivers would be relieved of her work at Andrews hospital for the Alabama State Board of Heath and assigned as a scientific assistant to the Venereal Disease Program of the Macon County Health Department (Gray, 1998, pp. 43–44, 46, 47, 52). She also acted as the liaison for the study director and staff and the participants and their families. She worked on the Study from its start until it was terminated in 1972. In 1958, she received the third annual Oveta Culp Hobby Award, the highest commendation the Department of Health, Education and Welfare (HEW) could bestow on an employee.

On September 20, Surgeon General Cumming wrote a follow-up letter to Morton seeking his approval of the cooperation offered by Dr. Dibble. The proposed that a "study of the effects of untreated syphilis may have a marked bearing on the treatment, or conversely the nonnecessity of treatment of cases of latent syphilis" (Cumming, 2000). Like Clark, Cumming added that since the proposed study population was entirely without previous treatment, "the cooperation of your hospital offers an unparalleled opportunity to carry on this piece of scientific research which probably cannot be duplicated anywhere else in the world" (Cumming, 2000, p. 77).

At the very end of September 1932, Clark (2000) received a letter from Joseph E. Moore, head of the Department of Venereal Diseases in the medical clinics of the Johns Hopkins Hospital. Moore was interested in studying racial differences in neurosyphilis and would help guide the research design of USPHS syphilis study. Moore contended that syphilis in African Americans is a noticeably different disease from syphilis in Whites and that it was important to collect spinal fluid to understand the difference (Crenner, 2012, pp. 248, 261, 268).

In his letter, Moore (1933, pp. 77–39) was responding to Clark's questions about investigating the course of untreated syphilitic infections in African Americans in Macon County. He recommended focusing on males over 30 who report a history that includes an approximate date of the syphilitic infection of at least ten years earlier, and the presence of the lesions of secondary syphilis after initial genital sores. These men should be given a detailed survey, and the others, who have been previously treated, should be excluded. The selected patients should then have a complete medical history and physical examination, including asking about possible problems with their bone or cardiovascular systems, which are especially common in African Americans. Moore thought that Clark would then have perhaps two or three hundred males with an adequate history to be in the special study. The remainder should be completely disregarded. The actual number at the start of the study was 399 men with syphilis. Later, a comparison group of 201 men with syphilis would be added to the study.

In July 1933, Vonderlehr and Wenger exchanged letters marked "Personal and Confidential," which disclosed their concerns about the emerging study. Vonderlehr (2000) wrote that he had discussed the proposed study with USPHS officers in Washington, and everyone agreed that the study should involve a continuance of the observation of untreated syphilis cases among African American men, with the idea of eventually bringing them to autopsy. He expected those with advanced age and serious complications should only have to be followed for a few years. But he was also concerned that the Rosenwald Foundation was likely to discontinue funding. This meant that it was vital to obtain the cooperation of the state and local health departments and, most important of all, the Tuskegee Institute and Andrews Hospital.

A few days later Wenger, head of the Public Health Service Venereal Disease Center in Hot Springs, Arkansas wrote back. He thought that Vonderlehr had a good plan. However, he saw no need for part of his plan, which proposed hiring a nurse to make weekly calls on patients. This was because "we have no further interest in these patients until they die" (Wenger, 2000, p. 85). The question, in Wenger's view, was whether to secure the postmortems through signed death certificates or having doctors in Macon County turn over demonstration cases to Dr. Dibble, who could keep notes on the cases and persuade the families of participants to permit a postmortem.

Finally, Wenger wanted a pathologist at the US Veterans Bureau Hospital to do the postmortems to ensure their scientific value. He added that

> ...if the colored population becomes aware that accepting free hospital care means a post-mortem, every darkey will leave Macon County and it will hurt Dibble's hospital. This can be prevented, however, if the doctors of Macon County are brought into our confidence and requested to be very careful not to let the objective of the plan be known Wenger (2000, p. 85).

The full details of the Study, as this letter shows, were not to be shared with the potential subjects, their families or others not directly carrying out the Study.

Aware that the Rosenwald Foundation was ending its support for the syphilis treatment program, Clark planned an observation project of only six to eight months to assess the extent of medical deterioration from the first sign of infection among a group of untreated syphilitics. If syphilis could be shown to be a major public health problem and deadly disease among the poor and African Americans, perhaps government funding could be obtained for treatment (Gray, 1998, pp. 42–44; Jones, 2012, pp. 867–868).

4.2.5 *The Initial Study*

From 1932 through 1936, the USPHS conducted a study of treated and untreated cases of syphilis in Macon County. The medical examinations and procedures were conducted at the John A. Andrew Memorial Hospital of Tuskegee Institute. Surgeon General Cumming (2000) wrote Dr. Robert R. Moton, the President of Tuskegee Institute, stressing the value to be gained from the research and the necessity of having the assistance of the (African American) doctors at Andrew Memorial Hospital.

Notices of "blood tests" were distributed through the county extension services and posted in churches, schools and stores. The tests were to be held at churches, schools and outdoors under shade trees. Nurse Rivers believed people showed up eagerly because the screening was something out of the ordinary and in the hope of receiving any kind of medical attention (Gray, 1998, pp. 41, 49). Since the notices requested only men over 25 attend the clinics, many would not appear, suspecting a physical exam for the draft. Clark was therefore forced to test large numbers of women and men at considerable expense who did not fit the experiment's specifications (Brandt, 1978, p. 23).

Vonderlehr realized that only the offer of free care would attract the desired number of volunteers. Informed consent was not collected. Researchers only told the men they were being treated for "bad blood." Although syphilis was prevalent throughout the country, syphilis was not mentioned in polite conversations and was only mentioned occasionally in newspapers. Instead, the term "bad blood" circulated in American communities, including the African American communities (Reverby, 2009, p. 23). Johnson (1934, p. 188) found that not one of the 612 families interviewed seemed to connect syphilis with the sexual act. This suggests that sex education was lacking in these eight settlements. Under Parran, the USPHS had already abandoned providing sex education and prophylaxis (Jones, 1993, pp. 57–58).

Vonderlehr then brought on John R. Heller, a young physician, who had recently joined the USPHS, to assist him in assembling the control group of African American males, who matched the study group in age and socioeconomic status, but who tested negative for syphilis. These men also wanted free medical attention from government doctors. During November and December 1933, and again in February and March, Dr. Heller performed blood tests and physical examinations until he had two hundred controls. At this point, as noted above, the study consisted of 399 men with syphilis and 201 who were syphilis free (Jones, 2012, p. 781; Gray, 1998, pp. 55–56).

The best way to document the long-term complications of syphilis is to do an autopsy to determine the effects of the disease on vital organs, especially the brain, nervous system and spinal cord (Reverby, 2009, p. 161). Although funds were limited, they hoped to perform autopsies on the older subjects who might die over the next few years. To accomplish this, Vonderlehr and Heller contacted all local and state officials who were involved in any way with issuing death certificates. They also met with the medical societies of Macon and neighboring counties, which, given segregation, were all-White. Vonderlehr explained the study and gave them lists of participants. The White physicians were asked not to provide any syphilis treatments to the men, but to report any critical illnesses and deaths. If the men received terminal medical care, this would facilitate conducting an autopsy (Gray, 1998, p. 56).

The problem, in the view of the proponents of observational study, was that many people died at home without the benefit of terminal medical care and were buried without autopsies. The recently passed 1935 Social Security Act provided for a lump sum death benefit to survivors of individuals who died prior to their retirement age of 65. However, the 600 men in the Study were not likely to participate in the Social Security system. On November 29, 1935, Vonderlehr wrote the New York-based Milbank Foundation, which supported medical research. Milbank agreed to provide a grant to pay $50 dollars for each autopsy. The money was to be split, with $15 allocated to the pathologist and the remainder going to the survivor's family for the burial. This was a particularly strong inducement as funeral rites constituted an important component of the cultural life of rural African Americans. Throughout the study, Nurse Rivers would give the study participants with untreated syphilis transportation and hot meals on the days of their examinations (Brandt, 1978, p. 25).

The documentary evidence suggests the doctors informed the participants at annual meetings held around the county in 1935 that continued participation in the program would include burial insurance and treatment of other conditions disclosed by the physical exams (Gray, 1998, p. 57).

Vonderlehr then assigned Nurse Rivers to approach the families and gain their consent for an autopsy. The community knew about the payments and $35 was enough to get individuals to report the deaths of participants (Lederer, 2000, p. 267). For 30 years, from 1935 to 1965, the Milbank Memorial Fund would spend approximately $16,500 or $550 per year on the Tuskegee Study (Gray, 1998, p. 71). In 1958, the participants were given another incentive in the form of an elaborately printed 25-year certificate of participation signed by the Surgeon General and accompanied by $25, one dollar for each year of the Study (Gray, 1998, p. 58).

4.2.6 The 1936 Report

Vonderlehr, Clark, Wenger and Heller presented a paper at the May 1936 meetings of the AMA entitled "Untreated Syphilis in the Male Negro: A Comparative Study of Treated and Untreated Cases" (Vonderlehr et al., 1936). They compared the 399 syphilitic and 201 control subjects in the USPHS Tuskegee Study after two years, with the nine-year retrospective study from the five CCG clinics of patients with syphilis who received varying amounts of treatment during the first two years of their disease.

Approximately one-fourth (26.1%) of 399 untreated syphilitic males had either clinical or serologic evidence of central nervous system involvement, compared with only 2.5 percent of the 201 nonsyphilitic males who had any disease of the central nervous system. Definite cardiovascular disease was found in 46.6 percent of the Study's syphilitic males, compared with 23.9 percent in nonsyphilitic males. Neurosyphilis among the CCG patients peaked at six years at 36.0 percent for those receiving no treatment and 18.4 percent for those inadequately treated during the first two years of infection. In contrast, cardiovascular manifestation among the untreated increased from 7.7 percent at three years to 41.9 percent at nine years, but for the inadequately treated rose from 1.2 percent at three years to 6.9 percent at nine years. The authors suggested that an observation period of at least 20 or more years is necessary to give a true picture of the value of therapy. This seems to indicate their intention for a study that would continue into the 1950s.

4.2.7 The Chicago Syphilis Control Program

In his 1936 report to Congress, Surgeon General Thomas Parran noted that the Social Security Act made money available to states that could be used to improve the ability of state, city and private laboratories to perform accurate, efficient tests for syphilis and gonorrhea. He had met with Dr. Herman Bundesen, the Chicago Board of Health Commissioner, about syphilis control. Bundesen then submitted a budget request to the state of Illinois for a share of its funds for venereal disease testing for the Chicago Syphilis Control Program.

In December 1936, Parran assigned the then-Assistant Surgeon General Vonderlehr and Dr. Wenger as special consultants to the Chicago Program. In his 1936 report to Congress, Surgeon General Thomas Parran noted that the Social Security Act made money available to states which could be used to improve the ability of state, city and private laboratories to perform accurate, efficient tests for syphilis and gonorrhea. Chicago was one of 17 states to receive such funds and was considered to be the flagship city for this effort. Chicago received additional funds from the PHS, Works Progress Administration, Illinois Department of Public Health and Chicago Board of Health (Poirier, 1995, pp. 2, 7–8, 11–12).

In contrast to the USPHS Tuskegee Study, the Chicago Program was located in a racially and ethnically diverse urban city of 3.3 million, of which approximately ten percent were African American. It began with two surveys of physicians and medical facilities in spring and summer of 1937. The second survey was designed to record the age, sex and dates of visits of all people being treated for syphilis. The data was analyzed on an IBM Central Tabulating Unit, the only machine supplied through the USPHS for the exclusive purpose of recording information about syphilis. Data for gender, race, disease, age on admission and date of infection was coded and entered on a summary punch card. Cards could be sorted by people's age, race or political ward and studied by public health statisticians to determine which age, sex and racial groups had the highest incidence of reported syphilis (Poirier, 1995, pp. 106, 111–112).

The Program had the support of the mayor and the *Chicago Tribune*, which printed the word "syphilis," as opposed to the euphemism "bad blood," on its pages. Letters were sent on stationary bearing the letterhead of the Treasury Department, USPHS, and embossed with the seal of the Office of the Chicago Board of Health to a million Chicago households asking if they might be interested in having their entire family tested for syphilis to prevent its spread. In November 1937, the Board of Health began distributing cards to area parents requesting permission to give their high school aged children a free blood test for syphilis. By April 1938, students at four of Chicago's then 47 high schools had been tested. Two of the four schools were predominantly African American (Poirier, 1995, pp. 14–15, 132–133).

The program found a higher incidence of syphilis in African American than White men and adolescents.

African American women frequently were highest of all groups for gonorrhea, while Anglo-American women were lowest for all venereal diseases. That being said, the participation rates for African Americans were always proportionately higher as they presumably showed up for the free testing. Much of the data came from clinics located in poor, largely African American neighborhoods. When the program did not report social or economic information in its results, Chicago's African American community issued a swift critical response (Poirier, 1995, p. 118).

Although the Chicago Program had provided the best statistical data available from mass blood testing, Wenger concluded that the find and treat method alone would prove inadequate, expensive and time consuming, and that more direct methods were needed (Poirier, 1995, pp. 120–121). Almost 30 years later, and without any direct reference to the Chicago Program, sociologist Odin Anderson (1965, p. 48) observed that routine serological testing in high schools provides for an attractive captive audience. However, the highest incidence is thought to be among high school dropouts, resulting in a low yield of cases relative to the time and effort necessary.

Both Vonderlehr and Wenger remained involved in the Tuskegee study. Vonderlehr was the onsite director until 1943 and Wenger continued to advise and assist the study. Perhaps the availability of treatment and lack of follow up data collection in Chicago precluded a comparison analysis in the late 1930s. But such an analysis would not have shortened the longitudinal study which was designed to follow the syphilitic subjects to autopsy.

4.3 The USPHS Tuskegee Longitudinal Study

In the end, the USPHS Tuskegee longitudinal study, a cohort study of men with late-stage syphilis, lasted over 40 years. The men were periodically examined, and autopsies were performed when they died to identify the presence of cardiovascular or neurological complications. A second cohort of men without syphilis were also followed; if they contracted syphilis, they were moved into the first cohort to maintain the number of men with syphilis. Each year, the men in the first cohort were given a blood test and offered various incentives to continue their participation in the study: free medical care except for syphilis treatment, free hot meals on the day of the examination, transportation to and from the hospital and an opportunity to stop in town on the return trip to shop or visit with friends (Rivers et al., 1953, p. 303).

USPHS doctors from Washington D.C. conducted follow-up surveys in 1938, 1948 and 1952, and wrote periodic reports (Gray, 1998, p. 58) and publications such as the *Archives of Dermatology and Syphilology*. Doctors were able to examine 409 of 600 or 68.2 percent of the men in the 1938–1939 follow-up. The examinations revealed that 10 of the 201 nonsyphilitic controls had acquired syphilis between 1933–1934 and 1938–1939. In addition, a proportion of the syphilitics had received small amounts of treatment, with 12 individuals receiving as many as 10 injections. Several of the men had died between the two examinations. To maintain a reasonable number of syphilitic subjects, 14 young untreated men were added to the study in 1938–1939, raising the syphilitic group to 431 men. This was an attempt to ensure that this group embodied only completely untreated cases (Deibert & Bruyere, 1946, pp. 302–303; Olansky et al., 1956, p. 516). The researchers did not compare the results of the first and second examinations of the same individuals because the number of such cases was too small for statistical analysis (Deibert & Bruyere, 1946, p. 303).

Study records indicate that by the end of 1944, 101 syphilitics and 28 without syphilis had died. Of these, 93 or 72.1 percent were autopsied. Those not autopsied either lived outside the area or the news of their death was not received in a timely fashion (Heller & Bruyère, 1946, p. 34). In 1948–1949, a quarter (26%) of the syphilitics and a little over a third (35%) of those without syphilis, who were presumably living, were not examined (Gray, 1998, p. 63). Nurse Rivers (Rivers et al., 1953, p. 393) noted that some of the men refused their examinations because they did not consider themselves sick and did not see any benefits from being examined. They did not want a doctor to tell them that were not as healthy as they felt.

By 1953–1954, about 280 had died, of which 145 or 51.8 percent had been autopsied. Over the 20 years, Nurse Rivers reported only one refusal to conduct an autopsy. She would assure families that the body would not be harmed, that they would learn the reasons for the death and that the information gained might aid them if another family member had the same malady (Rivers et al., 1953, p. 394). Of the 331 known to be living, only 66 (20%) had moved out of Macon County. More than half had migrated north to Chicago, Detroit and Cleveland. But many came back on vacations and family visits. Not surprisingly, the migrants were on average younger compared to those who stayed in the county, 49 versus 61 years of age (Olansky et al., 1954, p. 963).

The 1963 30th-year follow-up made a concerted effort to account for the Study participants. Almost all (96%) of those examined had received some therapy other than an incidental antibiotic injection, and perhaps as many as one-third (33%) had had curative therapy. But the follow-up could not locate or account for 128 of the 630, or 20.3 percent of all the men ever in the study (Rockwell et al., 1964, pp. 794–795, 797). Some may have died but the Study had no record of their deaths. I surmise that those who wanted or needed curative therapy for their syphilis were able to get it and others were able drop out despite repeated efforts to locate them.

Participants were warned that leaving the study would end benefits including burial insurance.

4.3.1 Penicillin

In September 1943, the Subcommittee on Venereal Diseases of the Committee on Medical Research of the Office of Scientific Research and Development appointed a Penicillin Panel to study the effects of penicillin in human beings (Moore et al., 1944). Moore, the lead author, was an advisor to the Study and had worked closely with Parran when he headed the USPHS Division of Venereal Disease (Thomas, 2016, p. 39).

Preliminary results were published in the September 1944 issue of the *Journal of the American Medical Association*, one on penicillin treatment of early syphilis (Mahoney et al., 1944) and the other on action of penicillin in late syphilis (Stokes et al., 1944). The first, on early syphilis, could have called for giving penicillin to men in the control group who would contract syphilis. The second, on late syphilis, could have informed the treatment of those with late-stage syphilis.

Some penicillin research was conducted outside the United States. In 1946, a 12-member USPHS Syphilis Study Section chaired by Moore approved a grant proposal for a project in Guatemala directed by John C. Cutler. Cutler was a highly committed public health investigator persistently seeking long term solutions to treating syphilis by documenting the best time to administer treatments for venereal diseases. He joined the USPHS soon after graduating from Western Reserve University medical school. He directed his first study, the Terre Haute prison experiment, to determine the effectiveness of treatments for gonorrhea. In 1943–1944, prisoners consented to participate and received $100 and a letter of commendation to the parole board at the end of the study. They were injected with various strains of gonorrhea. However, it proved difficult to infect the prisoners and the experiment ended.

Between 1946 and 1948 Cutler directed the Guatemala Syphilis Experiment, in which prisoners, mental patients and soldiers were to be infected with syphilis though sex with prostitutes or an injection of syphilitic tissue directly from syphilitic humans (Thomas, 2016, pp. 49–50). The project was supported by the USPHS, the NIH, the Pan American Sanitary Bureau and the Guatemalan government (Cutler, n. d.). They were treated with penicillin if they showed symptoms. But again, exposure did not always lead to infection and penicillin did not always cure the infection. Cutler never published his Guatemala research. However, historian Susan Reverby (2011, p. 9) was able to reconstruct the study from records in the University of Pittsburgh archives.

His third attempt was at Sing Sing Prison in New York State in 1954. He inoculated prisoners with a vaccine and then exposed them to syphilis to see if it would protect them. Cutler became a lead researcher on the USPHS Tuskegee Study from the mid-1960s until it ended in 1972.

On November 6, 1951, Sidney Olansky, then director of the Venereal Disease Laboratory in Georgia, responded to a letter from Cutler, then Chief of the Division of Venereal Disease, dated October 22, 1951 (Reverby, 2000, pp. 99–101). Olansky and Stanley H. Schuman, an examining physician during the 1952 Tuskegee survey, agreed that follow ups were important and should include clinical examinations. Olansky enclosed an Outline of Problems to be considered in USPHS Tuskegee Study which Cutler had requested. Olansky justified the Study, writing, "We have an investment of almost 20 years of Division interest, funds and personnel; a responsibility to the survivors both for their care and really to prove their willingness to serve, even at the risk of shortening of life, as experimental subjects" (Olansky, 1951, p. 3). The Outline assumed that complete studies will be done, i.e., physical and history, with attention to intercurrent illness (diseases occurring during syphilis) and the administration of penicillin (Olansky, 1951, p. 100). Although Olansky believed that the men should be receiving penicillin treatments, this was never implemented.

4.4 The Exposé

As Reverby (2009) documented, the USPHS Tuskegee Study continued, although it was not because no one in the USPHS expressed criticism of it before 1950 or for a lack of effort by whistleblowers and journalists beginning in 1965. The Study would not become public until Jean Heller's 1972 exposé appeared in the *Washington Star*.

4.4.1 Sociology of Whistleblowing

How and why did the USPHS Tuskegee Study continue for 40 years before becoming public knowledge? One answer can be found in Armand Mauss's (1975, pp. 57–71) excellent review and summary of the literature on social problems as social movements. Social problems are identified and may become social movements by moving through several stages: incipiency, coalescence, institutionalization, decline and legacy. American social values and priorities changed with respect to race and segregation, with the rise of the civil rights movement in the mid-1950s, culminating with the 1965 Civil Rights Act and Voting Rights Act. Americans began questioning clinical research after Henry Beecher's (1966) article in the *New England Journal of Medicine* revealed ethical issues in 22 medical research studies carried out by mainstream researchers and institutions. By 1972, these had coalesced and the time was right for Heller's article exposing institutional racism and quoting Senator William Proxmire, calling the Study "a moral and ethical nightmare." As sociologist Sydney Halpern (2001, pp. 69, 77) pointed out, "moral entrepreneurs" used this moment to shift the moral boundaries in order to gain influence over the public discussion of research ethics.

The other answer to the question of how the study continued for so long lies in Mark Granovetter's (1973) paper on the strength of weak ties. He argued that information can reach a larger number of people and transverse greater social distances when passed through weak rather than strong ties. Strong ties exist in groups like the family, churches and work places in which members interact regularly, usually on a face-to-face basis. In contrast, weak ties link a person to a string of friends of friends or acquaintances who interact occasionally. We will see how a whistle blower, through a friend of a friend, was able to transmit his findings to Jean Heller, whose article brought an end to the Tuskegee experiment.

4.4.2 USPHS's Early Internal Critics

As Reverby has noted (2009, p. 58), Assistant Surgeon General Austin V. Deibert and Albert P. Iskrant, Chief of the Office of Statistics, were two USPHS employees who expressed criticism of the study. When Vonderlehr was assigned to the Chicago Syphilis Study, he sent Deibert to study syphilology at Johns Hopkins in 1937. Deibert went to Tuskegee in 1938 and quickly familiarized himself with the study. His questions were primarily methodological. He discovered that fully 40 percent of 163 men had received some sort of treatment between 1932 and 1934. He told Vonderlehr that this meant the study could not be compared with the Oslo study without being subject to criticism.

To remedy this, Deibert divided the Study subjects into two groups, with inadequately treated men in one, and strictly untreated men of comparable ages and infection dates in the other. After checking with statisticians, Vonderlehr agreed that adding more untreated men was a good idea. Deibert needed to do spinal taps on the new men to complete their examinations and check for any neurological complications. But word had spread about the spinal taps, and fewer men were volunteering. Deibert was sympathetic and listened to the participants. He told Vonderlehr that the men simply do not like spinal punctures. After Deibert promised not to give them, he easily recruited the needed volunteers (Reverby, 2009, pp. 58–60).

In 1948, after reading three recent articles on the USPHS Tuskegee Study, Iskrant concluded that the Study was not what he thought it would be. He expressed his concerns in a letter to Lida J. Usilton, Director of Program Operations, Division of Venereal Disease USPHS. He pointed out several procedural and conceptual weaknesses, and specifically asked if the subjects had been tested in accordance with Alabama law, and if they had been placed in treatment. He also noted that the articles failed to reference recent syphilis studies that reported higher rates of neurological damage in "nonwhites" than in Whites. No response to his letter has been found (Reverby, 2009, p. 63; Jones, 1993, p. 181).

Another internal critic was Olansky, who left the PHS in 1955 for a career at Duke and Emory Universities. While he long defended the program, he eventually publicly stated, "I'm terribly sorry, I wish it had never started" (Warren, 1993). Schuman, who was an epidemiologist on the faculty of the University of Michigan, agreed with Olansky about providing penicillin to the men in the USPHS Tuskegee Study.

4.4.3 External Critics

Count D. Gibson, Jr., MD, was perhaps the first non-USPHS physician to raise ethical issues about the Study. He earned his medical degree at Emory University and joined the US Army Medical Corps, where he became Chief of Laboratory

Service in the 110th Station Hospital in Vienna, Austria. While in Europe, he observed the Nuremberg trials in 1946 (*Stanford Report*, October 29, 2003).

In 1955, Gibson was an associate professor at the Medical College of Virginia focusing on the treatment of infection using newly developed antibiotics, including penicillin. He went to a talk by fellow Emory graduate Sidney Olansky, one of the lead researchers on the Study. Gibson learned that treatment was being withheld from Study participants and talked with Olansky about penicillin treatment. Olansky replied that at the stage it became available, the mortality between the men with and without the disease had evened out, so no real therapy was indicated.

Gibson then read all available reprints of the Study. He wrote a letter to Olansky in which he pointed out that the ethical problem in the Study was that it never mentioned specifically that the syphilitic men were not aware that treatment was being deliberately withheld. He concluded that the continued practice of withholding treatment cannot be justified on the basis of any accepted moral standards such as the Hippocratic Oath and the AMA Code of Ethics (Reverby, 2009, pp. 70–72). Gibson went on to help create a model for community health centers that reached out to impoverished communities. He was engaged in the civil rights movement, and in 1965 marched with Dr. Martin Luther King Jr. from Selma to Montgomery, Alabama (Kim, 2002).

Another external critic was Irwin J Schatz, a young physician who was four years out of medical school when he read "The USPHS Tuskegee Study of Untreated Syphilis; the 30th Year of Observation" in the *Archives of Internal Medicine* (Rockwell et al., 1964). He was shocked and wrote the article's senior author, Dr. Donald H. Rockwell, a surgeon at the USPHS VD research laboratory "I am utterly astounded by the fact that physicians allow patients with potentially fatal disease to remain untreated when effective therapy is available" (Gray, 1998, p. 68).

Rockwell then sent the letter to coauthor, Dr. Anne R. Yobs of the Centers for Disease Control, who wrote a brief memo to her supervisor: "This is the first letter of this type we have received. I do not plan to answer this letter" and stapled it to the top of the letter. After the exposé appeared in 1972, a *Wall Street Journal* reporter found Schatz's letter through a Freedom of Information Act request (Kaplan, 2015). A few months later in April 1965, Yobs attended a meeting regarding the Study at which several doctors from USPHS and the Centers for Disease Control discussed what to do with the data from the Study. According to notes summarizing the meeting, Dr. Yobs observed, "If you can't evaluate it somehow, you better call it quits right now because it is not getting any clearer as time goes on" (Gray, 1998, p. 68).

A notable external critic who was racially representative of the community targeted by the study was Bill Jenkins. Jenkins graduated from Morehouse, a historically African American college in Atlanta, GA, with a degree in mathematics in 1967. He was among the first group of African American students who were recruited straight out of college into the Public Health Service Commission Corps, where he worked as a statistician. Describing himself as "a somewhat Black radical," (Smith, 2019) he started an underground newspaper called *The Drum* to end racism in the Department of Health Education and Welfare (HEW).

Jenkins went to his advisor, a statistician on the Study, who told him it was an important study, adding, "Don't worry about it." Instead, Jenkins read several of the Study's publications and discovered it was well known within the syphilology community because it was so well documented. He talked with some friends at Morehead and after several weeks of investigation they concluded that something was terribly wrong with the Study. They decided to write an article about it in *The Drum*. Finally, they put all the articles they had read in a package and sent it to newspapers including *The Washington Post*, but nothing was ever published. Jenkins went on to join the Centers for Disease Control and Prevention Division of Sexually Transmitted Disease in 1980, where he managed the participants in the health benefits program that ensured health services to the survivors (Seeley, 2019).

4.4.4 The Whistleblower

Peter J. Buxtun, the Tuskegee Study's whistleblower, earned a political science degree at the University of Oregon. He had some experience as a psychiatric social worker and was doing graduate work in history in 1965 when he chanced across a job flyer. He was hired as an interviewer/investigator by the USPHS and assigned to the Venereal Disease Clinic operated by the city of San Francisco. His job was to distribute information on the effects of untreated syphilis to doctors and the public (Buxtun, 1973, p. 1223).

One day in the coffee room, he overheard a conversation in which an older worker was discussing a syphilis patient in Alabama. The patient was insane, and the family had taken him to a private physician who diagnosed tertiary syphilis and gave the patient a shot of penicillin. The older worker added that the USPHS was annoyed because the patient had seen a doctor who had not been notified about the Study and this would jog their statistics (Elliott, 2018).

Part of Buxtun's job was to write a report on a subject related to his work. He requested information on the USPHS Tuskegee Study and received ten reports of what were called roundups—the occasions when the subjects were found and brought in for examination. He discovered the researchers were not treating the men but simply following them until they died, at which point they conducted an autopsy.

Buxtun was the son of a Jewish Czech father and a Catholic Austrian mother, and the family had moved to America in 1937. He was aware of the Nuremberg Trials and the resulting code of ethics. In his report, Buxtun compared the Study with what the Nazis had done. He showed the report to his boss and said he planned to send it to William Brown, the head of the USPHS Venereal Disease Section. Elliott asked Buxtun not to mention his name because he had a family to support and wanted to keep his job. In addition, Buxtun wrote Brown a letter asking whether the men knew the true nature of the study and that they were being followed for autopsy. Brown's response, which apparently was never sent, maintained that the men were volunteers and completely free to leave the study at any time. As mentioned earlier, study participants were able to leave the study but would lose their burial insurance.

Buxtun was invited to meet with Brown in Atlanta at the 1967 annual conference for health care workers specializing in venereal disease. After the first session, Buxtun was taken to a meeting room where he was confronted by Assistant Surgeon General John Cutler. Readers will recall that Cutler had conducted the Guatemala experiment and was now one of the leaders of the USPHS Tuskegee Study. He began by telling Buxtun that the USPHS was doing serious work and that the men were volunteers. Buxtun replied by reading from one of Cutler's reports that the men would not have volunteered without the incentive of compensation for burial expenses. Cutler responded that one of his colleagues must have written that. As mentioned above, some of the free benefits were developed by Nurse Rivers, and the burial benefits were provided through a grant from the Milbank Foundation. A year later Buxton left the USPHS to enter law school in San Francisco (Elliott, 2018; Buxtun, 1973, pp. 1229–1231).

After law school, Buxtun remained in San Francisco. He became friends with a group of recent Stanford graduates. Among them was Edith Lederer, who, in 1972, had just taken a job as an Associated Press reporter. One night, he and Lederer went out for pizza with other reporters. When he started talking about the Study, a friend of Lederer's told him, "Give us a break, we just want to have pizza" (Elliott, 2018). A month later he met Lederer at a dinner party and brought up the Study. When she asked if he had any documentation, they drove to his apartment. After looking at his files, she asked if she could borrow and copy them. She took them to her bureau chief who had her send the material to Jean Heller, an investigative reporter in Washington, DC. Buxtun's identity was protected. His name did not appear in Jean Heller's 1972 exposé, nor was he mentioned in Brandt's (1978) *Hastings Center Report* (Elliott, 2018).

Here, it is useful to apply insights from the theory of whistleblowing, which would consider the USPHS and its Division of Venereal Diseases to be a group with strong ties. They worked together, learned about and commented on each other's projects, and published together, first in a specialty journal (*Journal of Venereal Disease Information*), and later in more widely read journals (*Public Health Reports* and *Archives of Internal Medicine*). When an insider questioned or criticized the Study, they were told it was an important study and not to worry about it. Critics were usually given several research publications to look over. As Mauss (1975, p. 62) pointed out, such boundary testing is a rejection of the compromises and co-optations of the group. As long as those concerned about the ethics and morality of the Study were few and far between, they could not effectively challenge the group's existing prejudices or attract the attention of the emerging civil rights movement in the late 1950s and early 1960s.

Similarly, inquisitive outsiders were sent publications on the Study. If the outsider wrote a letter, it was usually filed and not answered. Some outsiders had a weak link to an individual within the USPHS. They met and talked with their inside contact but were told that penicillin was not readily available until the 1950s and that, given the condition of the syphilitic men, there was no real indication for therapy. Buxtun was a marginal member of the USPHS Venereal Disease Section. Buxtun was warned by his boss about possibly losing his job and got that message when he went to the meeting in Atlanta. His weak link through a group of Stanford graduates was Lederer, who brought his work to the attention of her boss, who in turn had her send it on to Jean Heller in Washington, DC.

4.5 After the Exposé

Heller's article jumpstarted federal government efforts to address the problem. Within five months, the Department of Health, Education, and Welfare (HEW) established the USPHS Tuskegee Syphilis Study Ad Hoc Advisory Panel to investigate the circumstances surrounding the study. The Senate held hearings and passed the National Research Act of 1974, which created the National Commission for the Protection of Human Subjects of Biomedical and Behavioral Research. The Commission's *Belmont Report* (1979) institutionalized research ethics in the United States. A 1974 class action lawsuit awarded $10 million to living survivors and their heirs. In 1996, the Tuskegee Legacy Committee was formed. It encouraged President Bill Clinton to issue a public apology and established the Tuskegee Legacy Project to help investigators conduct ethically responsible research on the impacts of the Study.

4.5.1 The Ad Hoc Advisory Panel

To constitute the Ad Hoc Advisory Panel, the Assistant Secretary for Health and Scientific Affairs appointed nine members from the fields of medicine, law, religion, labor, education, health administration and public affairs who were not full-time government employees. Five of the members were African Americans. Panel members were to review the study and expected to serve until December 31, 1972, but that was extended. The HEW final report was issued on April 28, 1973. The whole process took seven months (DHEW, 1973, p. 1).

While acknowledging that both ethical rules for research and social standards had changed significantly since the Study began in 1932, the Panel identified several shortcomings. The Study lacked a definitive protocol and its experimental design for a long-term study was of questionable value. It should have been proposed as a follow-up to the 1929 six southern county prevalence studies in order to learn more about the course of syphilis, especially in its latent phase. The protocol should have included procedures to ensure the scientific validity and reliability of the Study. The Panel asserted that the participants should have been given penicillin starting in 1953 when it became generally available. Withholding treatment only added to the injustices suffered by the participants. The Panel could not find any evidence that consent was obtained from the participants in the study (DHEW, 1973, pp. 6–8, 12).

The Panel recommended that the study be terminated immediately and that arrangements be made for health assessment, treatment and care of all persons included in the study in a suitably adequate and easily accessible facility. This would require locating all surviving participants as well as others who may have subsequently been infected. The USPHS was to inform all surviving participants of the nature of the Study and its desire to assess their current health status. The Panel called for creating a group of physicians along with a dentist and social worker, to oversee the treatment and referral of the participants for the range of required health care in cooperation with appropriate medical societies and health departments. The men were to continue to receive any promised benefits for participating in the study and arrangements would be made to maintain their standards of living to minimize economic barriers to receiving the health care they required.

Six years later, Alan Brandt, a history graduate student doing bioethics research at the Hastings Center, a nonpartisan, nonprofit organization that was critical to establishing the field of bioethics, pointed out errors in the Final Report (Brandt, 1978). The Panel believed that the men had volunteered for the experiment but the records in the National Archives make clear that the men did not submit voluntarily to participate in the study. They were told and believed that they were getting free treatment from expert government doctors for a serious disease.

Brandt also criticized the Panel's discussion of penicillin, arguing that it betrayed a basic misunderstanding of the experiment's purposes and design. He noted that while medical authorities in the 1930s firmly believed in the efficacy of arsenotherapy for treating syphilis, nontreatment was an essential aspect of the study. Providing syphilitic treatment of any kind would have violated the rationale to study the natural course of the disease until death. Further, he could find no evidence that the USPHS had ever considered providing penicillin.

4.5.2 The Institutionalization of Research Ethics

This chapter has discussed the Tuskegee Study in the context of how social problems become social movements. Here, it turns to the next step in the life cycle of social movements, namely, their institutionalization. This may occur in two ways (Mauss, 1975, p. 63). The first occurs when the mass media takes the movement seriously and government officials acknowledge the problem through public hearings that lead to legislation to address and manage the problem. The second occurs when the movement's goals and objectives are widely adopted and implemented in a society. Mauss noted that this second type is frequently accompanied by a decline in the movement itself. However, in the case of the USPHS Tuskegee Study, it jumpstarted a spin-off social movement in research ethics.

According to Mauss, the last two stages in a social movement are decline and legacy. With respect to the Tuskegee Study, these stages were marked, as noted above, by a class action lawsuit, Presidential apology and the Tuskegee Legacy Committee.

4.5.3 The Class Action Lawsuit

The men who lived to see the end of the Study received some degree of justice and compensation through the efforts of attorney Fred D. Gray. After graduating from the Alabama State College for Negroes, he was encouraged to apply to law school. At the time no law schools in Alabama would accept African Americans, so he graduated from Case-Western Reserve in 1954. He returned to Alabama, passed the bar exam and began his practice. In February 1956, he filed *Browder v. Gayle* to challenge bus segregation in Montgomery, AL. Among the five plaintiffs were Claudette Colvin and Rosa Parks, who refused to give up their seats on a public bus.

In July 1972, Gray (1998, pp. 80–99) met with Charlie Pollard, a Macon County farmer who told him about his involvement in the Study beginning in the 1930s. Gray agreed to represent Pollard in a class action lawsuit (*Pollard v. United States of America*) against the government and any others legally responsible for operating and maintaining the study. The amended complaint was on behalf of living syphilitics and those in the nonsyphilis cohort, and personal representatives of the estates of deceased study participants. The defendants included the Civil Division of the US Department of Justice, the State Health Officer of Alabama and members of the Alabama State Committee of Public Health.

When Gray asked the defendants to produce documents covering the early years of the study, it responded that as far as it knew, no records were available. Gray then met James H. Jones, who had located records of the study from 1931 through 1939 in the National Archives in Washington, DC (Gray, 1998, p. 90). Jones, a history professor at the University of Houston, published *Bad Blood: The Tuskegee Syphilis Experiment* in 1981 after the case was settled.

Gray (1998, pp. 87–89) argued that the defendants had breached their duty to the participants by failing to obtain informed consent by not telling them of the nature and purpose of the study and possible hazards that might result from their participation. Because the Study lacked established protocols, the participants were subject to unnecessary risks. the doctors failed to treat those who had syphilis once penicillin became available. Finally, the defendants violated the civil rights of the plaintiffs by denying them their constitutional rights of equal protection, due process and privacy.

The case was settled in 1974 for $10 million, with living syphilitics receiving $37,500; heirs of deceased syphilitics, $15,000; those living without syphilis, $16,000; and heirs of deceased without syphilis, $5000. In addition to the financial settlements, the defendants were ordered to continue providing other benefits, including free health care for living participants and the families of syphilitic participants, as well as free burial expenses for participants based on the cost-of-living index at the time of their deaths (Gray, 1998, p. 98).

4.5.4 The Legacy Committee

In 1994, James Jones and Susan Reverby spoke at a symposium at the University of Virginia entitled "Doing Bad in the Name of Good? The Tuskegee Syphilis Study and its Legacy." Afterward, a group met in Tuskegee in 1996 and created the Tuskegee Legacy Committee. The committee's first goal was to persuade the nation's President, at that time Bill Clinton, to apologize to the surviving Study participants, their families and to the Tuskegee community.

Clinton issued his apology for the USPHS Tuskegee Study in the East Room of the White House on May 16, 1997. Present were five survivors including Charlie Pollard, family representatives from the other three survivors, and Fred Gray, who brought the successful class action suit. "We can finally say on behalf of the American people, what the United States government did was shameful, and I am sorry" (Clinton, 1977). He went on to announce that the Department of Health and Human Services would award a planning grant to Tuskegee University for a center for bioethics in research and health care. He also committed to providing postgraduate fellowships to train bioethicists, especially among African Americans and other minority groups.

As a follow-up to Clinton's statement, the Legacy Committee (2008) supported the development of a professionally staffed center at Tuskegee for public education about the Study, training programs for health care providers, and a clearinghouse for scholarship on ethics in scientific research. The National Center for Bioethics in Research and Health Care at Tuskegee University was established in 1999. The Center's Legacy Museum features exhibits on the USPHS Tuskegee Syphilis Study and on Henrietta Lacks, whose cancerous cells were taken without her consent and used for polio vaccine testing and other research projects.

The committee also established the Tuskegee Legacy Project to address and understand the range of issues related to the recruitment and retention of African Americans and other minorities in biomedical research studies. One of the first studies was to compare the self-reported willingness of African Americans, Hispanics and Whites in four US cities to participate in research studies (Katz et al., 2006). The study found no differences on likelihood to participate, although African Americans were 1.8 times more likely than Whites to have a higher fear of participation in such studies.

4.6 Discussion and Conclusions

Three key lessons learned are the absence of ethical research protections for the study participants, the lack of moral responsibility of the USPHS and the presence of racism in health research and care that has continued into the twenty-first century.

4.6.1 Ethical Research

The USPHS Tuskegee Study raises ethical issues on informed consent, inducements to participate, and incentives not to leave a study. Providing informed consent faced several challenges. The potential participants understood that they had "bad blood" but not that it was syphilis or sexually transmitted. Today, they would be recognized as a vulnerable racial minority population who were economically and educationally disadvantaged. The observational nature of the Study meant that both syphilitics and nonsyphilitics would not receive treatment related to syphilis. Today, a Data Safety Monitoring Board (DSMB) would require and review a plan to assure the safety and welfare of the research subjects. If a DSMB existed in the early 1950s, it would have challenged the withholding of penicillin to control group men who had contracted syphilis.

Study participants received a series of inducements to continue to participate. The offer of burial insurance proved to be the most persuasive and one that most could not afford to turn down. This was on top of a set of reasonable benefits that covered the costs of transportation for follow-up examinations as well as medical treatment for nonsyphilitic conditions.

Despite the detailed recordkeeping, and efforts by Nurse Rivers and others to maintain contact with the 630 participants, approximately one-fifth (20.3%) were unaccounted for in 1963. They may have been able to leave the study alive, or at least the USPHS had no record of their deaths. As a result, these men could no longer receive burial insurance or other benefits to which they may have been entitled. The records did facilitate the identification of survivors and the families of the deceased for inclusion in the successful class action law suit.

4.6.2 Moral Responsibility

A difficult moral decision is made in the context of a real or hypothetical ethical dilemma (APA, n.d.). The public health leaders making decisions concerning the USPHS Tuskegee Syphilis Study were doing so in a real and evolving social, cultural and professional context over half a century. Medical, public health and social behavioral research ethics also advanced from "do no harm" and self-regulation to the Common Rule (45 CFR 46) and IRBs. Of those leaders involved in the Study's decision making processes, some made more stringent moral decisions while others were more lenient.

The physicians in the USPHS were trained to practice medicine. They were expected to treat and heal others, which requires an ability to interact with patients, listen to their accounts of their medical problems and persuade them to follow their physician's orders and change their health behaviors. These physicians also became public health researchers and investigators, which requires persistence in problem solving through scientific observations and experiments to document new knowledge and improve the lives of individuals, groups and societies.

The physicians and researchers who worked on the Tuskegee Study had to balance their degree of guilt or responsibility for any of their unethical decisions or actions. Some acted morally given the ethical standards at the time they worked there. But several defended the project after the exposé. John Heller stated that "There was nothing in the experiment that was unethical or unscientific" (*New York Times*, 1972), and "there was absolutely no racial overtone, and this was not an attempt to exploit the Negroes. We told them what they had" (Reverby, 2009, p. 91).

As readers will recall, John Cutler, who conducted the Guatemala syphilis experiments, became a lead researcher on the USPHS Tuskegee study during the 1960s until 1972. In "The Deadly Deception," a 1993 Nova documentary about the Tuskegee experiments, Cutler states, "It was important that they were supposedly untreated, and it would be undesirable to go ahead and use large amounts of penicillin to treat the disease, because you'd interfere with the study" (Strait, 1993; Goodman, 2010). Perhaps, they were both experiencing the cognitive dissonance that can occur when someone realizes she or he has behaved in a questionable way but continue believing they were doing the right thing. One way to relive cognitive dissonance between one's values and actions in the Tuskegee Study is to convince others of its beneficial aspects (see *When Prophecy Fails*, Festinger et al., 1956).

Opportunities for career change after a controversy such as this one includes becoming administrators within the health sector, and academic appointments teaching, conducting research or serving as a chair or dean. Both Raymond Vonderlehr and John Heller applied their administrative and leadership skills to health problems beyond venereal diseases. Vonderlehr was head of the USPHS Venereal Disease Division from 1933 to 1943. He then moved to Atlanta, where he helped establish and become the third director of the Centers for Disease Control and Prevention (CDC) from 1947 to 1952. Heller succeeded Vonderlehr as Chief of the Division of Venereal Diseases and directed wartime venereal disease control programs. In 1948, Heller became Director of the National Cancer Institute and later President and Chief Executive Officer of the Memorial Sloan-Kettering Cancer Center in New York.

Thomas Parran had political savvy as well as administrative and leadership skills. He received his initial commission as Assistant Surgeon General in 1917, was appointed Surgeon General in 1936 and retired 31 years later in 1948 with the rank of Vice Admiral. He served as the first dean of the University of Pittsburgh School of Public Health until 1958. The building housing the Graduate School of Public Health was renamed for Parran in 1969. However, his name was removed in 2018 because of his role in both the Tuskegee and Guatemala syphilis studies.

John Cutler was a highly committed public health investigator persistently seeking long term solutions to treating syphilis by documenting the best time to administer treatments for venereal diseases. He became a lead researcher on the USPHS Tuskegee Study from the mid-1960s until it ended in 1972. When the experiment ended in 1967, he became a professor of International Health, serving as Chair of the Department of Health Administration and acting Dean of the

Graduate School of Public Health at the University of Pittsburgh. The University started a lecture series in his name after his death but discontinued it in 2008.

The United States finally apologized for its involvement in the Guatemala syphilis experiment on September 30 and October 1, 2010, when Secretary of State Hillary Clinton and President Barak Obama called Guatemalan President Alvaro Colom (McNeil, 2010).

4.6.3 Racism and Health

A growing body of research reveals that centuries of racism have profoundly and negatively impacted communities of color. It has created inequities in access to housing, education and employment as well as to health services (CDC, 2021). The NIH (NIH, n.d.) has recognized that structural and institutional racism has contributed to a disproportionate burden of morbidity and mortality from COVID-19 in communities of color. It calls for practicing science in a way that includes the full breadth of talent with attention to research that might reduce health disparities.

The initial syphilis study from 1932 through 1936 sought out and included the Andrew Memorial Hospital of Tuskegee Institute and its African American physicians and staff. Except for then-contemporary syphilis treatments, which are now known to be ineffective if not detrimental, the men in the Study received health care and other benefits that they otherwise might not have had. But by the end of World War II and certainly by the early 1950s, participation became disadvantageous. The failure to offer penicillin to the men, and Cutler's three experiments with prisoners between 1943 and 1955, are examples of racism in health care at its worst. Fortunately, the 1972 exposé of the USPHS Tuskegee Syphilis Study and the subsequent reports, class action suits and official apologies have evidenced the role of racism in the Study.

One persistent myth is that the Tuskegee participants were intentionally infected with syphilis. As mentioned earlier, alternative facts concerning the Study were promulgated by African American leaders, a Yale Law School professor and a Detroit radiation oncologist. Although less well known, Cutler's Guatemalan subjects were infected but not the Tuskegee subjects. Reverby thought that "Tuskegee is often raised as a metaphor for structural racism. That is what is at issue, not the Tuskegee study itself" (Carroll, 2016).

The Kaiser Family Foundation (KKF) conducted a survey on Race, Health and COVID-19: The Views and Experiences of African American Americans (Hamel et al., 2020). The survey of over 1700 US adults included an oversample of nearly 800 African Americans. When asked over the last 12 months where they felt they were treated unfairly because of their race, 40 percent of African Americans responded in stores while shopping; 28 percent at their place of work; 26 percent, when dealing with police in a traffic incident; and 20 percent, when getting health care for themselves or a family member. When asked if they can trust a group to do what is right for them or their community, almost all of the time or most of the time, over half said doctors (59%) and local hospitals (56%). Only 30 percent said the police and 25 percent said the courts. They were also asked an open-ended question about why they would not get a COVID-19 vaccine; 39% of African Americans mentioned safety concerns and side effects, while 35 percent said distrust of the health system, government or vaccines in general. Almost 50 years after the USPHS Tuskegee Syphilis study made national headlines, the health care system, however, no longer has the predominant negative impact on African Americans that it previously had.

Acknowledgments I appreciate the comments, advice and suggestions from Cliff Broman, Jan Marie Fritz, Andrea Lowe, Greg Pavela, Susan Reverby, Henry Schaffer, Dianne Schaffer, Zachery Schrag and Ron Westrum.

References

Anderson, O. W. (1965). *Syphilis and society: Problems of control in the United States, 1912–1964*. University of Chicago, Center for Health Administration Studies, Research Series 22.

APA. (n.d.). American Psychological Association. *Dictionary of psychology*. Retrieved August 12, 2021, from https://dictionary.apa.org/ethical-judgment

ASA1. (n.d.). *Franklin Henry Giddings*. Retrieved June 28, 2021, from https://www.asanet.org/about/governance-and-leadership/council/presidents/franklin-h-gidding

ASA2. (n.d.). American Sociological Association. *Robert Ezra Park*. Retrieved March 1, 2023, from https://www.asanet.org/robert-e-park/

Ascoli, P. M. (2006). *Julius Rosenwald: The man who built Sears, Roebuck and advanced the cause of black education in the American south*. Indiana University Press.

Bender, W. (2017, July 20). Did a U.S. surgeon general come up with the idea of the notorious Tuskegee syphilis experiment? *The Philadelphia Inquirer*. Retrieved August 26, 2020, from https://www.inquirer.com/philly/news/thomas-parran-tuskegee-syphilis-hornblum-experiment-20170720.html

Benedek, T. G., & Erlen, J. (1999). The scientific environment of the Tuskegee study of syphilis, 1920-1960. *Perspectives in Biology and Medicine, 43*(1), 1–30.

Blackman, K. (2014). *Public power, private matters: The American social hygiene association and the policing of sexual health in the progressive era* [Master's thesis, University of Montana]. Retrieved June 15, 2021, from https://scholarworks.umt.edu/cgi/viewcontent.cgi?article=5318&context=etd

Brandt, A. M. (1978). Racism and research: The case of the Tuskegee syphilis study. *The Hastings Center Report, 8*(6), 21–29.

Brandt, A. M. (1987). *No magic bullet: A social history of venereal disease in the United States since 1880*. Oxford University Press.

Buxtun, P. J. (1973). *Quality of health care: Human experimentation, 1973- Hearings before the subcommittee on health of the committee on labor and public welfare* (pp. 1223–1228). https://babel.hathitrust.org/cgi/pt?id=uiug.30112108474856&view=1up&seq=51&q1=Buxtun

Carroll, A. E. (2016). A Mistrust of Doctors That Runs Deeper Than One Study. *New York Times*, June 23, 2016, Section A, Page 3.

CDC. (2021). Center for Disease Control. Racism is a serious threat to the public's health. Retrieved March 13, 2022, from https://www.cdc.gov/healthequity/racism-disparities/index.html
Clark, E. F., & Danbolt, N. J. (1955). The Oslo study of the natural history of untreated syphilis: An epidemiologic investigation based on a restudy of the Boeck-Bruusgaard material a review and appraisal. *Journal of Chronic Disease, 2*(3), 311–344. https://doi.org/10.1016/0021-9681(55)90139-9
Clark, T. (1932). The control of syphilis in southern rural areas. In D. H. Rockwell, A. R. Yobs, & M. B. Moore. (1964). The Tuskegee study of untreated syphilis: The 30th year of observation. *Archive of Internal Medicine, 114*(6), 792–798. https://doi.org/10.1001/archinte.1964.03860120104011
Clark, T. (2000). Letter to Dr. J. N. Baker 8/29/1932. In S. M. Reverby (Ed.), *Tuskegee's truths: Rethinking the Tuskegee syphilis study* (p. 73). University of North Carolina Press.
Clark, T., Parran, T., & Cole, H. N. (1932). Cooperative clinical studies in the treatment of syphilis I: Introduction. *Venereal Disease Information, 13*, 135–139.
Clarke, C. W. (1955). The American social hygiene association. *Public Health Reports, 70*(4), 421–427.
Crenner, C. (2012). The Tuskegee syphilis study and the scientific concept of racial nervous resistance. *Journal of the History of Medicine and Allied Sciences, 67*(2), 244–280. https://doi.org/10.1093/jhmas/jrr003
Cumming, H. S. (2000). Letter to Dr. R. R. Moton, 9/20/32. In S. M. Reverby (Ed.), *Tuskegee's truths: Rethinking the Tuskegee syphilis study* (p. 77). University of North Carolina Press.
Cutler, J. C. (n.d.). *John C. Cutler, Tuskegee and Guatemalan syphilis doctor, in his own words*. History News Network. Retrieved August 2, 2021, from https://historynewsnetwork.org/article/132061
Davis, M. M. (1960). Michael Marks Davis [sound recording]: An oral history/interviewed by Theodore Wiprud, May 26, 1960. (National Library of Medicine). WorldCat record id: 62430024.
Deibert, A. V., & Bruyere, M. C. (1946). Untreated Syphilis in the Male Negro. *Journal of Venereal Disease Information, 27*, 301–314.
DHEW. (1973). *Final report of the Tuskegee syphilis study ad hoc advisory panel*. Department of Health, Education and Welfare. US Government Printing Office. Retrieved August 11, 2021, from https://biotech.law.lsu.edu/cphl/history/reports/tuskegee/complete%20report.pdf
Dibble, E. H., Jr. (2000). Letter to Dr. R. R. Moton, 9/17/1932. In S. M. Reverby (Ed.), *Tuskegee's truths: Rethinking the Tuskegee syphilis study* (pp. 75–76). University of North Carolina Press.
Dunne, M. W. (1998). Next steps: Charles S. Johnson and southern liberalism. *The Journal of Negro History, 83*(1), 1–34. https://doi.org/10.2307/2668553
Elliott, C. (2018). Tuskegee truth teller. *The American Scholar, 87*(1), 44–56.
Festinger, L., Riecken, H. W., & Schachter, S. (1956). *When prophecy fails*. University of Minnesota Press.
Gamble, V. N. (1997). Under the shadow of Tuskegee: African Americans and health care. *American Journal of Public Health, 87*(11), 1773–1778. https://doi.org/10.2105/AJPH.87.11.1773
Goodman, A. (2010). From Tuskegee to Guatemala via Nuremberg. *Democracy Now!*. Available at: https://www.democracynow.org/2010/10/6/from_tuskegee_to_guatemala_via_nuremberg. Accessed 25 July 2023.
Gray, F. D. (1998). *The Tuskegee syphilis study: The real story and beyond*. NewSouth Books.
Halpern, S. A. (2001). Constructing moral boundaries: Public discourse on human experimentation in twentieth-century America. In B. Hoffmaster (Ed.), *Bioethics in social context* (pp. 69–89). Temple University Press.

Hamel, L., Lopes, L., Muñana, C., Aartiga, S., & Brodie, M. (2020). *Race, Health, and COVID-19: The views and experiences of Black Americans.* Kaiser Family Foundation (KKF). Retrieved July 19, 2022, from https://files.kff.org/attachment/Report-Race-Health-and-COVID-19-The-Views-and-Experiences-of-Black-Americans.pdf

Hanchett, T. (1988). The Rosenwald Schools and black education in North Carolina. *The North Carolina Historical Review, 65*(4), 387–444. Retrieved July 20, 2020, from www.jstor.org/stable/23520778

Harrison, L. W. (1956). The Oslo study of untreated syphilis review and commentary. *British Journal of Venereal Diseases, 32*(2), 70–78.

Harter, C. (n.d.). *Julius Rosenwald Fund (1917-1948).* Amistad Research Center. Retrieved July 17, 2020, from http://amistadresearchcenter.tulane.edu/archon/?p=creators/creator&id=154

Hawkins, B. (2020, January 15). *Photo-history—The incredible true story of how Booker T. Washington & the president of Sears built 5000 schools for generations of southern black students.* Retrieved July 19, 2020, from https://www.the74million.org/article/photo-history-the-incredible-true-story-of-how-booker-t-washington-the-president-of-sears-built-5000-schools-for-generations-of-southern-black-students

Heller, J. R., & Bruyère, P. (1946). Untreated syphilis in the male Negro; mortality during 12 years of observation. *Journal of Venereal Disease Information, 27*, 34–52.

JAMA. (1970). Boeck's sarcoidosis. *Journal of the American Medical Association, 211*(9), 1537–1538. https://doi.org/10.1001/jama.1970.03170090053013

Johnson, C. S. (1934). *Shadow of the plantation.* University of Chicago Press.

Jones, J. H. (1993). *Bad blood: The Tuskegee syphilis experiment.* The Free Press.

Jones, J. H. (2012). Bad blood thirty years later: A Q & A with James H. Jones- interview by Nancy M. P. King. *Journal of Law, Medicine & Ethics, 40*(4), 867–872. https://doi.org/10.1111/j.1748-720X.2012.00716.x

Kaplan, S. (2015). Dr. Irwin Schatz, the first, lonely voice against infamous Tuskegee study, dies at 83 *Washington Post.* April 20, 2015.

Katz, R. V., Kegeles, S. S., Kressin, N. R., Green, B. L., Wang, M. Q., James, S. A., Russell, S. L., & Claudio, C. (2006). The Tuskegee Legacy Project: Willingness of minorities to participate in biomedical research. *Journal of Health Care Poor Underserved, 17*(4), 698–715. https://doi.org/10.1353/hpu.2006.0126

Kim, R. (2002). Count D. Gibson Jr.—physician and activist. SFGate. Available at: https://www.sfgate.com/bayarea/article/Count-D-Gibson-Jr-physician-and-activist-2815655.php. Accessed 25 Sept 2020.

Lederer, S. (2000). The Tuskegee syphilis study in the context of American medical research. In S. M. Reverby (Ed.), *Tuskegee's truths: Rethinking the Tuskegee syphilis study* (pp. 266–275). University of North Carolina Press.

Lombardo, P. A., & Dorr, G. M. (2006). Eugenics, medical education, and the public health service: Another perspective on the Tuskegee syphilis experiment. *Bulletin of the History of Medicine, 80*(2), 291–316. https://doi.org/10.1353/bhm.2006.0066

Mahoney, J. F., Arnold, R. C., Sterner, B. L., Harris, A., & Zwally, M. R. (1944). Penicillin treatment of early syphilis. *Journal of the American Medical Association, 126*(2), 63–67.

Mauss, A. L. (1975). *Social problems as social movements.* J. B. Lippincott Co.

Mayo Clinic. (2020). *Syphilis: Patient care & health information, diseases & conditions.* Retrieved July 2, 2020, from https://www.mayoclinic.org/diseases-conditions/syphilis/symptoms-causes/syc-20351756

McNeil, D. G. Jr. (2010). U.S. Apologizes for Syphilis Tests in Guatemala. *The New York Times.* October 1, 2010. Retrieved March 10, 2023, from https://www.nytimes.com/2010/10/02/health/research/02infect.html

Mills, C. W. (1959). *The sociological imagination.* Oxford University Press.

Moore, J. E. (1933). Letter to T. Clark. In S. M. Reverby (Ed.), *Tuskegee's truths: Rethinking the Tuskegee syphilis study* (p. 44). University of North Carolina Press.

Moore, J. E., Mahoney, J. F., Schwartz, W., Sternberg, T., & Wood, W. B. (1944). The treatment of early syphilis with penicillin. *Journal of the American Medical Society, 126*(2), 67–73.

New York Times. (1972). Ex Chief Defends Syphilis Project. *New York Times*, July 28, 1972, p. 29.

NIH. (n.d.). National Institutes of Health. *Ending structural racism*. Retrieved March 13, 2022, from https://www.cdc.gov/healthequity/racism-disparities/index.html

Olansky, S. (1951). *Letter to Cutler with Outline of Problems*. Retrieved August 05, 2021, from https://secure-media.collegeboard.org/digitalServices/pdf/yes/Document24.pdf

Olansky, S., Harris, A., Cutler, J. C., & Price, E. V. (1956). Untreated syphilis in the male Negro: Twenty-two years of serologic observation in a selected syphilis study group. *AMA Achieves of Dermatology, 73*(5), 516–522. https://doi.org/10.1001/archderm.1956.01550050094017

Olansky, S., Simpson, L., & Schuman, S. H. (1954). Untreated syphilis in male Negro: Environmental factors in Tuskegee study. *Public Health Reports, 69*(7), 691–698.

Osler, W. (1897). *Internal medicine as a vocation: An address to the New York Academy of Medicine*. Creative Media Partners.

Parascandola, J. (2008). *Sex, Sin, and Science. A history of Syphilis in America*. Praeger Publishers.

Poirier, S. (1995). *Chicago's War on Syphilis, 1937-40: The times, the "trib," and the clap doctor*. University of Illinois Press.

Reverby, S. M. (2000). *Tuskegee's truths: Rethinking the Tuskegee Syphilis study*. University of North Carolina Press.

Reverby, S. M. (2009). *Examining Tuskegee: The infamous Syphilis study and its legacy*. University of North Carolina Press.

Reverby, S. M. (2011). Normal exposure and Inoculation Syphilis: A USPHS "Tuskegee" doctor in Guatemala, 1946-48. *Journal of Policy History, 23*(1), 6–28.

Rivers, E., Schuman, S. H., Simpson, L., & Olansky, S. (1953). Twenty years of follow-up experience in a long-range medical study. *Public Health Reports, 68*(4), 391–395. PMID: 13047502 PMCID: PMC2024012.

Rockwell, D. H., Yobs, A. R., & Moore, M. B., Jr. (1964). The Tuskegee Study of Untreated Syphilis, the 30th year of observation. *Archives of Internal Medicine, 114*(6), 792–798. https://doi.org/10.1001/archinte.1964.03860120104011

Rosenwald Foundation. (n.d.). *What is the Julius Rosenwald Foundation*? Retrieved October 11, 2021, from http://www.searsarchives.com/people/questions/rosenwaldfoundation.htm

Seeley, K. Q. (2019). Bill Jenkins, Who Tried to Halt Tuskegee Syphilis Study, Dies at 73. *New York Times*. Retrieved February 9, 2023, from https://www.nytimes.com/2019/02/25/obituaries/bill-jenkins-dead.html

Selected Letters. (2000). Letter to Taliaferro Clark 9/23/1932. In S. M. Reverby (Ed.), *Tuskegee's truths: Rethinking the Tuskegee syphilis study* (pp. 74–75). University of North Carolina Press.

Smith, H. (2019). Bill Jenkins, epidemiologist who tried to end Tuskegee syphilis study, dies at 73. *The Washington Post*. 2/27/2019.

Snyder, L. P. (1995). The career of Surgeon General Thomas J. Parran, Jr., MD, (1892–1968). *Public Health Reports, 110*(5), 630–632.

Stokes, J. H., Sternberg, T. H., Schwartz, W. H., Mahoney, J. F., Moore, J. E., & Woods, W. B. (1944). The action of Penicillin in late Syphilis including Neurosyphilis, Benign Late Syphilis and Late Congenial Syphilis: Preliminary report. *Journal of the American Medical Association, 126*(2), 73–80. https://doi.org/10.1001/jama.1944.02850370011003

Strait, G. (1993). The Deadly Deception. *Nova*. PBS. January 26, 1993.

The Chicago Commission on Race Relations. (1922). *The Negro in Chicago: A study of race relations*. University of Chicago Press.

Thomas, K. K. (2016). *Health and humanity: A history of the Johns Hopkins Bloomberg School of Public Health, 1935-1985*. Johns Hopkins University Press.

Thomas, S. B., & Quinn, S. C. (1991). The Tuskegee Syphilis Study, 1932 to 1972: Implications for HIV education and AIDS risk education programs in the black community. *American Journal of Public Health, 81*(11), 1498–1505. https://doi.org/10.2105/ajph.81.11.1498

Tuskegee University. (n.d.). *History of Tuskegee University*. Retrieved June 28, 2021, from https://www.tuskegee.edu/about-us/history-and-mission

University of Iowa. (n.d.). *Continuing review of IRB-approved research*. Human Subjects Office. Retrieved June 10, 2021, from https://hso.research.uiowa.edu/institutional-review-boards-irbs

Usilton, L. J. (1930). Prevalence of venereal disease in the United States. *Venereal Disease Information, 11*(12), 543–562. Retrieved July 13, 2020, from https://babel.hathitrust.org/cgi/pt?id=uc1.$b158525&view=1up&seq=19

Vonderlehr, R. A. (2000). Letter to O. C. Wenger 7/18/1933. In S. M. Reverby (Ed.), *Tuskegee's truths: Rethinking the Tuskegee Syphilis study* (p. 84). University of North Carolina Press.

Vonderlehr, R. A., Clark, T., Wenger, O. C., & Heller, J. R., Jr. (1936). Untreated Syphilis in the male Negro: A comparative study of treated and untreated cases. *Journal of the American Medical Society, 107*(11), 856–860. https://doi.org/10.1001/jama.1936.02770370020006

Warren, J. (1993, May 20). Too little, too late. *Chicago Tribune*. Retrieved August 5, 2021, from https://www.chicagotribune.com/news/ct-xpm-1993-05-20-9305200354-story.html

Wenger, O. C. (2000). Letter to R.A. Vonderlehr 7/21/1933. In S. M. Reverby (Ed.), *Tuskegee's truths: Rethinking the Tuskegee Syphilis study* (p. 84). University of North Carolina Press.

Zimmermann, E. L. (1921). A comparative study of Syphilis in Whites and in Negroes. *Archives of Dermatology and Syphilology, 4*(1), 75–88. https://doi.org/10.1001/archderm.1921.02350200078008

Chapter 5
The Wichita Jury Study: Violating a Sacred Trust

> Now, Jurymen, hear my advice—all kinds of vulgar prejudice I pray you set aside:
> With stern judicial frame of mind, from bias free of ev'ry kind, This trial must be tried!—
> W. S. Gilbert, *Trial by Jury*

5.1 Introduction

In 1954, researchers at the University of Chicago were able to tape-record actual jury deliberations in six civil trials in the federal district court in Wichita, Kansas. Although the judge and the attorneys agreed to the tapings, the jurors were not aware that their deliberations would be taped and did not give their consent. When this became known, it made national headlines. A subcommittee of the US Senate Committee on the Judiciary (United States Senate, 1955, 1956) held hearings on the matter, and subsequently Congress passed Public Law 84-919, an Act designed to further protect and assure the privacy of grand or petit juries in the courts of the United States while such juries are deliberating or voting.

The Subcommittee to Investigate the Administration of the Internal Security Act of 1950 (Public Law 81-831), also known as the Subversive Activities Control Act, required Communist organizations to register with the federal government (Katz, 1972). The subcommittee hearings that took place at the end of the McCarthy red scare era make for fascinating reading, especially with respect to the University of Chicago study. Those involved in the research were subpoenaed and testified on October 12 and 13, 1955. Law School Dean Edward H. Levi and lead researcher Harry Kalven Jr. were questioned about their subversive political affiliations and religious beliefs. Levi was asked about his possible involvement in the National Lawyers Guild, the American Civil Liberties Union (ACLU) and the Hillel Club, and Kalven, about his advocating clemency for Ethel and Julius Rosenberg, who were convicted for spying for the Soviet Union (United States Senate, 1955; Drury, 1955a, 1955b; Cornwell, 2010, p. 62).

H. Perlstadt, *Assessing Social Science Research Ethics and Integrity*, Clinical Sociology: Research and Practice, https://doi.org/10.1007/978-3-031-34538-8_5

In 1956, the Internal Security Subcommittee of the Senate Committee on the Judiciary held public hearings in order to assess the impact of the Wichita Jury Study upon the integrity of the jury system. These hearings led to Public Law 84-919 (1956) which prohibited any recording of jury deliberations. This law reinforced existing legal opinions. In *McDonald v. Pless* (1915), the US Supreme Court found that the courts of each jurisdiction, state and federal, must be in a position to adopt and enforce their own self-preserving rules. In *Clark v. US* (1933, p. 16), Justice Benjamin Cardozo wrote that:

> Freedom of debate might be stifled, and independence of thought checked if jurors were made to feel that their arguments and ballots were to be freely published to the world. The force of these considerations is not to be gainsaid. But the recognition of a privilege does not mean that it is without conditions or exceptions.

State exceptions would permit videotaping of jury deliberations for documentary films and television broadcasts with the approval of the courts and consent of the counsels and jurors. As this chapter will discuss, the Wichita Jury Study became a negative example of social science research ethics but contributed to scientific jury selection and jury consultants.

5.2 The Chicago Jury Project

In 1952, the University of Chicago Law School applied for and received a large grant from the Ford Foundation to conduct research on three topics: the jury system, commercial arbitration and public attitudes toward taxation. In England, the use of civil trials by jury had diminished enormously since the early 1900s because they were more expensive, time consuming and unpredictable regarding the amount of damages awarded, compared with a civil trial by a judge without a jury (See Devlin, 1956, p. 129; Zander, 1978). The Chicago Jury Project would investigate how juries reached decisions in both civil and criminal cases. The study of the American jury system became the largest of the three projects, eventually claiming over $1.4 million, more than half of the Ford Foundation funds given to the law school (Cornwell, 2010).

The law school's interest in empirical research can be traced back to University President and Chancellor Robert Hutchins. Hutchins had been dean of the Yale Law School from 1927 to 1929. In his first report as dean, Hutchins expressed interest in learning how the judicial system actually works and how it may be improved (Schlegel, 1979, p. 493; Zimring, 2003, p. 2).

Just before he left Yale for the University of Chicago, Hutchins secured funding for the Institute of Human Relations, which brought social scientists to Yale's law school. Among them was sociologist Dorothy Swain Thomas, who was hired as a consultant in the summer of 1929 to help decide what the Institute should be doing.

She officially joined the Institute in 1930 and served as director of Social Statistics (1935–1939). She would become the first woman president of the American Sociological Association.

In 1951, Hutchins left the University of Chicago to become an associate director of the Ford Foundation; a year later, Dean Levi applied for a grant to create a graduate research and clinical center at the law school (Schlegel, 1995, pp. 238–239; Zimring, 2003, p. 3). The grant application stated that the subject matter of law is human behavior and identified five research topics: the youthful offender, obscenity, the association between beliefs about tax burden and attitudes toward government spending, the jury system and arbitration. He thought that empirical research studies could suggest solutions and improvements for these social problems and legal practices (Schlegel, 1995, pp. 239–240).

With respect to the jury system specifically, the University of Chicago researchers hoped to learn how jurors understand the judge's instructions, the types of evidence presented, the length of a trial and the order of presentation of a case and how lawyers can influence the behavior and decisions of juries (United States Senate, 1955). They proposed several methodologies for their study. One was to interview jurors after a verdict was returned. Journalists often do this after a high-profile case; the Chicago researchers proposed interviewing jurors, with the permission of the courts, under conditions assuring anonymity and other safeguards (United States Senate, 1955, p. 161; Meltzer, 1953). They also proposed having a simulated jury observe an actual trial or holding a mock trial and then recording the jury's deliberations and conducting subsequent interviews with the mock jurors.

Overall, the Chicago Jury Project conducted four studies. One study collected and analyzed data on trials where the judge disagreed with the jury's verdict. The second compared juries' first ballot vote and its final verdict. A third observed a series of trials and then interviewed the judges, the attorneys and the jurors at the end of the trial. The fourth explored how juries interpreted judicial instructions (Strodtbeck et al., 1954; Kalven, 1955; Ferguson, 1955, pp. 79–80).

5.2.1 *The Mock Jury Studies*

The University of Chicago hired Fred Strodtbeck, an assistant professor of sociology at Yale, to serve as director of experimental research of the University of Chicago Law School's American Jury Project from 1953 to 1959 (Kalven & Zeisel, 1966). He received his Ph.D. from Harvard in 1950 and from 1947 to 1950 had worked with social psychologist Robert F. Bales as a research assistant conducting small-group experiments. Bales (1950) developed Interpersonal Process Analysis (IPA), a method of measuring the types of interactions that occur in small face-to-face groups. Group discussions were tape-recorded. The researchers listened to the tapes and counted every time a participant did one of the following:

(A) showed positive social-emotional actions by praising another, joking or agreeing
(B) worked on the task by giving suggestions, opinions or information
(C) participated in the task by asking for information, assessments or directions
(D) showed negative social-emotional actions by disagreeing, withholding help, or being antagonistic or warding off criticism (Madge, 1962, pp. 432–434).

Then and now, a jury is comprised of a small group of 6 to 12 people who are asked to reach a decision, preferably unanimous. Strodtbeck planned to tape-record mock juries to understand the relationship between judicial instructions in civil cases concerning negligence and possible juror bias toward the injured party. The IPA system did not, however, measure the content of the interactions, that is, what information was asked for or given and what was agreed upon in reaching a verdict. Instead, Strodtbeck et al. (1954) developed a salience score, based on Bales's IPA method, which would compare an ideal or rational jury deliberation to the observed deliberations of the mock jury. The salience score would indicate the importance or centrality of a concept or wording of a juror's statements in the trial deliberation transcripts. They could then compare an ideal or rational jury deliberation to the observed deliberations of the mock jury.

An ideal jury would consider those portions of the law that, according to the judge's instructions, were applicable to the resolution of the case at hand. It would evaluate all the relevant evidence applicable to those facts in dispute in order to apply the law. The ideal jury would not consider facts or testimony the judge told them to disregard. It would accurately remember what had happened during the trial and logically appraise the evidence. Finally, it would be logical in its application of the law to the presented facts in reaching its verdict.

In late 1953, Strodtbeck discovered an auto negligence case that had been tried in a federal district court in Chicago. The case was closed and renamed *Doyle v. Miller* to protect the identities of the plaintiff and defendant. The plaintiff, Miss Doyle, a 40-year-old stenographer, was injured when the car in which she was a passenger collided with a car driven by the defendant Miller (Strodtbeck, 1953a, 1953b; Broeder, 1959). Strodtbeck created a 70-minute audio tape based on the transcript of the court proceedings. The recording included the opening statements, the testimony of eyewitnesses, medical personnel, the plaintiff and defendant, the closing arguments and the judge's instructions to the jury. Participants were jurors drawn by lot from an existing jury pool.

Strodtbeck's experimental design consisted of six mock juries. Each would each hear slightly different versions of the trial. These versions allowed the researchers to assess the influence of attorney objections to particular points of law on a juror's determinations of liability, the amount of monetary reward and how well the jurors followed the judge's instruction to disregard evidence about the defendant's liability insurance.

After hearing one of the six versions of *Doyle v. Miller*, each of the 12 mock jurors filled out a first ballot indicating their beliefs concerning the defendant's guilt and the appropriate amount, if any, to award to the plaintiff. They then met and deliberated in a room with a recording machine and one observer until a verdict was reached. Afterward, the jurors completed a postdeliberation questionnaire which asked about the credibility of witnesses, the impartiality of the judge and the contributions of fellow jurors to the deliberations. This questionnaire also asked about their attitudes and bases of actions, and their final estimate of how much they personally believed the plaintiff should recover (Strodtbeck, 1953b; Mikva, 1954).

5.2.2 *Access to Actual Jury Deliberations*

It was only after the jury study was underway that the researchers decided to include a limited number of actual jury deliberations to check the results of their experimental methods and findings (Ferguson, 1955, p. 79). Paul Kitch was a trial attorney and member of the Wichita, Kansas, Bar Association's public relations committee. The committee wanted to combat a series of articles in a local newspaper that claimed people were able to hire a lawyer who would trick juries and win their cases (United States Senate, 1955, pp. 152–153). As an alumnus of the University of Chicago Law School, Kitch received a pamphlet describing the proposed jury study and pointing out that the risk of distortion inherent in the simulated situation (i.e., mock juries) would be appraised in light of experiences with both real and simulated juries (United States Senate, 1955, p. 159).

Kitch (1972), a classmate of Dean Levi, wrote Professor Bernard Meltzer in May 1953 suggesting that the researchers could directly obtain information about what goes on in a jury room if courts would permit the installation of a secret transcribing device (Kitch, 1953a). The University of Chicago researchers agreed that if Kitch could get a court to consent, they would be interested in a study that might involve the recording of an actual deliberation (United States Senate, 1955, pp. 115, 153).

In November 1953, Kitch (1953b) wrote a letter to Orie L. Phillips, Chief Justice of the Tenth Federal Circuit Court of Appeals, which included Kansas, as a follow-up to a discussion they had had about a possible research project to study the jury system. Phillips was a well-known and respected jurist who exhibited leadership as a judicial administrator and had served on several Judicial Conference Commissions (Tepker, 1992, pp. 330–338). In 1950, he received the American Bar Association's Gold Medal for "Conspicuous Service to the Cause of American Jurisprudence."

Kitch envisioned a three-year study of 500 jury deliberations in various federal courts across the country. The study would not include any criminal cases, and transcriptions would only be made with the consent of the trial counsels for the respective litigants (United States Senate, 1955, p. 177). He suggested that the study could be started in the Tenth Circuit comprising the states of Oklahoma, Kansas, New Mexico, Colorado, Wyoming and Utah, which he believed contained a typical cross section of community life. In 1950, its major metropolitan areas included Denver, Oklahoma City, Salt Lake City, Tulsa and Wichita, while approximately half the population in New Mexico and Wyoming lived in rural areas. In addition, District Judge Delmas C. Hill of Wichita was willing to assist in the proposed project. Hill had been a prosecutor in the 1945 war crimes trial of General Yamashita and was a member of the special three judge district court panel that heard *Brown v. Board of Education of Topeka* in the summer of 1951 (Tepker, 1992, pp. 402–408).

In his letter to Judge Philips, Kitch suggested a detailed set of procedures resembling a research protocol that a researcher might submit to an IRB. Microphones would be placed in the jury room and be wired to a recording device located in the judge's office. The judge would be the sole custodian of the key and would designate a person to operate the machine. The recordings would be made only in civil cases with the explicit permission of the trial judge and the counsels for both parties. No one would be allowed to monitor the taping of the ongoing jury deliberations, and the recordings would be kept under lock and key until the case had been decided and all appeals terminated (United States Senate, 1955, p. 178).

According to Kitch, the recording would then be forwarded to a designated person who would oversee its transcription, after which the original recording would be destroyed. The transcript would then be edited to remove all personal names, geographical references and other identifying information. The edited and original transcripts would be sent to the clerk of the circuit court of appeals for final review. If approved, the edited transcript would be returned to the research committee and the original transcript destroyed. These procedures would ensure both the confidentiality and security of the data. Finally, the entire project, insofar as it involved the recording of jury deliberations, would receive no publicity from any source until after the project was completed (United States Senate, 1955, p. 178).

Judge Hill did not want the jurors to be informed that their deliberations would be recorded because he did not want that fact to affect the jury deliberations (United States Senate, 1955, p. 192). Social scientists have established that if research subjects are aware that they are being studied, they may change their behavior to perform according to expectations. This phenomenon, the Hawthorne Effect, is named for a study that took place in Hawthorne, Illinois, outside Chicago. Employees at a Western Electric Plant located there knew they were being studied. The result was that workers in three shops at the plant increased their productivity when the level of workplace lighting was increased, but when lighting was restored to its normal level, output did not fall back to its original rate (Mayo, 1933; Madge, 1962, p. 169).

For the jury study, Judge Hill would allow the Chicago researchers to personally interview the jurors only after they had been finally discharged from jury duty. He stipulated that the jurors should not learn that any recordings had been made. The copies of the interviews would be sent to him, and he would forward them to Judge Phillips (United States Senate, 1955, p. 1193).

Throughout the negotiations, Judge Philips repeatedly stated that he was still of the opinion that the jurors should be informed, but eventually indicated that he might not object if it was tried out on an experimental basis in a limited number of cases. Kitch then informed the University of Chicago researchers that the need to disclose the taping to the jurors had been waived for the proposed set of trials (United States Senate, 1955, p. 194).

5.2.3 *Taping Jury Deliberations*

In the spring of 1954, recordings were made of jury deliberations using concealed microphones in Judge Hill's jury room (United States Senate, 1955, p. 194). All six trials were civil cases: two automobile damage suits, two government land condemnations, one breach of promise to marry and one damage suit arising from alleged underground water seepage (United States Senate, 1955, p. 192). Prior to the trials, both plaintiff and defendant attorneys met with Judge Hill in his chambers. They were fully informed about the project and that an audio recording would be made but not heard by anyone until after all posttrial matters were disposed of by the court and it was clear that the case would not be appealed. The jury deliberations were only to be recorded if the attorneys agreed to the conditions of the study. They had the legal right to do so on behalf of their clients (United States Senate, 1955, pp. 148, 175).

After the trial was completed and the jury discharged, the research team planned to interview the jurors. Lawyers may interview jurors after any trial is over unless explicitly prohibited from doing so by the trial judge, and jurors may talk with the media once the jury is dismissed. The researchers also planned to interview some of the attorneys.

The two keys to Judge Hill's office, where the recording machine was placed, were held by Hill, and Abner Mikva, a Chicago attorney and University of Chicago Law School graduate. Mikva had clerked for US Supreme Court Justice Sherman Minton in 1951–1952. He would serve in Congress from 1969 to 1973 and 1975 to 1979. He was appointed to the US Court of Appeals for the District of Columbia in 1979 and was chief judge from 1991 to 1994. Judge Hill's coat closet was kept locked at all times except to start and stop the machine. Mikva took all of the recordings back to Chicago, which Dean Levi kept under lock and key. Transcripts were made of each case when it was finally disposed.

By mid-April 1954, the jury deliberations were recorded for three of the trials. At that point, Strodtbeck (1954a) sought to reduce the costs of purchasing an official trial transcript by making a full recording of the actual trial. Mikva spoke with Judge Hill and reported that the judge was willing to have recordings made of the trial proper if the microphones could be concealed. The microphones were located under the judge's bench and the clerk's desk. This additional taping of the courtroom proceedings may explain why, after the Wichita Jury Study was made public, the federal law would go on to prohibit all recordings of courtroom procedures as well as jury deliberations.

Judge Hill requested, however, that the researchers conduct no interviews with the jurors until May 2, when the entire jury pool was to be dismissed. The judge set no guideline concerning the number of persons who could be interviewed. Strodtbeck and Mikva agreed that one or two people should be sent down with Mikva around May 3 to complete the interviews of the 36 jurors who had participated in the deliberations recorded so far. The taping of the final three trials and jury deliberations was completed by mid-June.

Meanwhile, the Wichita Bar Association independently conducted a mail survey of all jurors who, during the previous year, had served in the Tenth Circuit (Kitch et al., 1954). Their research questions asked jurors the following questions: if they followed the judge's instructions? Their impression of the system? and What suggestions they had for improving the jury system? Over 1100 surveys were mailed to jurors by the clerks of the respective districts within the Tenth Circuit, and 620 were returned in time to be included. The 56.4 percent response rate would have been higher had the Colorado questionnaires been mailed out by the district court clerks in a timely fashion.

Kitch presented the results at a meeting of the Tenth Circuit in Estes Park, Colorado, in July 1954. The survey found that 86.6 percent of responding jurors felt they fully understood the court's instructions. However, 41.6 percent reported a dispute among the jurors as to the meaning of these instructions. Of those reporting a dispute, 63.0 percent indicated that the jury decided to ask the judge for more information. Almost two-thirds (64.5 percent) of the jurors thought it would have helped if they had been provided with a written copy of the court's instructions for use in the jury room. Today, many jurisdictions require that final instructions be issued in writing and at least one copy be provided to the jury.

5.2.4 Presenting Preliminary Findings

The American Bar Association met in Chicago the third week of August 1954. Strodtbeck (1954b) saw the meeting as an opportunity to present some findings from the mock jury deliberations in the *Doyle v. Miller* automobile injury case. Within a week, Mikva received an urgent call from Judge Hill in Wichita requesting the return of all tape recordings, the summaries of the jury deliberations and the interviews with 30 jurors that had been completed from four of the six cases (United States Senate, 1955, p. 193). Since three of the cases had gone to appeal, Judge Hill wanted to know if those tapes had been listened to and if the jury interviews had been read (Strodtbeck, 1954c).

On August 26, 1954, Strodtbeck returned all the materials from the six trials. His cover letter to Judge Hill read in part:

> We exhibited charts and played recordings from our mock trial experimentation program. Many of our visitors listened to these simulated trial deliberation recordings. We consistently stressed that our materials were drawn from 18 repetitions of the same trial. . . . The attendant at the exhibit took particular pains to explain that the deliberations were from a mock-trial with a hung jury. (Strodtbeck, 1954d)

Judge Hill returned all the materials to the University of Chicago almost a year later (Inventory, 1955).

In the spring of 1955, Chief Justice Phillips was preparing the program for the Judicial Conference of the Tenth Circuit scheduled for July in Estes Park, Colorado. The judge asked Kitch if he wished to have his committee participate in the program.

In addition to presenting the findings from the Wichita Bar Association's survey of jurors, Kitch suggested having a session featuring a portion of one of the recordings of the Wichita jury deliberations, and Judge Phillips agreed (United States Senate, 1955, pp. 190–191). Kitch contacted Dean Levi, who objected. But Kitch successfully argued that since the Tenth Circuit had cooperated in facilitating the research, the Dean could not deny the judge's request (United States Senate, 1955, p. 182). They agreed to using an edited tape with all identifiers removed, including those of the University of Chicago. Judges Phillips and Hill reviewed the tape the day before the session.

The session, entitled "A Study of the Functioning of Juries," was held on July 7. The program began with a statement by Judge Hill explaining the purpose and conditions of the experiment. He noted that little to no effort had been made to scientifically study the jury system with the aim of improving its efficiency. Such a study would require the full cooperation of the bench and bar. Judge Hill then read the list of safeguards and conditions that had been agreed to by the court and the researchers. The audience was told that the unidentified case concerned an automobile accident in which a driver swerved to avoid hitting a pedestrian. An abbreviated version of the trial was presented with Judge Hill playing the part of the trial judge and two members of the Wichita bar playing the attorneys. At the end of the trial, Judge Hill read the actual instructions given to the jury (Program of 10th Circuit Conference, 1955; Strodtbeck, 1955).

Strodtbeck was introduced as "Mr. X," the representative of a large eastern university conducting the research. He played sections of the recording, commented on what was happening after each section and read his concluding comments (United States Senate, 1955, p. 132; Strodtbeck, 1955). This was followed by a group discussion of the procedures used and the desirability of future studies (Program of 10th Circuit Conference, 1955). Someone asked what would have happened if one of the jurors had discovered the jury room was wired and reported that to the Court? A few minutes later, Judge Sherman Christensen from Utah asked how the knowledge that jury rooms were bugged would affect juries and jurors in the cause of justice in general? To this, Judge Hill replied he thought it would be very bad. Someone then defended the study, suggesting that a few instances of bugging seemed unlikely to have any adverse effect on our jury system at all, and gave his opinion that the study would ultimately be beneficial (Marson, 1955).

5.3 The Scandal

The first press report on the session appeared in the *Rocky Mountain News* on Friday July 8 under the headline, "Court Rules on Criminal Insanity Opposed." The piece focused on US Solicitor General Simon E. Sobeloff's address, but went on to report that:

> Attorneys and judges . . .were taken into the jury room by recording . . .for the first time at any such meeting. The recording of a jury's deliberation in a case was made secretly as part of the study of the jury system being undertaken in the 10th Circuit. All geographical references and the names were deleted from the recording, which was made with the consent of the attorneys, under supervision of the judge, but without knowledge of the jurors. The recording was sealed until after all possibility of appeal had passed and then was studied as part of the inquiry as to whether the jury system was working. (Margolin, 1955)

News of the events at the Estes Park conference slowly made its way around judicial and legal circles. In a September 29 letter to Judge Phillips, Federal District Judge Richard Hartshorne of New Jersey wrote that he had heard about Kitch's 1954 mail survey of Tenth Circuit jurors and that he had wanted to have a similar survey done in the Third Circuit. But he had also been told of the jury recordings and playback at the 1955 Tenth Circuit Judicial Conference. Hartshorne (1955) wrote that while recognizing the laudable purposes of the project and the restrictions imposed by Phillips, if jurors can no longer consider their deliberations to be secret, further violations could set a possible precedent. He sent copies of his letter to, among others, US Supreme Court Chief Justice Earl Warren, Chief Justice Arthur T. Vanderbilt of the New Jersey Supreme Court and an ABA past president, and Will Shafroth, Chief of the Division of Procedural Studies and Statistics of the Administrative Office of the United States Courts.

A week later, on October 5, the story broke in the *Los Angeles Times* with the headline "Eavesdropping on Jury Under Probe by US" (Cornwell, 2010, p. 56). No one has identified how the Washington bureau of the *Los Angeles Times* learned of the recordings. By that evening, US Attorney General Herbert Brownell Jr. denounced any eavesdropping on juries and indicated that he would ask Congress for a law to prevent any such intrusions upon jury privacy (*Chicago Sun Times*, 10/6/55).

Warren Olney III (1955), an assistant attorney general in the Justice Department's Criminal Division, was concerned that the Justice Department was not aware of, and had not given its consent to, the recording of the two condemnation suits to which it may have been a party. He asked Professor Kalven, Judge Hill and Dean Levi for the names and case information for the two condemnation cases, but they refused to divulge them. The Justice Department considered the taping of jury deliberations an obstruction of justice and stated that such taping would be prosecutable were it not for the absence of any corrupt motive. He enclosed a draft of a proposed bill the department intended to submit to Congress to prevent such intrusions upon the privacy of the deliberation of juries in federal courts by any persons and by any means.

Meanwhile, the story exploded into a national scandal, with editorials, columnists, cartoonists and letters to the editor accusing the project and researchers of threatening the jury system and democratic government (Cornwell, 2010, pp. 56–57). Several called for legal action of some sort against the researchers, the university and the foundation that funded it (Burchard, 1958, p. 687).

In a press release, the ACLU noted that even if the jurors themselves had consented, the threatened damage to civil liberties would be far greater than the scientific knowledge, however beneficial (United States Senate, 1955, pp. 189–190).

On the other side of the political spectrum, George E. Sokolsky, a conservative radio broadcaster and syndicated columnist, raised a set of pointed questions about social behavioral research:

> What can the Chicago professors with a fat grant from the Ford Foundation learn about the behavior of ordinary Americans from their casual conversation even in the jury room? And what is the object of all these behaviorist studies, starting with the Kinsey reports on the most private of occupations to this peep-holing of a jury room? What are the objectives of the Rockefeller and Ford Foundations in underwriting these behaviorist studies? Is it to prove that we are not all professors and most of us act all too human? (Sokolsky, 1955).

After the hearings, Senators James Eastland (D-MS), chair of the Internal Security Subcommittee and William Jenner (R-IN) introduced legislation that passed both the House of Representatives and the Senate without opposition and signed by President Eisenhower on August 2, 1956. Public Law 919 provided for a fine of not more than $1000 and/or imprisonment of not more than one year for anyone not a member of the jury who records, observes or listens to the proceedings of a US jury while it is deliberating or voting. By 1996, only seven states explicitly prohibited recording of jury deliberations (Abramovsky & Edelstein, 1996).

5.4 Subsequent Studies

Despite the political and ethical condemnation of the Wichita Jury Study, audio and visual recording of jury deliberations continued, usually with the jurors' explicit knowledge and consent. One example from the academic sector is the work of University of Wisconsin law professor Stephen Herzberg, who taught trial advocacy and conducted research on jury selection at the University of Wisconsin Law School. While working for a Milwaukee public television station in 1977, he broadcast the first gavel to gavel coverage of a murder trial in the United States. He planned to make a documentary on the jury process to educate both attorneys and the public.

In 1985, he asked Judge Ralph Adam Fine if he could film jury deliberations in the Milwaukee County Circuit Court. He wanted a victimless crime since he did not want a victim to testify on camera. Victor Manian, the chief circuit judge, proposed using a case in which the defendant, a felon, had purchased a gun in violation of the letter of a Wisconsin law (Vidmar and Diamond, 2001). Potential jurors were told their deliberations would be filmed and only three of the 40 potential jurors consequently declined to serve. Judge Fine allowed the defense attorney to argue for nullification in front of the jury which is not permitted in many jurisdictions (Diamond, 2007). But he instructed the jury that although they could acquit for any reason, they could not nullify the law (Nichols 1996). It took 11 jurors two and half hours to convince the lone holdout that the defendant should be acquitted because the prosecutor did not prove beyond a reasonable doubt that the defendant had committed the crime. The jury's filmed deliberations aired on PBS on April 13, 1986 (Abramovsky & Edelstein, 1996, pp. 867–868).

Other examples of documenting jury decision making processes can be found in the media. For instance, when a set of high-profile cases in the early 1990s rekindled interest in how juries reached their decisions, CBS television decided to produce a documentary on civil and criminal cases that would include trial coverage, jury deliberations and commentary by a panel of experts. The American Bar Association's Section on Litigation agreed to sponsor the project. The Arizona Supreme Court approved CBS's application in a unanimous decision in March 1996. CBS was able to select any case in which the parties, including the jurors, gave full consent to be filmed. In consultation with a superior court judge in Phoenix, jury proceedings were filmed in three criminal trials. The three cases involved manslaughter, burglary and possession of narcotics for sale. In April 1997, portions were shown on *CBS Reports: Enter the Jury Room* (Abramovsky & Edelstein, 1996, p. 872).

In August 2004, ABC aired a special program called *In the Jury Room*, which featured the case of a drug addict on trial for killing two people with lethal cocktails of prescription drugs. The Ohio Supreme Court granted ABC permission to film, if the defendant, his lawyers, the judge, the prosecutors and prospective jurors all agreed. Ten of the 60 potential jurors did not want to be filmed and were excused from the jury panel.

On the first vote in the jury room, half the jurors favored a guilty verdict; after several days of deliberations, that became unanimous. But when discussing the death penalty, one juror, who had originally favored acquittal, opposed a life sentence and insisted on parole after 30 years. This resulted in a hung jury and the judge proceeded to impose a sentence of two consecutive life terms. In posttrial interviews, six jurors said the filming had not affected their behavior or the case's outcome. Several other jurors thought the lone holdout was showboating by playing to the cameras. The holdout claimed that other jurors were inhibited by the cameras (Rosenberg, 2004).

As part of a public awareness effort, the Arizona Supreme Court sanctioned a videotaping project of 50 civil juries in Pima County (Tucson). Discussions and deliberations for all cases were recorded by two unobtrusive cameras and microphones mounted in opposite corners of the jury rooms at ceiling level, so that all jurors could be seen on a split screen seated around the jury table. An on-site technician was instructed to tape the conversations in the jury room whenever at least two jurors were present (Diamond et al., 2003, pp. 5, 18).

The tapes reveal that the jurors, who, unlike those in the previous examples, had not been informed they would be recorded, were aware of the unobtrusive cameras. When one juror arrived late, another juror jokingly asked, "Did everybody smile and wave at the camera?" (Diamond et al., 2003, p. 22). In another trial, a juror remarked, "Three days and nine people for this. No wonder the court system is so backed up. It's ridiculous. For being educated professionals [the lawyers], (excuse me if the camera's on or not) they're disorganized" (Diamond et al., 2003, p. 22). The jurors were brutally honest. They talked about the weight of a litigant, the obnoxiousness of a lawyer and that the judge was not paying close the trial proceedings. In their deliberations, the jurors occasionally spoke sharply to one another about their opposing views. Diamond et al. (2003, pp. 22–23) concluded that, overall, jurors were probably not altering their behavior in the presence of the cameras, and once they were focused on the trial task before them, they forgot about the cameras.

5.4.1 Entertainment and Jury Consulting

The public is curious to know what is really going on behind the curtain, and popular and cultural answers have ranged from Plato's *Allegory of the Cave* to the *Wizard of Oz*. Reginald Rose wrote *Twelve Angry Men* based on his jury service on a manslaughter case in New York City in the early 1950s. The play is set entirely in the jury room. Juror #8 is the last holdout on the first ballot but eventually persuades everyone to choose acquittal. In September 1954, CBS broadcast *Twelve Angry Men* (Westinghouse Studio One, 1954; Ferguson, 1955, p. 83). Rose won the 1955 Primetime Emmy Award for Best Written Dramatic Material. A motion picture adaptation was released in 1957 which received Oscar nominations for Best Picture, Best Director and Best Writing/Screenplay from another medium. Like the expert studies explored in this chapter, the play and film hold the actions and responsibilities of jurors under the microscope.

More than half a century later, public curiosity about jury deliberations remained strong. In 2016, CBS (2022) began a successful television series, *Bull*, about a trial consulting firm based on the early career of Dr. Phil McGraw, the founder of a successful trial-consulting firm. Bull's firm uses psychology, high tech data and investigative research to select jurors, find and work with witnesses and monitor the reactions of a mock jury observing the trial proceedings.

As Strodtbeck has shown, the Chicago Jury Study has had long-term effects, including, in this case, contributions to understanding jury selection and providing a basis for the practice of jury consultation. In one of two articles based on the mock jury deliberations in the *Doyle v. Miller* automobile negligence case, Strodtbeck considered sex role differences in jury deliberations (Strodtbeck & Mann, 1956). The data suggested that men were more likely to give opinions and orientation directed at the solution of the problem, while women tended to react to and support the contributions of other jurors. In civil trials, some states require only a majority verdict, but a unanimous verdict is required if the claim is for money and is above a certain amount. Based on these findings, a jury consultant might want to select men who would understand and back their client's case and women who would favor the amount being claimed.

The second article based on the Chicago Jury study (Strodtbeck et al., 1957) found that men and jury members in higher status occupations were more likely than women and jury members in lower status occupations to have higher participation, influence and perceived competence for the jury task. They also found that the foreman was more likely to be a male of higher occupational status, but that that outcome may result from the early impressions other jury members make based on dress and speech. These findings, in turn, have come to enable jury consultants to assess a juror's status as a potential foreman.

Jury consultants provide a variety of services for trial lawyers. In many cases, the consultant prepares witnesses, attorneys and even the accused for trial. A consultant with a background in psychology might develop a questionnaire to identify which potential jurors would be most sympathetic to their client's case. A consultant with a background in sociology might organize and conduct focus groups before the trial to gather opinions about the case (APA, n.d.).

The first known use of jury consultants was in the 1972 trial of Daniel and Philip Berrigan, who were accused of conspiring to plan violent demonstrations against the Vietnam War. The defense attorneys decided to poll those persons likely to qualify as jurors in Harrisburg, PA, the site of the trial. The results led the defense attorneys to conclude that Protestants with a fundamentalist outlook and college graduates would favor the prosecution. As a result, the defense was successful in having a jury selected that consisted entirely of blue-collar workers. This jury deadlocked at 10–2 in favor of acquittal. The government afterward declined to retry the case (USLegal, 2019).

5.5 Discussion and Conclusion

The Wichita Jury Study appears in training and educational materials for both social science researchers and IRB members and staff. The issue here is not the need for human research protection, but rather the accuracy of these materials, which highlight the lack of informed consent. The larger Chicago Jury project contributed to a better understanding of the nature of juries, the complexity of social science research ethics and the integrity of the jury system.

5.5.1 Research Ethics

The earliest ethical discussions of the Wichita Jury Study concern whether social science researchers should conduct jury studies, the impact of the secret recording of actual juries on social science research and the need for laws prohibiting the taping of jury proceedings (Amrine & Sanford, 1956; Burchard, 1957, 1958; Vaughan, 1967). The study became a prominent subject in human-research protections through the work of legal-medical ethicist Jay Katz, who included source materials on the jury study in his encyclopedic work *Experimentation with Human Beings.* He provided the following summary of the case:

> In 1954 a group of law professors and social scientists, with the approval of judges of the Tenth Judicial Circuit, recorded the deliberations of juries in six civil cases in the United States district court in Wichita, Kansas. The investigators did not inform the jurors that microphones had been concealed in the jury room. The litigants were also unaware of the research project, although their attorneys had consented to the recordings Katz (1972, p. 67)

He then asked the reader to consider several questions about the study. Two that are pertinent here include:

- What values are preserved or undermined by delegating decision making power to each participant respectively?

- Under what circumstances should the extent of actual or potential harm and benefit to subjects or society affect the authority of each participant in the human experimentation process? (Katz, 1972, pp. 67, 10).

The problem of delegating decision-making power was a central concern of Judge Philips and Dean Levi, with Kitch acting as a proactive mediator who promoted taping actual jury deliberations. The judges and university researchers were aware of the actual and potential harm to the jury system and to a lesser extent to the jurors themselves. The US senators, most newspaper editors, columnists and citizens writing letters to the editor feared serious potential harm to the sanctity of the jury system and American democracy.

The *Institution Review Board Member Handbook*, now in its fourth edition (Amdur & Bankert, 2022, p. iii), provides IRB members with valuable information on the structure and processes involved in carrying out their responsibilities to protect the rights and welfare of research subjects, to understand the complex issues and to make difficult decisions about biomedical and social behavioral research. The *Handbook* begins with a brief history of the IRB system. Unfortunately, its cursory reviews of main milestone research studies, including the Wichita Jury Study, contain several factual errors.

All four editions state that:

> The study involved audio-taping jury deliberations in criminal trials in Wichita, Kansas. To avoid influencing their behavior, the jurors where not informed that they were subjects of a research project or that their discussions would be recorded. The investigators completed the study as planned and presented the results in respected academic forums." (Amdur, 2003, pp. 11–12; Amdur & Bankert, 2007, pp. 8–10; Amdur & Bankert, 2011, pp. 8–9; Amdur & Bankert, 2022, pp. 8–9) The investigators did not inform the jurors that microphones had been concealed in the jury room. The litigants were also unaware of the research project, although their attorneys had consented to the recordings. (Katz, 1972, p. 67)

In fact, all six jury deliberations recorded in Wichita were civil cases.

The Chicago Jury Project researchers interviewed, with the consent of courts in Chicago, IL, and Brooklyn, NY, 700 jurors at the conclusion of their service in 225 criminal trials to determine the relationship between first-ballot votes and the final verdict.

All four editions also state:

> Congressional hearings were held on the subject, and eventually Congress passed a federal law that prohibited the recording of jury deliberations in any setting.

While it is reasonable to assume that federal law preempts state law, this did not apply to state and local courts. The US Constitution does address the secrecy of jury deliberations. In addition to the 1956 federal law, only seven states make recording jury deliberations a misdemeanor, and in most of them, it appears that the law was not intended to apply to court sanctioned recordings (Harawa, 2021, pp. 598, 617).

The first two editions of the *Institutional Review Board Member Handbook* (Amdur, 2003, p. 11; Amdur & Bankert, 2007, pp. 8–9) stated that

> A motivation for this study was the concern that showmanship on the part of trial attorneys might have a major influence on the jury verdict. One can only imagine the cynical comments this kind of discussion would elicit today!

This was dropped in the third edition (Amdur & Bankert, 2011, pp. 8–9).

Readers will recall that the Chicago study of how lawyers influenced the behavior and decisions of jurors focused on the *Doyle v. Miller* automobile injury mock jury deliberations. They analyzed to what extent an attorney's objections to particular points of law influenced the jury's determinations of liability and monetary compensation. Although two of the Wichita cases involved automobile damage suits, attorney behavior was not analyzed.

Twenty-five years after the Wichita Study became a scandal, Strodtbeck (1980) addressed the rumors alleging that after the Wichita jury taping incident, the government would not permit publication of parallel studies. These rumors were in fact erroneous, the result of confusing the experimental mock-jury studies with the actual jury deliberations recorded in Wichita. He noted that the scandal surrounding the clandestine taping of Wichita juries consumed a great deal of the Chicago researchers' time and embarrassed the Ford Foundation when Congress was rewriting the tax codes governing nonprofit organizations.

In terms of research ethics, the Wichita Jury study was conducted 16 years before the 1971 *Department of Health and Education HEW Institutional Guide to HEW Policy on Protection of Subjects*, known as "The Yellow Book," and 24 years before the 1979 *Belmont Report*. As mentioned earlier, Katz (1972, p. 16) correctly noted that jury deliberations were recorded in six civil cases. In contrast, all four editions of the *IRB Handbook* mistakenly claimed that six criminal, not civil trials, were taped.

5.5.2 Research and Jury Integrity

In the 1970s, the Wichita Jury Study was used to justify the establishment of federal regulations for the protection of human subjects in research (45 CFR 46). By 1991, this became the Common Rule, when, as has been noted, 15 federal departments and agencies agreed to follow it to protect the privacy of subjects and maintain the confidentiality of data. In the Wichita Jury Study, both the researchers and judges involved established and followed procedures that ensured the confidentiality and privacy of the jurors. Only a few individuals had access to the data; the names, geographical locations and other identifiers were deleted; and the tapes and transcripts of the jury deliberations destroyed. Although the location was revealed in the press and Senate hearings, Kalven, Judge Hill and Dean Levi refused to name the cases when asked by an assistant attorney general in the federal Justice Department's Criminal Division.

Given the strict confidentiality, the Wichita Jury Study involved a low probability of harm and low magnitude of harm, that is, minimal risk to the individual jurors. Although the jurors were not asked to give their personal informed consent to be taped, the trial judge and counsel for both parties, readers will recall, consented to the taping of jury deliberations in specific cases.

Like newspaper and media reporters, social scientists can interview or survey jurors after their service without presenting an ethical threat to jury research or the integrity of the jury system. The ethical issues under discussion after the Study was published focused on the justification for deceiving the jurors and compromising the integrity of the jury system.

Ferguson (1955, pp. 86–87) defended the deception and failure to inform the jury. At that time, he was studying law and international relations at the University of Chicago; he would become an American Ambassador and university president. Ferguson argued that if the prevailing doctrine in common law requires secrecy in the jury room, then individual jurors are entitled to personal privacy but the jury as a body is not. A juror cannot testify to matters occurring in the jury room and this guarantees impartial jury deliberations. If jury members are not able to consent to a recording without affecting their deliberations, then the judge has the authority to grant or deny the consent. Subsequent filming of jury deliberations suggested that when jurors were aware of the cameras, almost all remained on task during the deliberations. Only a few showboated by drawing attention to themselves and their opinions.

During the discussion following the presentations at the 1955 Tenth Circuit Judicial Conference, as noted above, Judge Christensen from Utah asked how the knowledge that jury rooms were bugged up would affect juries and jurors in the cause of justice in general. This question was on the minds of many lawyers. But was it on the minds of social scientists?

To answer this question, sociologist Waldo Burchard (1957, 1958) conducted a survey in 1956 of lawyers, political scientists and sociologists, comparing their views on concealing microphones to study jury deliberations. He sent a total of 900 questionnaires, 300 each, to lawyers, political scientists and sociologists with response rates of 42.7 percent from lawyers, 38.0 percent from political scientists and 57.0 percent from sociologists.

The questionnaire asked respondents to agree or disagree with a series of statements. Question 24 asked respondents to agree or disagree with the following statement: "The use of a concealed microphone in a jury room for study purposes cannot be compared to 'wiretapping' to get evidence, since the purposes for which the information is to be used are entirely different." Sociologists were more likely to agree (76 percent) compared with political scientists (58 percent) and lawyers (49 percent).

Question 13 stated, "The use of concealed devices for purposes of studying the jury in action will destroy public confidence in the jury system." Lawyers were most likely (65 percent) to agree, compared with political scientists (32 percent) and sociologists (27 percent) (Burchard, 1957, pp. 114, 115). Sociologists, then, were more likely to distinguish between wire-tapping and concealed microphones to describe jury research, were less likely to believe that using concealed microphones for research purposes will destroy public confidence in the jury system, and were least likely to believe that taping would destroy public confidence in the jury system.

Another survey question asked whether a researcher should surrender information when ordered to do so by a judge. Lawyers were more likely to agree (39 percent), compared with political scientists (19 percent) and sociologists (10 percent).

And another question that reveals similar response patterns asked, "Is it better to face prosecution than to risk identifying informants." This time sociologists were more likely to agree (80 percent), compared with political scientists (53 percent) and lawyers (39 percent) (Burchard, 1958, pp. 688, 690, 691). The sociologists favored following the lead of journalists who were reluctant to reveal sources. Borden (2007:16) suggested that virtue theory requires doing one's role related work well. An occupation's purpose provides it with moral justification and its member's standards of excellence. According to Plaisance, (2021), a professional social science association's ethics try to balance the goals of conducting research within the guiding principles for ethical research of the federal government and nonprofit Foundations.

Buchard's findings reveal differences among lawyers, political scientists and sociologists, with sociologist closer to holding journalist practice ethics, while political scientists are closer to the ethical practices of attorneys and presumably judges.

The decision not to ask the Wichita jurors to consent to having their deliberations audio taped may have taken the following into consideration. As we have seen, some were concerned that the jurors would be uncomfortable and unwilling to speak their mind if the deliberations were taped. However, several subsequent studies and television programs indicate that jurors were both aware of the cameras and occasionally spoke frankly to one another about their opposing views. I assume that IRBs would approve taping where legal, if the jurors gave their informed consent.

5.5.3 *Ownership of Data*

During the Wichita Jury Study, the question of who owned and had control of the data and findings arose at two points. The first was when Judge Phillips wanted to play a small section of one deliberation, but Dean Levi objected. The second was when the US Justice Department's Criminal Division requested the names and case information for the two condemnation cases and Professor Kalven, Judge Hill and Dean Levi all refused to divulge them.

Funders also factor into questions about data ownership and control. Biomedical and social science research is primarily funded by federal, state and local government agencies; nonprofit foundations, e.g., the Ford Foundation; and private industry, e.g., tobacco or pharmaceutical companies. The ownership of the data and findings, along with publication rights, depends on whether the research project is grant or contract based (see Steneck, 2007, pp. 888–889). A research grant usually specifies that the researcher must carry out the research as planned and submit reports, with the institution that receives the grant having control of the data. The institution may choose to require approval before presenting or publishing the findings. Government agencies and many philanthropic foundations may also require a review of research presentations and publications to ensure accuracy, protection of subject privacy and recognition of the funding source. Private companies seek to retain the right to the commercial use of the data for patent and property rights as well as advertising and lobbying purposes. Under a contract, the researcher delivers a product or service which is then usually owned and controlled by the private funder.

5.5.4 *Conclusion*

The Wichita Jury Study is a controversial social science research project. It asked what ethical principles should govern research in sacrosanct areas such as jury rooms, and what procedures should be followed to ensure moral actions and responsibilities on the part of researchers, judges, trial attorneys, litigants and jurors. The answers differed among and between judges, trial lawyers, sociologists, political scientists and ethicists.

The Wichita Jury Study was possibly the first empirical scientific effort to learn what actually happens in a jury room. As we have seen in Chap. 3, IRB members expect a research proposal to contain a set of clearly defined hypotheses, a research design that includes data collection from a population, a sampling methodology and the project's overall impact. Some IRB members accustomed to reviewing proposals for randomized clinical trials are accordingly uncomfortable with a proposal focused on the jury system that includes surveys, a mock jury, secretly taping jury deliberations and finally taping the actual trial.

The Wichita jury study had several unanticipated impacts. Congress passed Public Law Public Law 84-919 to further protect and assure the privacy of grand or petit juries in the courts of the United States while such juries are deliberating or voting. However, some states allow the recording of jury deliberations. The research methods and findings from such recordings enabled the development of jury consultants to advise trial lawyers on jury selection and preparing witnesses and their client to testify. Finally, it impacted the development of federal research guidelines to protect participants in human research, culminating in 45 CFR 46, the Common Rule.

Acknowledgments This chapter has benefited from comments and suggestions by Erin York Cornwall, Shari Diamond, Paula L. Hannaford, Valerie Hans, Chris Herrera, Ruth Homrighaus, Dan Menchik, Jerry Schatz, Zachary Schrag and Ruth Spivak. I am grateful for the assistance of the reference librarians at the University of Chicago Special Collection Research Center who facilitated access to the archived jury project materials. Archival materials consulted for this paper, including letters and memoranda from the Chicago Jury Project, can be found in the Joseph Regenstein Library of the University of Chicago. Finally, I want to thank Erica Harbatkin who went to the Library of Congress and found the correspondence between judges Richard Hartshorn of New Jersey, Orie L. Phillips of the Tenth Circuit Court and Earl Warren of the US Supreme Court.

References

Abramovsky, A., & Edelstein, J. I. (1996). Cameras in the jury room: An unnecessary and dangerous precedent. *Arizona State Law Journal, 28*(3), 865–892.

Amdur, R. J. (2003). *Institutional Review Board: Member handbook*. Jones and Bartlett Publishers.

Amdur, R. J., & Bankert, E. A. (2007). *Institutional Review Board: Member handbook* (2nd ed.). Jones and Bartlett.

Amdur, R. J., & Bankert, E. A. (2011). *Institutional Review Board: Member handbook* (3rd ed.). Jones and Bartlett.

Amdur, R. J., & Bankert, E. A. (2022). *Institutional Review Board: Member handbook* (4th ed.). Jones and Bartlett.

Amrine, M., & Sanford, F. H. (1956). Across the secretary's desk: In the matter of juries, democracy, science, truth, senators, and bugs. *American Psychologist, 11*, 54–60.

APA. (n.d.). American Psychological Association Trial Consultant Career. Retrieved December 26, 2022, from https://www.psychologyschoolguide.net/psychology-careers/trial-consultant/

Bales, R. F. (1950). *Interaction process analysis: A method for the study of small groups*. Addison Wesley.

Borden, S. L. (2007). *Journalism as practice: MacIntyre, virtue ethics and the press*. Ashgate.

Broeder, D. W. (1959). The University of Chicago Jury Project. *Nebraska Law Review, 38*, 744–760.

Burchard, W. W. (1957). A study of attitudes toward the use of concealed devices in social science research. *Social Forces, 36*(2), 111–116. https://doi.org/10.2307/2573844

Burchard, W. W. (1958). "Lawyers, political scientists, sociologists – and concealed microphones," The Profession: Reports and opinion. *American Sociological Review, 23*(6), 686–691. www.jstor.org/stable/2089057

CBS. (2022). *Bull*. (CBS Television Series 2016). Retrieved March 17, 2022, from https://www.cbs.com/shows/bull/

Chicago Sun Times (10/6/55). Brownell Assails U. of C. Jury Recording. p. 3.

Clark v. United States, (1933) 289 U.S. 1, 13.

Cornwell, E. Y. (2010). Opening and closing the jury room door: A socio-historical consideration of the 1955 Chicago Jury Project Scandal. *Justice System Journal, 31*(1), 49–73. https://www.jstor.org/stable/27977478

Devlin, P. (1956). *Trial by jury*. Stevens & Sons, Limited. Retrieved October 20, 2021, from https://socialsciences.exeter.ac.uk/media/universityofexeter/schoolofhumanitiesandsocialsciences/law/pdfs/Trial_by_Jury.pdf

Diamond, S. S. (2007). Dispensing with deception, curing with care: A response to Judge Dann on nullification. *Judicature, 91*(1), 20–25.

Diamond, S. S., Vidmar, N., Rose, M., Ellis, L., & Murphy, B. (2003). Juror discussions during Civil Trials: Studying an Arizona innovation. *Arizona Law Review, 45*(1), 1–81.

Drury, A. (1955a, October 13). *Secret jury room microphones defended before Senate Inquiry: Professor backs jury room 'mikes*. The New York Times.

Drury, A. (1955b, October 14). *2 Senators ask law to bar eavesdropping on juries: Ban on listening to juries sought*. The New York Times.

Ferguson, G. W. (1955). Legal research on trial. *Journal of the American Judicature Society, 39*(3–4), 78–87.

Harawa, D. S. (2021). Sacrificing secrecy. *Georgia Law Review, 55*(2), 593–655.

Hartshorne, R. (1955). Letter from Richard Hartshorne to Orie L. Phillips. Includes a cover letter from Hartshorne to Earl Warren Dated Sept. 29, 1955. Available in Library of Congress, Earl Warren Papers, Box 725, Jury Tapping 1955.

Inventory. (1955). An inventory of materials sent to Levi the law school. 6/17/1955. University of Chicago Joseph Regenstein Library: Chicago Jury Project Records (CJPR). Addenda Box 25 Jury Project Controversy File.

Kalven, H., Jr. (1955). Statement by Harry Kalven Jr. 12 October 1955. University of Chicago Joseph Regenstein Library: Chicago Jury Project Records (CJPR). Addenda Box 7 File 65.

Kalven, H., Jr., & Zeisel, H. (1966). *The American jury*. Little Brown and Co.

Katz, J. (1972). Th Wichita Jury recording case. In *Experimentation with human beings: The authority of the investigator, subject, professions, and state in the human experimentation process* (pp. 67–109). Russell Sage Foundation.

Kitch, P. R. (1953a). A report on a Survey of Tenth Circuit Jurors. Prepared for use at annual conference of Tenth Judicial Circuit Estes Pk CO July 12-14, 1954. University of Chicago Joseph Regenstein Library: Chicago Jury Project Records (CJPR). Addenda Box 7 File 62.

Kitch, P. R. (1953b). Letter to Judge Orie L. Phillips. 11/23/53. University of Chicago Joseph Regenstein Library: Chicago Jury Project Records (CJPR). Addenda Box 25 Jury Project Controversy File.

Kitch, P. R. (1972). Letter from Paul R. Kitch, Esq. to Professor Bernard D. Meltzer-5/1,53. In J. Katz (Ed.), *Experimentation with human beings; The authority of the investigator, subject, professions, and state in the human experimentation process* (pp. 71–72). Russell Sage Foundation.

Kitch, P. R., Stallwitz, G., Powers, G., Spradling, G., Coulson, W., & Robinson, W. I. (1954). *A report on a survey of tenth circuit jurors.* Prepared for use at annual conference of Tenth Judicial Circuit Estes Park, CO. 12-14 July 1954. University of Chicago Joseph Regenstein Library: Chicago Jury Project Records (CJPR). Addenda Box 7 File 62.

Madge, J. (1962). *The origins of scientific sociology.* Free Press of Glencoe.

Margolin, M. L. (1955, July 8). Court rules on criminal insanity opposed *Rocky Mountain News*, p. 20.

Marson, J. M. (1955). Proceedings of the Annual Conference of the Tenth Circuit. Denver, CO: Stenotype Transcription. University of Chicago Joseph Regenstein Library: Chicago Jury Project Records (CJPR). Addenda Box 25 Jury Project Controversy File.

Mayo, E. (1933). *The human problems of an industrial civilization.* MacMillan.

McDonald v. Pless, (1915). 238 U.S. 264, 267 68.

Meltzer, B. D. (1953). A projected study of the jury as a working institution. *Annals of the American Academy of Political and Social Science, 287*, 97–102. https://doi.org/10.1177/000271625328700115

Mikva, A. (1954). Memo to Levi and Strodtbeck. 14 June 1954. University of Chicago Joseph Regenstein Library: Chicago Jury Project Records (CJPR). Addenda Box 25 Jury Project Controversy File.

Nichols, B. (1996). The unseen jury. *University of San Francisco Law Review, 30*(4), 1055–1064.

Olney, W., III. (1955). Letter to Dean Edward H. Levi. Undated. University of Chicago Joseph Regenstein Library: Chicago Jury Project Records (CJPR). Addenda Box 25 Jury Project Controversy File.

Plaisance, P. L. (2021). The concept of moral ecology in media sociology research. *Communication Theory, 31*(3), 422–441. https://doi.org/10.1093/ct/qtz022

Program of 10th Circuit Conference. (1955). University of Chicago Joseph Regenstein Library: Chicago Jury Project Records (CJPR). Addenda Box 25 Jury Project Controversy File.

Rosenberg, D. (2004). Death Penalty, Cameras Report the Jury Decides. *Newsweek, 144*(6), 8.

Schlegel, J. H. (1979). American legal realism and empirical social science: From the Yale experience. *Buffalo Law Review, 28*, 459–588.

Schlegel, J. H. (1995). *American legal realism and empirical social science.* The University of North Carolina Press.

Sokolsky, G. E. (1955, October 11). Are foundations blameless for fund groups' actions? *The Milwaukee Sentinel.*

Steneck, N. H. (2007). *Office of Research Integrity Introduction to the Responsible Conduct of Research.* Retrieved October 17, 2021, from https://ori.hhs.gov/sites/default/files/2018-04/rcrintro.pdf

Strodtbeck, F. L. (1953a). Pilot Jury Deliberations Protocol. 10/15//53. University of Chicago Joseph Regenstein Library: Chicago Jury Project Records (CJPR). Addenda Box 7 File 59.

Strodtbeck, F. L. (1953b). Working Paper #1. 12/1/53. University of Chicago Joseph Regenstein Library: Chicago Jury Project Records (CJPR). Addenda Box 7 File 59 The Experimental Study of Jury Decision-Making Jury.

Strodtbeck, F. L. (1954a). Recapitulation of phone conversation between Strodtbeck and Mikva. 4/14/54. University of Chicago Joseph Regenstein Library: Chicago Jury Project Records (CJPR). Addenda Box 25 File 59 The Experimental Study of Jury Decision-Making Jury.

Strodtbeck, F. L. (1954b). Untitled memo with no date or addressee with Not for Publication stapled to top. 8/26/1954. University of Chicago Joseph Regenstein Library: Chicago Jury Project Records (CJPR). Addenda Box 25 Jury Project Controversy File.

Strodtbeck, F. L. (1954c). Handwritten memo from Strodtbeck to Mikva, Garfinkle, and Mendlowitz, undated. Chicago Jury Project Records (CJPR). Addenda Box 25 Jury Project Controversy file.

Strodtbeck, F. L. (1954d). Letter to Judge Hill. 8/26/ 54. University of Chicago Joseph Regenstein Library: Chicago Jury Project Records (CJPR). Addenda Box 25 Jury Project Controversy File.

Strodtbeck, F. L. (1955). Memo: Estes Park Trip. 7/11/55. University of Chicago Joseph Regenstein Library: Chicago Jury Project Records (CJPR). Addenda Box 25 Jury Project Controversy File.

Strodtbeck, F. L. (1980). Notes for Human Rationality: Juror Sympathy for the Injured. University of Chicago Joseph Regenstein Library: Chicago Jury Project Records (CJPR). Addenda Box 25 File Human Rationality Jury File.

Strodtbeck, F. L., James, R. M., & Hawkins, C. (1957). Social status in jury deliberations. *American Sociological Review, 22*(6), 713–719. https://doi.org/10.2307/2089202

Strodtbeck, F. L., & Mann, R. D. (1956). Sex role differentiation in jury deliberations. *Sociometry, 19*(1), 3–11. https://doi.org/10.2307/2786099

Strodtbeck, F. L., Mendlowitz, S., Haygood, N., & Robertson, M. (1954). Analysis of an individual mock jury deliberation: A portion of a paradigm for the Study for a fully recorded jury trial. 15 March 1954. University of Chicago Joseph Regenstein Library: Chicago Jury Project Records (CJPR). Addenda Box 7 File 59.

Tepker, H. F., Jr. (1992). The judges of the Circuit Court. In J. K. Logan (Ed.), *The federal courts of the Tenth Circuit: A history US Court of Appeals for the Tenth Circuit* (pp. 319–423). Government Printing Office.

United States Senate. (1955). Recording of Jury Deliberations: Transcripts of Hearings by the Subcommittee to Investigate the Administration of the Internal Security Act and Other Internal Security Laws. October 12 and 13, 1955. Washington, DC: U.S. Government Printing Office.

United States Senate. (1956). Recording of Jury Deliberations: Report of the Subcommittee to Investigate the Administration of the Internal Security Act and Other Internal Security Laws to the Committee on the Judiciary. March 20, 1956. Washington, DC: U.S. Government Printing Office.

USLegal. (2019). Use of jury consultants. Retrieved July 7, 2020, from https://courts.uslegal.com/jury-system/selection-process-at-the-courthouse/use-of-jury-consultants

Vaughan, T. R. (1967). Governmental intervention in social research: Political and ethical dimensions in the Wichita jury recordings. In G. Sjoberg (Ed.), *Ethics, politics, and social research* (pp. 50–77). Schenkman Books, Inc.

Vidmar, N., & Diamond, S. S. (2001). Juries and expert evidence. *Brooklyn Law Review, 66*(4), 1121. Retrieved June 10, 2020, from https://brooklynworks.brooklaw.edu/blr/vol66/iss4/5

Westinghouse Studio One. (1954). LIVE TV RESTORATION: *Twelve Angry Men* - Studio One (Original 1954 Broadcast) - YouTube Studio One (Original 1954 Broadcast). Retrieved February 27, 2023, from https://www.youtube.com/watch?v=HlaXebUi72A

Zander, M. (1978). Jury in England—Decline and Fall. *American Jury System—Final Report* by R.S. Jacobson and B. Morrissey. Retrieved October 20, 2021, from https://www.ojp.gov/ncjrs/virtual-library/abstracts/american-jury-system-final-report

Zimring, F. E. (2003). The American Jury Project and the Chicago Law School (Fulton Lectures). Retrieved June 10, 2020, from https://chicagounbound.uchicago.edu/cgi/viewcontent.cgi?article=1016&context=fulton_lectures

Chapter 6
Obedience to Authority: A Whirlwind of Controversy

To really ask is to open the door to the whirlwind.
The answer may annihilate the question and the questioner.
—*Anne Rice (1985).* The Vampire Lestat

6.1 Introduction

In 1963, Stanley Milgram published the initial findings from his study of obedience in the *Journal of Abnormal and Social Psychology*, an official publication of the APA. To begin, this chapter will briefly sketch the study's setup. A naïve subject, in the role of "Teacher," is told the study will concern the effects of punishment on memory. The Teacher will be ordered by the "Experimenter" to administer increasingly severe punishment every time the "Learner" failed to pick the correct matching word from a list of four choices. Both the Experimenter and the Learner were part of the research team. The Teacher watched as the Learner in an adjoining room was strapped into an "electric chair" apparatus and an electrode attached to his wrist.

The Teacher was seated in the main room in front of the "shock generator" and would administer a stronger shock to the Learner every time he gave a wrong answer. The Teacher could not see the Learner or hear his answers which he gave by pressing one of four buttons, which turned on one of four answer lights in an answer panel on top of the shock generator. The shock generator had 30 switches ranging from 15 V labeled 15 V "Slight Shock" to 375 V "Danger: Severe Shock" to 450 V "XXX." The Learner pounds on the wall after the 20th shock (300 V) and again on the following 315-V shock. But he is unresponsive and silent after that shock.

If the Teacher indicated he did not want to continue, the Experimenter gave four verbal prods in the following order: (1) "Please continue," (2) "The experiment requires you to continue," (3) "It is absolutely essential that you continue" and (4) "You have no other choice, you must go on" (Milgram, 1975:21). If the Teacher refused to obey after the fourth prod, the experiment was terminated. Subjects who quit administering shocks before the highest 250-V shock were considered defiant, while those who administered all 30 shocks were termed obedient. The primary

H. Perlstadt, *Assessing Social Science Research Ethics and Integrity*, Clinical Sociology: Research and Practice, https://doi.org/10.1007/978-3-031-34538-8_6

dependent variable was the maximum shock a subject administered (Milgram, 1975:373–374).

Milgram's finding that 65% of 40 subjects administered all 30 shocks, including the highest marked XXX, was reported in newspapers across the country. In his report, Milgram (1963:371) quoted C.P. Snow (1961:24), who wrote that during World War II the German Officer Corp in the name of obedience, participated in "the most wicked large-scale action in the history of the world." This would include Adolph Eichmann, who had organized the mass deportation of Jews to death camps. At his trial in Jerusalem in 1961, Eichmann claimed that he was just following orders and, along with other low-level officers, was a mere instrument of those in higher authority. By asking and answering the question of when orders were most likely to be obeyed, Milgram unleashed a whirlwind of controversy.

Much has been written on the Milgram experiment since its original publication in 1963. This chapter will first describe how Milgram conceived, designed and carried out his series of experiments. It will present the ethical and methodological questions and concerns raised by developmental psychologist Diana Baumrind known for her studies of authoritarian, permissive and authoritative parenting styles. It will discuss replications of the study both scientific and nonscientific including television games and prank calls.

6.2 Background

Stanley Milgram was born and raised in a working-class Jewish family in the Bronx. He was a political science major at Queens College/City University of New York (CUNY). He applied for the graduate program in the Department of Social Relations at Harvard but needed to have taken psychology courses in order to be considered as an applicant. He took five psychology classes at three different schools during the summer and was admitted as a special student. He took and passed the four required courses his first year and became a regular student in 1955 (Blass, 2004:71; Russell, 2011:142–143).

Milgram worked as a research and teaching assistant for Solomon Asch when Asch was a visiting professor at Harvard in 1955–1956. Asch (1951) was already well known for his work on group pressure to conform. In one of his experiments, a group of eight college students were shown a line segment and asked to choose the matching one from a set of three lines of different lengths. In 12 of 18 trials, seven confederates in the group were instructed to choose the wrong line, whereupon the naïve subject, who had to choose last, had to choose between conforming with the others or resisting the peer pressure and picking the correct matching line. Only 25% of the naïve subjects never conformed over the 12 trials.

After Asch left Harvard, Gordon Alpert became Milgram's major advisor for his dissertation, which was a cross-cultural comparison of conformity performed in Norway and France between 1957 and 1959. Milgram modified Asch's procedure using sound rather than visual stimuli. In each trial, subjects had to indicate which of a pair of tones was longer. This required the subject to rely on his memory of sound which is not the same as remembering a visual set of three lines. Milgram had almost 400 subjects and found that the Norwegians were more conforming than the French participants. In 1959 and 1960, he worked for Asch at the Institute for Advanced Studies at Princeton, helping Asch edit a book on conformity while drafting his dissertation (Blass, 2004:71; Russell, 2011:144–145).

In designing his obedience experiments, Milgram (1964a:137) wanted to learn under what conditions a naïve subject would take an action that may harm the well-being of another person, e.g., when a delinquent in a gang is pressured to throw a rock through a shop window. But Milgram needed to generate sufficient social pressure on an individual in a one-on-one situation (Miller, 1986:18).

Milgram adopted methods of persuasion from Alfred Binet and Victor Henri. Psychologist Alfred Binet, who invented the first practical IQ test, wanted to learn which students had difficulty learning in a regular classroom. He collaborated with Victor Henri, a physiologist and psychologist (Binet & Henri, 1894) on a study to discover what would happen if school children were given a suggestion so slight that they did not notice its existence. Children were shown a model line on one board which was then turned around. They then had to identify from memory the model line on a second board which contained several lines. When a child pointed to a line on the second board that he thought was the model line, the Experimenter would quietly ask: "Are you really sure? Is it not the next line?"

Milgram wanted to know how to prod subjects to obey a suggestion or command. During World War II, social psychologist Kurt Lewin tested various ways to get people to support the war effort by eating food they may not like. One of Lewin's students was Jerome Frank, who later became a psychiatrist. Frank designed an experiment with 12 unsalted soda crackers. College students were told it was an experiment in persuasion, and whether or not they ate all 12 was up to them and wouldn't affect the experiment. But if they chose not to eat the crackers, the Experimenter would try to make them eat the crackers anyway. Frank's Experimenter was variously situated with respect to the subjects: he could be seated across the table from the student, be standing across the table from the student, or come around the table and stand close to the student. In each case, the Experimenter prodded the student, saying, "please eat" or "go on eating" (Frank, 1944:45–46).

Frank found that resistance was less likely when continuing the activity appeared to imply that the subject had implicitly agreed to eat 12 unsalted soda crackers during the experiment. Milgram appears to have combined Binet and Henri's use of suggestibility with Frank's attempts to pressure the subject by coming physically closer and asking the subject to continue eating the crackers. As a result, he changed the proximity between the Experimenter and Teacher and created four prods compared to Frank's two (Milgram, 1975:21).

6.2.1 Developing Obedience to Authority

In June 1960, Milgram received his Ph.D. and that fall was hired by Yale as an Assistant Professor in the Department of Psychology. Obedience to Authority began that fall as a project in his Psychology of Small Groups class (Blass, 2004:67ff; Perry, 2013a:48–49). He wanted his students to have some hands-on experience in a social psychology laboratory with a one-way mirror that allowed others to observe interactions. The class developed several possible experiments and the students voted to conduct what would become the pilot study for Obedience to Authority. Twenty Yale undergraduates participated in the experiment, which was conducted in five different sessions.

The class's experiments revealed that the student participants readily accepted the reality of the situation—that they were giving extremely painful electric shocks to another person. They would obey commands even when these went against accepted standards of behavior. They exhibited signs of nervousness and anxiety—one pulled on his hair, another wiped his sweating palms and shook his head in dismay as he administered the shock. But they refused to sample the shock they had just administered. Milgram observed that during the class experiments, participants were often reluctant to look at the Learner and turned their heads to avoid seeing the painful consequences of their actions (Blass, 2004, 93).

If, for theories of persuasion, Milgram drew from Benet and Henri and Frank, for both the idea of his obedience experiment and its laboratory procedures, Milgram likely drew directly from Arnold Buss's (1961) *The Psychology of Aggression*, whose "investigations," he wrote, "promise to be a useful complement to the present research" (Milgram, 1965:59). This can safely be said to be an understatement. In Buss's study of aggression, the subject is told that he will train a second subject in a conceptual task. This would require the subject, playing the role of Experimenter, to administer an electric shock to a second subject, who was an accomplice, whenever the accomplice gave an incorrect response.

Buss built aggression machines for both the subject and the accomplice. The subject's aggression machine had 10 buttons of increasingly higher levels of shock and an accompanying control panel indicating the accomplice/Learner's response. The accomplice responded by pressing one button for a correct answer and another for an incorrect answer on his aggression machine (Buss, 1961:47–49).

Milgram used the class experiment as the basis for an application to the NSF, which he submitted in early 1961. In the proposal, Milgram included a special section titled "Responsibility to Participants," in which he acknowledged that participants would be placed in a difficult predicament and that strong feelings would be aroused. In order to ensure the well-being of the research participants before leaving the laboratory, Milgram planned to make every effort to set the participants at ease (Blass, 2004:70–71).

Ever the Experimenter, Milgram conducted both a deceptive and a full debriefing after three different experimental conditions with 32 obedient and 24 defiant Teachers. The deceptive debriefings began with the Teacher filling out a demographic questionnaire while the Experimenter brought the Learner from the adjacent room. The Experimenter told the Teacher that the Learner was too nervous although the machine has previously only been used to shock mice and rats, and that the amperage was adjusted to be only slightly more painful than the sample shock. The Learner showed his arm and said he was unharmed and not resentful. The Experimenter made sure the Teacher had his check for $4.50 and led him outside. The deceptive debriefing only took less than 5 min (Turowetz & Hollander, 2018).

The full debriefings took much longer. After the Teacher completed the demographic questionnaire, the Experimenter told the Teacher that the Learner was working with the Experimenter and didn't receive any shocks. The Experimenter explained that the experiment was about obedience to authority, not punishment's effect on memory and learning. When the Learner appeared, he told the Teacher that he had overreacted and was nervous. In one of the three conditions, Milgram reassured what he described as "panicked" female Teachers, next asking them, "How do you feel now?" In these ways, Milgram shifted the responsibility for administering the shocks from the Teacher to the experiment itself. It could possibly have improved the Teacher's initial evaluations of the experiment (Turowetz & Hollander, 2018).

Although later vilified, Milgram was ahead of his time. His experiments preceded both the 1964 Helsinki Declaration that called for a clearly formulated protocol review by an independent REC, and the 1966 statement by US Surgeon General William Stewart that required anyone receiving PHS extramural grants to have prior review of their experiments conducted by institutional associates to assure an independent determination of the protection of the rights and welfare of the participants (Katz, 1987:3). Stewart specifically included the behavioral and social sciences in this regulation, although no mention was made of Milgram's experiment. Four months after Stewart's statement, the *New England Journal of Medicine* published Henry Beecher's (1966) article on Ethics and Clinical Research listing 22 unethical or questionably ethical clinical research studies, most of which failed to mention informed consent.

Beecher did not mention Milgram's experiments, but many of Milgram's critics later retroactively applied biomedical and social science research declarations, rules and regulations to his work.

6.2.2 The Grant Proposal

The grant proposal included a description of the pilot research and its findings, accompanied by some photographs showing the reactions of the student participants when making their decisions (Blass, 2004:69). Out of concern for the research participants, the NSF decided to make a site visit, which was not always a part of the grant review process (Blass, 2004:71). In April 1963, a site-visit team led by Henry Riecken, head of the NSF Office of Social Sciences, met with Milgram and others at Yale. Milgram was able to convince the committee that he would adequately debrief the participants and make sure they were comfortable with the decisions and actions they had made during the experiment. Yale's General Counsel assured the committee that Yale would be legally responsible for any negative effects the participants might suffer. The NSF agreed to fund the research.

However, the review committee commented on the scientific content of the proposal. The committee wrote that it was clear that Dr. Milgram neither had, nor planned to have, an elaborate a priori theory. This lack of theory was also noticed by Edward E. Jones, editor of *Journal of Personality*, who rejected Milgram's manuscript. Jones dismissed the whole study as "a kind of triumph of social engineering" (Blass, 2004:114).

Gina Perry (2013a:205–208, 210) noted that Milgram admitted he had no theory and had difficulty explaining how and why he got his results. He was not interested in testing hypotheses that obedience depended on life experiences, culture or individual personality differences.

The participants were recruited from the New Haven, Connecticut, area, with the experiments taking place in the Yale University social psychology laboratory. The subjects were recruited from the general adult population via ads in local newspapers that read, "We Will Pay You $4.00 for One Hour of Your Time. Persons Needed for a Study of Memory" (Slater, 2004). Of these first 40 subjects, 15 (37.5%) were skilled or unskilled workers, 16 (40.0%) were sales, business and white-collar workers and 9 (22.5%) were professionals. They ranged in age from 20 to 50, with most being over 30 (Milgram, 1963:372). Milgram changed the proximity between the Teacher and Learner, as well as the relationship between the Teacher and the Experimenter (authority figure). The location of one experiment was moved from the Yale laboratory to a rundown office building in the downtown shopping district of Bridgeport, CT. In another variation, only women were subjects.

Although his debriefing of the Teachers included a demographic questionnaire as well as follow-up surveys and questionnaires, Milgram did not conduct an analysis of obedience or disobedience by occupation, age or other sociodemographics (Turowetz & Hollander, 2018). Perry (2013a:253) notes that in his 1975 book, Milgram would eventually develop his agentic state theory in which individuals embedded in an authority system readily obey the orders of others. These individuals do not see themselves as responsible for their actions but are merely carrying out orders. This would happen despite personality or background. Milgram considered himself to be an empirical scientist who carefully observed concrete behavior.

Milgram, then, conceived of himself as practicing what philosophers of science call exploratory experimentation. Theory driven experimentation is the normal way of developing an experiment, with an existing theory in mind from the initial idea to its design and carrying it out to find a new effect. In contrast, exploratory experimentation involves systematically testing a large number of variables to determine which combination creates a condition that is indispensable to bring about the desired effect. "The first aim here is to find out which of the various parameters affect the effect in question, and which of them are essential" (Steinle, 2002:419).

Steinle's (1997:S68–S69) example was how Michael Faraday discovered the conditions that lead to electromagnetic induction by systematically varying the form and nature of electric circuits.

Milgram wanted to find the laboratory conditions under which the largest percentage of subjects would totally obey the orders of the Experimenter to administer ever higher levels of shock. His ideas came from a combination of theories, empirical studies and essays on authority rather than any a priori theory. This may explain why his 1963 article about the obedience experiment did not have a literature review or a set of hypotheses. In a short section titled "Related Studies," Milgram (1963:372) cited philosophic analyses of obedience and authority by Hannah Arendt (1958), Carl J. Friedrich (1958), Max Weber (1947), an early experimental study of obedience by Jerome Frank (1944), studies in "authoritarianism" by Theodor Adorno et al. (1950) and Milton Rokeach (1961), a recent series of analytic and empirical studies in social power by Dorwin Cartwright (1959) as well as Alfred Binet (1900) and Jean-Martin Charcot's (1881) long concern with suggestion in social psychology. However, Milgram did not describe these studies in his article.

In his first article on the obedience study, Milgram failed to mention that the research involved 24 experimental conditions which resulted in many fewer subjects administering all 30 shocks. For example, in a series of proximity variations, when the Teacher and Learner were in the same room with the Learner seated 50 cm (18 in.) behind the Teacher, 40% administered the maximum 450-V shock. But when they were closer together and the Teacher was ordered to force the Learner's hand on a metal plate to receive the shock, only 30% administered all 30 shocks (Perry, 2013a:304–305). Other conditions changed the relationship between the Teacher and the Experimenter (authority figure), and the location of the experiment. One of the variations—Informed or Educated Opinion—involved no shocks. Milgram had asked 40 psychiatrists at a leading medical school to estimate how far persons would be expected to act in this experimental condition. They were shown a diagram of the shock generator with the shock levels marked. They predicted that most subjects would not go beyond the tenth shock (150 V) and only 3.7% would still be obedient at the 20th shock (300 V) (Milgram, 1965:72).

At the conclusion of all experiments in the summer of 1962, Milgram sent 856 participants a written report and a ten-item follow-up questionnaire regarding their participation in the research. With two follow-ups, he had a 92% response rate (Blass, 2004:124–25; Milgram, 1975:195). Milgram used the highly favorable feedback results to defend his methods and findings.

6.3 The Controversy

At the end of October, *The New York Times* (Sullivan, 1963) reported on Milgram's study under the headline "65% in Test Blindly Obey Order to Inflict Pain: Yale Experiment Shows Many Became Distraught over Cruelty but Did Not Stop." It was picked up by newspapers around the country. The *Times* had conducted a telephone interview with Milgram in which he discussed aspects of the study that were not included in the journal article.

He also played excerpts from tape recordings of the experiments. He told the *Times* that by the time the study is completed, almost 1000 subjects will have been studied under 24 different experimental conditions, and that one group tested at the off-campus site in downtown Bridgeport, CT, had a lower obedience rate. Milgram noted that:

> . . .from 1933 to 1945 millions of innocent persons were systematically slaughtered on command. Gas chambers were built, death camps were guarded, daily quotas of corpses were produced with the same efficiency as the manufacture of appliances. . . .The purpose of the study is to seek out the roots of blind obedience (Sullivan, 1963:10).

He also described the intense reactions of several subjects who administered all 30 shocks including the 450-V shock. Others made nervous smiles or laughed bizarrely. Among those who defied the order to continue, one said "Oh, I can't go on with this; no, this isn't right. The guy is suffering in there. No, I don't want to go on. This is crazy."

Although this was not front-page news, it did draw a scathing editorial in the *St. Louis Post Dispatch* which called the experiment "Open Torture" (Blass, 2004:22). But the controversy was really ignited by Diana Baumrind's (1964) critique in *American Psychologist*. Obedience to Authority would become a negative exemplar of human research protections, specifically with respect to the deception of participants (Clarke, 1999; Elms, 1982).

6.3.1 Diana Baumrind

Baumrind spent her entire academic career at the University of California, Berkeley. She earned her MA and Ph.D. in developmental, clinical and social psychology. She became affiliated with the Institute of Human Development and would serve as the lifelong director of the Family Socialization and Developmental Competence Project. It was a nontenured research position funded by grants from government agencies and private foundations. She trained graduate students to conduct valid and ethical research. Baumrind did not use experimental strategies involving the use of deception or to test hypotheses on variations in parental authority by manipulating independent variables that might lead to one of her three models of parental control—authoritarian, permissive and authoritative (Baumrind, 1966, 2013; Sorkhabi & Larzelere, 2019).

Baumrind's (1964) thoughts after reading Milgram (1963) study reflect her concern with preventing psychological research from causing the subjects pain or indignity and ensuring that it does not raise ethical problems for the Experimenter. She acknowledged that Milgram was addressing "a very important problem, namely, the social consequences of destructive obedience." She argued that when experiments are conducted in a laboratory and the relationship between the Experimenter and the subject is an independent condition, the researcher must take into account the quality of trust the subject holds for the Experimenter and the research setting, and the obedience. She wondered if the same results would be found if the study was conducted outside of Yale and questioned the representativeness of subjects who would voluntarily participate in such a setting. A laboratory setting may arouse feelings of anxiety and passivity, in which case the subject is more prone to behave in an obedient and suggestible manner. She thought that it was not the place to study the degree of obedience or suggestibility.

She was skeptical about Milgram's comparison between obedience to orders given by the German Officer Corps and SS and those given by Milgram's Experimenter. In the German case, those "obeying the orders to slaughter had no reason to think of his superior officer as benignly disposed toward himself or their victims . . .and had no need to feel guilt of conflict because within this frame of reference he was acting rightly." She expected "a naïve sensitive subject to remain deeply hurt and anxious for some time, and a sophisticated, cynical subject to become even more alienated and distrustful" (Baumrind, 1964:423).

What she found most unconvincing was Milgram's casual assurance that the intense tensions he described as the subjects contemplated administering a high-level shock were dissipated before they left the laboratory. She wrote:

> The subject's personal responsibility for his actions is not erased because the Experimenter reveals to him the means which he used to stimulate these actions. The subject realizes that he would have hurt the victim if the current were on. The realization that he also made a fool of himself by accepting the experimental set results in additional loss of self-esteem. Moreover, the subject finds it difficult to express his anger outwardly after the Experimenter in a self-acceptant but friendly manner reveals the hoax (Baumrind, 1964:423).

Baumrind (1964:422–423) also mentioned that Milgram thought that the discomfort felt by the subjects was minimal compared to the possible scientific findings. But she skeptically noted that the ends might justify the means if the findings were of "inestimable value to humanity." She essentially accused Milgram of violating the APA's Ethical Standards. Psychologists are justified in exposing subjects to emotional stress or other harms only when the problem is significant and can be studied in no other way. Unless the subjects are fully informed of the possible dangers and nevertheless volunteer, the researcher should include in the research design a point when the subject should be removed from the experimental situation.

Drawing on her research on parenting, she regarded "the emotional disturbance described by Milgram as potentially harmful because it could easily effect an alteration in the subject's self-image or ability to trust adult authorities in the future" (Baumrind, 1964:422). This is questionable, since Milgram's subjects were all adults and it is not clear how their participation in his experiment would affect their parenting practices. Milgram would address Baumrind's assertion that his experiments could alter a subject's ability to trust adult authorities in the future, writing that "a child's obedience differs from a soldier's obedience, or the love, honor and obey of the marriage vow" (Milgram, 1965:58).

6.3.2 Milgram's Reply

Milgram (1964b:848–850) begins his reply by admitting that while his article did not include sufficient information for a systematic assessment of his experiments, Baumrind could have looked at the references and footnotes to learn that the experimental condition described was only one of series. He believed she mistakenly thought that stress was an intended effect of the experiment, whereas the extreme tension displayed by some subjects was unexpected. Milgram had discussed the procedures with many colleagues and none of them anticipated the stressful reactions of the subjects. He acknowledged that as the experiments progressed, it became evident that some would experience stress. But he claimed that momentary excitement is not the same as harm.

Baumrind asserted that the subject cannot justify their behavior and must take responsibility for his actions. Milgram pointed out that both during and after the experiment, the subject believed he was just doing the task assigned by the person in authority. She suggested that the subjects received no benefit from the study. But in response, Milgram referred to his follow-up survey and questionnaire, which revealed that 84% of the subjects reported they were glad to have been in the experiment, and that a similar percentage believed that more experiments of this sort should be carried out. Furthermore, 74% had learned something of personal importance about themselves. He acknowledged that that his findings should be interpreted cautiously.

6.3.3 Gina Perry in the Milgram Archives

Gina Perry was a freelance journalist who delved through Milgram's unpublished papers and transcripts of his experiments in the Archives at Yale University Library. She won the 2009 Silver World Medal for history documentary at the New York Festivals Awards. In her book, Perry (2013a:216) provided previously unknown insights into Milgram's thinking and his personal struggles about what he was doing to his subjects.

Baumrind (2015:692) approved of Perry's journalistic sleuthing and careful fact-checking, which revealed deception not only in Milgram's informed consent procedure but also in his debriefing of participants in his published accounts of his experiments. Baumrind (1985, 2013) had criticized Milgram for unethically and intentionally using deception about the purposes and methods of the obedience experiments. This included the newspaper ads, which readers will recall stated the study was investigating memory and learning, and a deceptive debrief (see Perry, 2013b:82), which informed those who had just completed the experiment that the shocks were not as painful as they seemed, rather than truthfully informing them that the shock machine was only a prop.

According to Milgram, this deception was necessary to ensure the construct validity of obedience to authority, since he did not want those who had completed the experiment to contaminate any future subjects until he had completed his series of variations. It appears that Baumrind was not familiar with Milgram's 1975:328–329) comments in Appendix I: Problems of Ethics in Research in *Obedience to Authority*. He noted that she focused on the 65% of subjects who obeyed to the end but did not report that obedience varied enormously from one condition to the next, including one in which 90% of the subjects disobeyed. Milgram should have included this in his 1964 response, which only focused on the experiment described in his original 1963 article.

Milgram planned to send all subjects a written debrief to more fully inform them about the experiment, since most had only been "dehoaxed" before they left the laboratory (Perry et al., 2020:87, 91–92). But after a site visit to Yale in April 1962 to observe the experiments, the NSF decided to terminate funding. At that point, Milgram developed and mailed a ten-item questionnaire, noted above, as well as a five-page report, which he sent to all subjects in July 1962 after the experiments ended.

The report contained information on the purpose and nature of the experimental program including its origins and logic of its design. It described the results of a dozen of the experiments; the causes of tension, chiefly, having to administer high voltage shocks; and the possible significance of the experiments (Milgram, 1975: 237). Critics focused on the deception and lack of informed consent before the subjects agreed to participate, and the dehoaxing which was designed to assure the subjects that they had not harmed the Learner. The five-page report contained what today might be considered an ethics debriefing handout when deception is used.

A month after mailing the questionnaires and reports, Milgram received 730 returns for an 85% response rate. The NSF then gave him one-time funding to analyze the questionnaires and transcribe follow-up interviews. Participants' responses to the question about the reality of the shocks may reflect a combination of their reactions following the end of the experiment as well as having read the report. Nevertheless, their comments were quite candid. One respondent seriously questioned the wisdom and ethics of allowing subjects to remain deceived even if the deception was thought necessary to avoid contamination. Several described their stress over the weeks following their experience as Teacher. Another who really believed that his Learner was probably dead after the stronger voltages, wanted to look him up. The report put his mind at ease. A third, who had talked with other subjects, wrote that Milgram was "somewhat irresponsible in permitting disturbed subjects to leave without informing them that they didn't half kill the shockee." A fourth, despite meeting the Learner, had "spent the night in a cold sweat and nightmares because of the fear that I might have killed the man in the chair. This fear was aroused from the fact that I had to sign papers that I would bring no charges against Yale" (Perry et al., 2020:87–88). Although Yale assured the NSF site visitors that it would be legally responsible for any negative effects the participants might suffer, the subjects did sign a release agreement waiving their right to sue.

6.3.4 Credibility of the Cover Story

After reviewing the questionnaire responses and comments, Milgram wanted to know whether the deception was credible and how it affected the performance of the Teachers. The Milgram Archives contained "Reported Beliefs in Shocks and Level of Obedience" prepared by Taketo Murata, Milgram's research assistant (Perry et al., 2020:93–95). The questionnaire asked the subjects how real the shocks were on a five-point scale from 1 (subjects fully believed the Learner was getting painful shocks) to 5 (subjects were certain the Learner was not getting the shocks).

Murata compared the degree of belief for defiant and obedient Teachers in the conditions in which shocks were administered She unexpectedly found that 62.5% of the 369 survey respondents who fully believed the reality of the shocks (on a 1 to 5-point scale) became defiant and refused to continue at *lower* shock levels than those who doubted the reality of the shocks (4 and 5 on a five-point scale). However, in three conditions, those who fully believed in the reality of the shocks stopped at *higher* shock levels than those who doubted the reality of the shocks. These three were Group Pressure to Obey, Common Man Authority and Voice Feedback.

Group Pressure to Obey was one of Milgram's conditions adapting the Asch conformity experiments to study likelihood of obedience. Group Pressure to Obey contained a triad of Teachers—actors A and B and the naïve subject. Teachers A and B followed the Experimenter's instructions and mumbled their dissatisfaction when the naïve Teacher hesitated or refused to continue. Of the 40 subjects, 72% administered the 450-V shock. In a complimentary condition, Group Pressure to Disobey, Teacher A read the word pair questions, the naïve Teacher read the voltage and administered the shock, and Teacher B read the correct answer. After the 11th shock (165 V), Teacher A refused to continue. When the Experimenter could not convince him to go on, he instructed the naïve Teacher and Teacher B to continue, while Teacher A quietly observed. After the 14th shock (210 V), Teacher B refused to continue, and the Experimenter required the naïve Teacher to continue to conduct the experiment while Teachers A and B looked on. Of the 40 subjects, only 10% administered the 450-V shock. These two variations support the Asch conformity experiments in a triad that resembles an assembly line. The naïve subject readily succumbs to Group Pressure to Obey in the first variation and to Disobey in the second.

The Common Man Authority or Teacher in charge condition has two Teachers, one of whom is an actor.In this variation, the Experimenter purportedly received a call and left the room. Upon departing he asked the actor Teacher to plan the number and voltage of shocks to be given after each incorrect answer. In Part A, the actor Teacher instructed the naïve Teacher to increase the voltage with each wrong answer. In Part B, the Experimenter returned after a few minutes and urged the naïve Teacher to follow the actor Teacher's plan. With 20 subjects in each part, 55% of the subjects in Part A administered the highest 450-V shock compared with only 15% of the subjects in Part B. In this three-person hierarchy, over half the subjects obeyed their promoted Teacher/colleague but became more defiant upon the return of the Experimenter. Perhaps the naïve Teacher believed his promoted colleague should be obeyed but disobeyed the Experimenter after his return, perhaps because he was not initially asked to develop a plan for the actor Teacher to administer.

The Voice Feedback condition has the Learner in the adjoining room crying, shouting and demanding to be let out. Here, 25 of 40, or 62.5%, of the naïve Teachers administered the highest 450-V shock. This is slightly below the 65% shocks reported for the following conditions: (1) No Feedback from the adjoining room; (2) Coronary Trouble condition where the Learner mentions heart trouble at beginning of the experiment and protests about it later; (3) Women Teachers who followed the Coronary Trouble script and (4) Experimenter Becomes Learner, when one of two Experimenters agreed to become the Learner after a phone call informed them that the second Teacher, who would have been an actor, will not be coming. The Voice Feedback condition would have reached 65% if only one more subject had administered all the shocks—26 of 40 or 65%.

6.3.5 *Our Moral Compass*

Milgram was able to pressure 65% of his naïve Teachers to administer what appeared to be a dangerous and fatal electric shock of 450 V in 5 of 23 (21.7%) of his experimental conditions. One question that researchers, ethicists and people who have learned about the Milgram experiments ask is: Would I have disobeyed or been fully obedient? The underlying question is: How strong is my moral compass? Our moral compass is our sense of right and wrong in a specific situation that guides us in making ethical decisions.

Neera Badhwar, a professor of philosophy interested in normative ethics and moral psychology, noticed that 65% of the subjects in four of Milgram's experiments were fully obedient and deeply conflicted. She wrote that Milgram's experiments "make us aware of how easily unobtrusive situational factors can tap our susceptibilities to obedience, conformity, irresponsibility, cruelty, or indifference to others' welfare" (Badhwar, 2009:257).

Reflecting on the atrocities committed by US soldiers in Viet Nam, Milgram (1975:188; Levine, 2018) saw this as a fatal flaw built into people when they become part of an organization which "gives our species only a modest chance of survival." Badhwar (2009:281) wondered if 65% reflects a strong natural propensity to obey an authority figure in a stressful situation. Perhaps many people have a compelling natural propensity to feel helpless in specific situations. She cited Overmier and Seligman (1967) and Seligman (2002:20), who administered shocks to harnessed dogs. When the dogs were unleashed, they passively accepted their lot by not trying to escape. Interestingly, the dogs again began trying to escape after about 48 h. Similar studies were carried out on rats, cats, gerbils and guinea pigs (Peterson et al., 1993:27).

Badhwar (2009:282) was surprised to find that the percentage of human beings, dogs and other animals that became helpless during the shock experiments is almost exactly the same: two out of three, or about 66% (Seligman, 2002, p. 23). Approximately two-thirds of Milgram's naïve Teachers were temporarily embedded in an experimental condition which enabled them to lose their moral compass, but judging from their questionnaire responses, they were able to reset their moral compass within a day or two.

6.3.6 Scientific Replications

Given the ethics controversy over Milgram's experiments, it may be somewhat surprising to learn that the Milgram experiments have been replicated in various forms. In the 25 years following the initial publication, Blass (1999:966) listed studies replicating one or more Milgram conditions which had both male and female subjects in Australia, Austria, Jordan, South Africa, Spain and the United States.

In 1969, one such study asked whether outcomes similar to Milgram's could be obtained if the participants were not deceived about the administration of the shocks and knew that their behavior during the experiment would be studied. In essence, the participants were asked to role play and act as if they were administering real shocks and had not been informed. O'Leary et al. (1970) found that the voltage range of shocks administered by their informed but playacting student who read parts of Milgram's methodology and knew that the Learner was not being shocked. They asked their participants to estimate how painful the last few shocks were and found no significant difference in estimated pain between their participants and the responses of Milgram's participants to the same question. They also observed more nervous activity by the participants than they had anticipated. However, while Milgram reported that defiant participants exhibited highly agitated and angered states, the defiant participants in the role-playing replication did not act this way.

In 2009, psychologist Jerry Burger conducted two limited replications of Milgram's experiments. In Milgram's Voice Feedback condition, the naïve Teacher first heard the Learner's protests through the wall and his demands to be released after the 150-V shock. Burger concluded that since 79% of subjects who continued past 150 V went on to administer the highest shock (450 V), he could end his experiment after the administration of 150 V. Burger could thereby avoid exposing naïve Teachers to the intense stress they might have experienced if the experiment continued past 150 V. In addition, Burger informed his subjects at least three times that they could withdraw from the study at any time and still receive their $50 for participation (Burger, 2009:2).

His subjects consisted of 29 men and 41 women whose ages ranged from 20 to 81 years. In order to ensure that the participants would be treated in a humane and ethical manner, Burger developed a two-step screening process to exclude potential subjects who might negatively react to the experiment. As a result, he dropped over half of the potential volunteers, which is an unusually high proportion. The IRB at Santa Clara University in California approved his research proposal.

Burger's Base condition followed Milgram's Voice Feedback condition. The Teacher sees the Learner being strapped in a chair in an adjoining room with electrode attached to his arm. The Teacher's task was to administer a paired associate learning test to the Learner in an adjoining room through an intercom system. The Teacher sits in front of the shock machine and is told to administer the next highest shock for a wrong answer. The Learner cries, shouts and demands to be let out. Each time the naïve Teacher hesitated to administer a shock the Experimenter gave the first of Milgram's four prods. If the subject was still hesitant after the fourth prod, the Experimenter ended the study. Subjects were not allowed to go beyond the 150-V shock.

Burger's Modeled Refusal condition was similar to Milgram's Group Pressure to Disobey but with only one confederate Teacher. For the female subjects, the confederate Teacher was a white woman in her late 20s; for the male subjects, it was a white male in his mid-30s. After watching the Learner being strapped into the chair in an adjoining room, the Teachers were told to sit next to each other in front of the shock machine with the naïve Teacher on the right. The Experimenter asked the confederate Teacher to begin the procedure by reading the list of word pairs and administering shocks when the Learner gave a wrong answer. When the Learner said "ugh!" on receiving the 75-V shock, the confederate Teacher hesitated before continuing. After the 90-V shock drew an "ugh!" the confederate Teacher" said, "I don't know about this." The Experimenter responded with the first prod, "Please continue," whereupon the confederate Teacher said, "I don't think I can do this," and pushed their chair away from the shock machine. The Experimenter asked the naïve Teacher to take over for the confederate Teacher who silently sat by without making eye contact with the naïve Teacher.

In the Base condition, 70% continued after administering the 150-V shock, at which point the Experimenter ended the experiment. In the Modeled Refusal condition, 63.3% continued after the 150-V shock. Burger found no significant difference between the two conditions. In the Base condition, 66.7% of the male subjects and 72.7% of the female subjects were willing to continue after the 150-V shock, while in the Modeled Refusal condition, 54.5% of the men and 68.4% of the women were willing to continue. Burger reported that although women were slightly more likely to continue in both conditions, the difference were not significant in either condition. These findings support Badhwar's hypothesis that approximately 65% of subjects would lose their moral compass.

6.4 Nonlaboratory Replications

In her critique of Milgram, Baumrind (1964:421) wrote that the laboratory is not the best place to study degrees of obedience, since the base line for the degree of obedience is probably much higher than in most other settings. While only a few statistical comparisons of nonlaboratory replications of Milgram's findings are available, several television game shows adapted some of its variations as rules for game show contestants. In addition, individuals claiming to be police called fast food restaurants asking a manger to identify and question a young employee who is a possible suspect of a complaint.

Hofling et al. (1966)studied nurses in a psychiatric hospital who received calls from a staff doctor to administer a drug to one of their patients. (Milgram (1975:207–208) knew about this study and considered the possibility of an extended prank wherein a fabricated authority sends a letter to a young man claiming to be from his draft board.) The Experimenter, claiming to be a Dr. Smith, called 22 nurses on night duty at a nursing station and ordered them to administer 20 mg of Astroten, a fictional drug, to a patient in the hospital. A bottle labeled "Astroten" was in the drug cabinet and the label clearly stated that 10 mg was the maximum daily dose. "Astroten" was a fictitious drug and not on the hospital's approved drug list. The Experimenter said that he would do the paperwork as soon as he got to the hospital. None of the nurses in the study questioned the telephone request. All but 1 of the 22 nurses entered the request on the patient's chart and went to the patient's room to administer the drug, where a senior nurse stopped them. A subsequent questionnaire revealed that in the past, 10 of the 22 nurses had actually administered an excessive dose of some other drug on a doctor's orders. But when the experiment was repeated with Valium, a well-known drug, 16 of the 18 nurses refused to administer it, and 12 attempted to contact the doctor to verify the dosage.

6.4.1 The Experiment as Entertainment

Social experiments are not limited to laboratories with one-way mirrors, cameras and microphones. Perry (2021) compared social psychology experiments with reality television shows. Both involve subterfuge, trickery and manipulation that are ethically problematic for scientific research. However, some TV shows hire psychologists as expert advisors.

A reality show may transform human behavior into a public spectacle, featuring competition and the weeding out of weak or unproductive team members. The television game show, *The Weakest Link,* originated in England on BBC Two in August 2000 and spread around the world within a year. In most versions, eight or nine contestants work together to answer general knowledge or trivia questions. After each round, the contestants vote on who is the worst player; this person then becomes "The Weakest Link." In contrast to previous game show hosts who were sympathetic to losing contestants, Anne Robinson, the first host, was cold and mean to the loser who was made to exit, passing the other contestants, in a walk of shame as Robinson announced, "You are the Weakest Link: goodbye!" (IMDB, 2017).

After watching an episode of the French version of *The Weakest Link* (*Le Maillon Faible*), producer Christophe Nick decided to make a documentary exploring how far people would go to win in a game-show setting. As in most other versions of the show, the French program featured an authoritarian female host dressed in black, who badgered the players. Nick consulted Jean-Léon Beauvois, a clinical psychologist and academician, for help designing and implementing a scientifically valid variation of Milgram's experiments in the framework of a fictional pilot television game show. Their project became the show *La Zone Xtreme* (The Extreme Zone).

Beauvois (2010) thought that by changing the social context from a scientific laboratory to a television studio, the nature of the power being tested would be based not on the authority of a scientist/Experimenter asking a participant to contribute to knowledge, but on the authority of a game-show hostess asking a participant to do what he or she thought best to win the game. The hostess of *La Zone Extreme* was a female weather forecaster for a French national TV station. In the game show, she dressed in a tailored white blazer that didn't quite resemble a lab coat, a black camisole and black slacks. The contestant/Learner, an accomplice, was strapped into an electric chair in an isolation booth by an assistant in a bright pink cocktail dress. The hostess told the naïve questioner/Teacher to ask the contestant/Learner to answer a set of 27 questions and, if they gave the wrong answer, to administer increasingly strong electric shocks. Both the hostess and the studio audience of about 100 persons recruited to view the pilot, were to encourage the questioner/Teacher to administer the next highest shock.

To ensure that the authority of the hostess/Experimenter was limited to prodding the questioner/Teacher to continue administering shocks, a television program producer/accomplice, rather than Milgram's Experimenter, greeted each participant. The producer informed them that they would be filmed during the game show and that the pilot show might be broadcast. He explained the rules of the game and obtained informed consent from the subjects after they, like Milgram's subjects, were deceptively told that the game involved delivering electric shocks. The producer had the participants draw straws, but the drawing was rigged so that the naïve subject was always the questioner. After the straws were drawn, the producer asked the players if they still wanted to participate in the pilot. No one refused (Beauvois et al., 2012:114–115).

Participants were recruited by an independent company that conducts opinion polls and market studies. Persons who had health problems, were taking any kind of medication or were familiar with Milgram's research were excluded. Each participant received 40 euros. All were from the metropolitan Paris area. Of the 76 subjects, 40 were men and 36 women, with a mean age of 39. Two-fifths (40.2%) were supervisory, or junior managerial, administrative, or professional workers, and 31.2% were working-class skilled manual workers. About one-fourth (23.7%) of the participants were avid watchers of reality TV (Beauvois et al., 2012:112–113). The research was approved by the French Society of Information Science and Communication Science (SFSIC) (see Oberlé et al., 2011).

The Standard condition was similar to Milgram's Voice Feedback. The contestant/Learner could be heard but not seen. When the contestant/Learner gave an incorrect answer (according to a predetermined schedule of 24 incorrect answers out of 27), the questioner (Teacher) was to penalize the Learner by delivering an (alleged) electric shock. The shocks ranged between 20 and 460 V, and were to be increased by 20 V. The gameshow host had five prods at her disposal for encouraging reluctant subjects to continue: four were similar to the ones used by Milgram, but the fifth had the hostess (Experimenter) ask the audience to intervene.

In the Social Support condition, when the voltage reached 120, the production assistant/accomplice rushed out on stage and asked that the game be stopped because it was too immoral. The hostess ignored the assistant and continued with the game. This was a single individual raising an ethical objection in the hope of getting the questioner to disobey, but differed from Milgram's Group Pressure to Disobey condition, in which two confederate Teachers disobeyed and then observed the naïve Teacher who was asked to take over and continue administering shocks. In the gameshow, the production assistant/accomplice was on stage for only a few moments.

The TV Broadcast condition was similar to the Standard condition but differed in that the producer told the participants the TV stations would broadcast the pilot show and that they would be on TV but could not win any money. The percent of questioners who were totally obedient and administered all shocks was 81% of 32 in the Standard condition, 74% of 19 in the Social Support condition and 72% of 18 in the TV Broadcast condition. All three did not differ statistically from Milgram's Voice Feedback condition of 62.5%. This means that the differences have a very low chance of occurring due to random factors. However, one must be cautious given the small number of respondents in each sample.

After the experiment, the questioners (Milgram's Teachers) were asked to assign responsibility among the producer (the principal researcher), the questioner/naïve subject (him or herself), the host (Experimenter), the audience and the contestant (Learner). All 71 questioners assigned 39.8% of the responsibility to the producer and 31.6% to themselves. However, 43.1% of the 51 obedient questioners assigned responsibility to the producer, compared with 30.5% of the 20 disobedient questioners, while 25.2% of the obedient questioners assigned responsibility to themselves compared with 40.1% of the disobedient questioners. No difference was found in blaming the host (Experimenter): 19.3% of the obedience questioners and 18.3% of the disobedient questioners (Beauvois et al., 2012:113–117).

Baumrind (1964:422) thought that participants would not be able to justify their own behavior and would bear the full brunt of their actions. This was true for the obedient questioners who placed more blame on the producers (PI) than themselves, but the disobedient questioners were more likely to accept their responsibility. Milgram contended that the same mechanisms that allowed the participants to obey to the very end would also justify their behavior because they would tell themselves they had been "carrying out the tasks assigned by the person in authority" (Milgram, 1964b:850).

The program was broadcast on French television as a documentary entitled *Le Jeu de la Mort* (The Game of Death) on March 12, 2010, followed by a heated debate. It was shown again on March 17, 2010, followed by a panel discussion. Afterward, Beauvois (2010) reported that he had received many e-mails, some of which were incredibly violent. His response was that he wanted to present a situation that compelled obedience and made viewers aware of the potential power of television. He defended himself by stating that if a way of behaving is not ethical, it should be banned not only for researchers but any authority figures, such as plant managers and Teachers.

Ethicists seeking to comprehend Milgram's experiments might look to the eighteenth-century Enlightenment philosopher Immanuel Kant, whose idea of the moral imperative continues to have lasting traction in decision-making today, including in the social and behavioral sciences and in bioethics. According to Kant, the moral imperative compels a person to act rationally. Philosophers add that people should treat each other as not as a means only, but always as an end it itself (Johnson & Cureton, 2022). It appears that the Milgram experiments revealed that the situations in which people find themselves enable some of them to reverse Kant's imperative and treat others as a means to an end.

6.4.2 Prank Calls

Scenarios replicating Milgram's key variables have been carried out not just in research and media settings, but in informal settings, by amateurs, as well. Take for example the scenario, noted above, in which an individual pretending to be a law enforcement official calls a fast food restaurant and asks the person who answers the phone to identify and question a young employee who is a possible suspect of a complaint. In Milgram's terms, the caller is the Experimenter, the person answering the call is the Teacher and the person under suspicion is the Learner or victim.

A set of such phone calls was uncovered by Andrew Wolfson (2005), a reporter for the Louisville, Kentucky, *Courier-Journal.* He discovered that someone claiming to be a police officer investigating a crime, had placed a phone call to a supervisor at a McDonald's in Kentucky. Early one evening in April 2004, the caller asked a female supervisor to question a small female employee about stealing a purse from a customer. The supervisor asked an employee fitting this description to come back to her office. The caller then told the supervisor to have the young woman, who happened to be 18 years old, empty her pockets and surrender her car keys and cell phone, which she did. Finally, the caller demanded that the supervisor have the young woman remove all her clothes to see if she was hiding anything. When the young woman did, the supervisor gave her a small apron to cover herself.

The supervisor told the caller that she had to leave the room to check on the restaurant. The caller demanded that another employee be brought in to watch the young woman until the police arrived. The supervisor called her fiancé to come over to the restaurant. For 2 h, the fiancé obeyed the caller's commands, ordering the young woman to drop her apron and do jumping jacks, after which he spanked her. The caller even talked directly to the young woman, demanding that she obey if she wanted to keep her job and avoid further punishment. During this time, the supervisor came back into the room periodically, but the fiancé had the young woman put the apron back on and told her to say nothing. The young woman reported that she begged the supervisor to get her out of there. Eventually, the supervisor called the store manager at home. Though the caller claimed the store manager was talking to him on another line, the manager said she had been sleeping and the supervisor finally realized that the call was a hoax. The victim pressed charges. The supervisor cooperated with police and the prosecutor's office but continued to deny some things that appeared on tape. The supervisor was convicted of a misdemeanor and placed on probation, and her fiancé received a 5-year prison sentence.

A subsequent police investigation uncovered a string of hoax phone calls to least 68 fast-food restaurants in 32 states over a 10-year period. Some police departments traced the calls to a prison guard living in Panama City, FL. Philip Zimbardo, who conducted the Stanford Prison Experiment speculated that the caller was "was very skilled in human psychology—he may have even read about Milgram" (Wolfson, 2005; Zimbardo, 2007:279–281).

ABC News (2006) interviewed clinical psychologist Jeff Gardere, who explained that the caller targeted fast-food restaurants because they are regimented with tasks done by the book. If something outside the book was requested, the employees had a difficult time responding and were likely to comply. This view is supported by the work of sociologist Ester Reiter (1996:165), a participant-observer who worked in a fast-food restaurant. She found that loyalty and obedience to authority were the most valued traits in fast-food workers.

6.5 Discussion and Conclusions

By asking the question, under what conditions will people continue to obey authority and harm others, and finding that in some situations, two-thirds of subjects would administer apparently fatal shocks Milgram's research became engulfed in controversies. These controversies center on his research ethics, theoretical explanations and his interest in the Holocaust. The Holocaust was the genocide, carried out by the German Nazi regime between 1941 and 1945, of more than 6 million European Jews as well as political dissidents, Romani, gay and disabled people and ethnic Poles and Ukrainians. However, these controversies should not overshadow his explanation of the systemic forces contributing to obedience and our understanding of the darker side of human behavior.

6.5.1 Ethics

Diana Baumrind first raised questions about Milgram's research ethics in 1964 and continued to do so throughout her long career. The Department of Health Education and Welfare (HEW) and the Federal Drug Administration published a proposal to revise regulations governing informed consent and listed dates for public hearings and written comments in August 1979. In October of that year, Baumrind (1979:3) published an article in which she cited Milgram as an example of deception. For Baumrind, by labeling as "destructive obedience" the actions of subjects who thought they were fully compliant by inflicting painful shocks on another, Milgram was imposing his individualistic bias upon the subjects. Further, his debriefing would not restore the subject's self-image or ability to trust adult authorities in the future.

In her view, Milgram's use of deception violated the fiduciary obligation of psychologists to be trustworthy and respectful in their dealing with research subjects. She criticized the APA's Code of Ethics, writing:

> In contrast to my condemnation of deception research, the utilitarian cost-benefit algorithm of the APA Code of Ethics (APA, 2002) permits deception when soliciting consent to participate and throughout the experimental procedure, requiring only that the deception, in the researcher's view, have prospective value, inflict no harm, and have no effective alternative. An "effective alternative" may be interpreted by the researcher as one that is as convenient and thrifty as the deceptive procedure, and "harm" is not defined to include lying to the participant (Baumrind, 2015:691–692).

From an ethical perspective, Baumrind firmly believed that individuals should be held responsible for their moral actions, because these are consciously and willfully determined (Vande Kemp, 1999). But she acknowledged that the participants were entrapped by a trusted individual, the researcher, into committing acts that they considered not representative of how they would normally behave (Blass, 2004:123–24).

Baumrind was the first of many to hold Milgram accountable for violating professional and government research ethics that did not exist when he conducted his experiments. In fact, Milgram's 1963 and 1964a, 1964b publications stimulated the development of research ethics in the United States. At that time, researchers tended to use their own judgment about whether their research posed an ethical problem and ethical questions took a back seat to scientific value (Blass, 2004:70–71). It was not until 1974 when Milgram's book was published, that the 1966 USPHS policy to assure an independent determination of the protection of the rights and welfare of the participants.

Readers will recall that Milgram's proposal to the NSF included a section on Responsibility to Participants, in which he promised to make every effort to put the participants at ease. At the April 1963 NSF site visit, he told the committee that he would adequately debrief the participants. The ethical issues involved with the Milgram experiment are as follows: the initial newspaper ads stating that the study concerned memory and learning, the experiments use deception in the informed consent procedure, withholding from participants the information that the shock machine was a prop and they were not administering actual shocks, and dehoaxing the participants (Baumrind, 1985, 2013, 2015).

These issues were addressed in a report by a Panel on Institutional Review Boards, Survey and Social Science Research and approved by the Governing Board of the NRC. The panel examined the structure, function and performance of the IRB system as it related to social, behavioral and economic research and recommended ways to improve the system. *Protecting participants and facilitating social and behavioral sciences research* (Citro et al., 2003) considered Milgram's experiments, noting that many subjects were distressed by what they were asked to do:

> Milgram's experiments aroused intense controversy about the conditions under which it appropriate to use deception, particularly when the consequence is intense (although apparently transitory) psychological stress and even when subjects are informed about the deception at the conclusion of the experiment. Milgram subsequently resurveyed his original subjects, most of whom said they supported the experimentation because it provided important information about how ordinary people could be induced to behave in reprehensible ways in response to a recognized authority, but this finding did not stop the controversy. (Citro et al., 2003:66)

Not only did it not stop the controversy, it did not stop scientific replications or cultural and entertainment engagements with the experiment.

6.5.2 Theoretical Explanations

As noted above, Milgram's initial research was not designed to confirm any a priori theory (Blass, 2004: 71). Nor did he present any philosophical and theoretical discussion of obedience in his 1963 article beyond a list of related studies. For Milgram (1963:372), obedience was an obvious and observable social fact that he considered a direct, ubiquitous and indispensable feature of social life. His concept of the Agentic Shift within the framework of a hierarchy, which he elaborated on a decade after his initial account of the obedience experiments, could have provided the foundation for a possible theory (Milgram, 1975:161–163). According to this concept, humans exist in two modes of operation. One is the self-directed or autonomous mode in which the individual meets his or her own internal needs; the other is the systemic mode or agentic state within an authority system in which a person acts as an agent executing the wishes of another who is higher in the organizational chain of command. Milgram argued that the burden of moral responsibility shifts from the individual in an autonomous mode to the person in an agentic mode to an authority.

He then raised three key questions or hypotheses:

1. Under what conditions will a person move from an autonomous to an agentic state (antecedent conditions)?
2. Once the shift has occurred, what behavioral and psychological properties of the person are altered (consequences)?
3. What keeps a person in the agentic state (binding factors)? (Milgram, 1975:264).

Milgram (1975:172) realized that a legitimate source of social control was a necessary prerequisite for a shift to the agentic state. For this reason, he conducted one experiment, described above, in a run-down office building in downtown Bridgeport, CT, rather than at Yale University. As expected, the obedience rate was lower—47% compared to 65% in four experiments conducted at Yale. He concluded that legitimacy depended on a justifying ideology that supported administrative authority.

Regarding administrative authority, political scientist and politician Conrado Santos (1978) identified two schools of thought. One is the Chester Barnard (1938) and Herbert Simon (1965) behaviorist approach that considered administrative authority as an observable interaction between members within an organizational hierarchy. The other is the Max Weber (1947) and Peter Blau (1964) structuralist approach, in which the position of individuals within an organization and its rational goals of efficiency and effectiveness create and reinforce power in a bureaucracy and social life.

Milgram was well aware of real-world examples of obedience within bureaucratic structures, and he included Weber in his list of related studies in his 1963 article. However, his review of studies on bureaucracy in *Obedience to Authority* (Milgram, 1975:159, 263) is limited to political scientist Simon (1965) on administrative behavior, and sociologist Robert Bierstedt (1954), who wrote on the problem of authority. It is surprising that Milgram did not reference Barnard (1938), who proposed that authority is confirmed only when it is accepted by a person to whom it has been addressed, and that disobedience of such a communication is a denial of authority. In a note, Milgram (1975:259) cited Simon's (1965) concept of "zone of indifference," which means that workers will comply with orders if they are indifferent to them, whether or not they agree with or support the orders. I note that it was Barnard, not Simon who coined the term.

Most commentators focus on the definition of the agentic stare rather than the shift into and out of it. Psychologist Walter Mischel (2009:288) started a debate in 1968 over the relative importance of persons and situations when he asked, "How can individuals be agentic and proactive, able to change the power of 'hot' situations and to influence their own fate?" David Funder (2009:120) proposed that personality theory and research include not only personality measures and traits but behaviors and situations. He thought that it was important to empirically predict behavior in new and unique situations. Milgram was most likely aware of this debate when he wrote:

> It is surprising how difficult it is for people to keep situational forces in mind, as they seek a totally personalistic interpretation of obedience, divorced from the specific situational pressures acting on the individual, which .... we know to be crucial in determining whether the person will submit or rebel (Milgram, 1979:9).

6.5.3 The Holocaust

It would seem prudent for both individual and public safety to further understand how obedience to authority operates, how to prevent blind obedience and how individuals may be empowered to walk away from situations in which authority is being abused. Milgram (1963, 1975) found that the physical presence of the authority figure, that is, when the Experimenter is in the room with the Teacher, resulted in the highest percentage of participants who obeyed until the very end. He concluded that obedience occurs in its most essential form when a person views himself as the instrument for carrying out another person's wishes and ceases to regard himself as responsible for his actions.

Milgram's findings challenge the belief that only those from the sadistic fringe of society would severely harm a stranger on the instructions of an unfamiliar authority figure. As discussed above, Milgram's participants were ordinary people drawn from the working, managerial and professional classes, and in certain conditions, over half administered the highest shock. He supported Hannah Arendt's (1963) contention that Adolph Eichmann was not a sadistic monster, but rather an uninspired bureaucrat who simply sat at his desk and did his job. For her part, Arendt (1979) stated that she always hated the notion that there is an Eichmann in each one of us, but "This doesn't mean that there are not quite a number of Eichmanns."

Psychologist Arthur G. Miller (1995:44–45) discussed historian Christopher Browning's analysis of interrogation transcripts of German police who were sent to Lublin, Poland as a battalion to exterminate Jews toward the end of World War II. The men were over 30 years old and middle or lower class. Very few were members of the Nazi party or the S.S. Browning found that:

> Direct proximity to the horror of the killing significantly increased the number of men who would no longer comply. On the other hand, with the division of labor and removal of the killing process to the death camps, the men felt scarcely any responsibility at all for their actions. As in Milgram's experiment, without direct surveillance, many policemen did not comply with orders when not directly supervised; they mitigated their behavior when they could do so without personal risk but were unable to refuse participation in the battalion's killing operations openly. (Browning, 1992:175–176)

Miller considered Browning's thoughtful analysis to be far more than a background metaphor for destructive obedience. Browning's effort to integrate the processes identified by Milgram with a remarkably detailed set of historical records is insightful:

> Everywhere society conditions people to respect and defer to authority. ... Everywhere people seek career advancement. In every modern society, the complexity of life and the resulting bureaucratization and specialization attenuate the sense of personal responsibility ...If the men of Reserve Police Battalion 101 could become killers under such circumstances, what group of men cannot? (Browning, 1992:189)

Reicher and Haslam (2006) noted that the Holocaust has cast a long shadow over social psychology. Studies were designed to understand how people come to hate and to discriminate against members of other groups, and to see others as less human and less deserving than themselves, as well as how authoritarianism, social dominance and power abuse arise. Although such studies cannot resolve ethical dilemmas, they can contribute to descriptive or empirical ethics of how people behave under given conditions and can suggest ethical prescriptions for what people ought to do under such conditions. Some studies have focused on individual characteristics of those who are prejudiced or discriminatory, but others concentrate on the nature of group processes and social conditions that can induce the most inoffensive of individuals to commit offensive acts. I suggest that these latter studies come much closer to revealing the social realities of oppression, discrimination and genocide than explanations based on individual-level subconscious processes or cognitive neuroscience perspectives.

Polish sociologist and philosopher Zygmunt Bauman (1989, 152) contended that the lessons of the Holocaust were not only that it could be done, but that we could do it. Milgram's findings unambiguously confirmed this reality, and that we may again do it if the conditions are right. He found that cruel and inhumane acts could be carried out by ordinary men and women who felt it was their duty to obey and that it would contribute to a desired end. Milgram showed that inhumanity was a function of social relationships and social distance which can be rationally manipulated to produce inhuman actions.

Milgram himself recognized that the results of his obedience to authority experiment were very provocative, when he wrote, "If everyone had broken off at slight or moderate shock, this would be a very reassuring finding, and who would protest?" (1975:194). Unfortunately, Milgram died of a heart attack in 1984 at the age of 51. Had he lived longer, he might have more explicitly stated that his experiments created a quasibureaucratic environment in which individuals, like Eichmann, become agents within a rational system of action that permits them act impersonally and harm other people.

6.5.4 The Importance of Milgram's Experiments

The *Institutional Review Board: Management and Function* (Bankert & Amdur, 2002) is a reference manual containing short pieces by over 90 contributors addressing core issues that IRB members and staff can turn to on how to run an efficient and effective IRB in compliance with federal regulations. It includes a chapter on Deception of Research Subjects which reads in part:

> The Milgram experiments are also widely cited as some of the most important ever conducted in social psychology. This is because they provide striking insights into an aspect of human behavior held to be responsible for some of the worst atrocities of the twentieth century: unquestioned obedience to authority as witnessed in the horrors of the Holocaust. As a consequence, these obedience studies place, in stark contrast, arguments for and against the use of deception in research on human behavior ...
>
> Simply asking participants to "role play" how they would act in a particular situation does not produce the same behavior as that actually observed by "naïve" participants. ...
>
> However, few would claim that these behaviors are governed by the same processes that yield spontaneous behavior when confronting actual situations ...
>
> The argument is made that to build a base of knowledge on what causes people to act certain ways, one must examine their behavior in situations they regard as "real." This often requires deception. (Slone & Hull, 2006:210–211).

Miller (1995:33, 38) noted that both students and researchers learn about the Milgram experiments in textbooks in psychology and other social sciences, as well as philosophy and manuals for IRB members and administrators. The accounts may range from a few summary paragraphs to a whole chapter. This chapter has attempted to provide a more detailed history of the several controversies and hopefully will stimulate constructive discussions about the importance and impact of Milgram's obedience experiments.

Acknowledgments I was fortunate to receive help from the following: Kristin Fermaglich, Chris Herrara, John Kennedy, Stan Kaplowitz, Dan Menchik, Arthur G. Miller, Bill Morgan and David Segal. In 2013, I presented a paper at a conference in Bracebridge, Ontario, marking the 50th anniversary of Milgram's 1963 article where I learned about the early work of Gina Perry and Nestar Russell. As a result, I made a few trips to explore the Stanley Milgram Papers at the Yale University Sterling Memorial Library.

References

ABC News. (2006, December 10). *Restaurant shift turns into Nightmare.* Accessed March 20, 2022, from https://abcnews.go.com/Primetime/story?id=1297922&page=1

Adorno, T. W., Frenkel-Brunswik, E., Levinson, D. J., & Sanford, R. N. (1950). *The authoritarian personality.* Harper & Brothers.

Arendt, H. (1958). What was authority? In C. J. Friedrich (Ed.), *Authority* (pp. 81–112). Harvard University Press.

Arendt, H. (1963). *Eichmann in Jerusalem: A report on the banality of evil.* Viking Press.

Arendt, H. (1979). On Hannah Arendt. In M. A. Hill (Ed.), *Hannah Arendt: The recovery of the public world.* St. Martin's Press.

Asch, S. E. (1951). Effects of group pressure upon the modification and distortion of judgments. In H. Guetzkow (Ed.), *Groups, leadership and men; research in human relations* (pp. 177–190). Carnegie Mellon University Press.

Badhwar, N. K. (2009). The Milgram experiments, learned helplessness, and character traits. *The Journal of Ethics, 13*(2/3), 257–289. http://www.jstor.org/stable/40345404

Bankert, E. A., & Amdur, R. J. (2002). *Institutional review board: Management and function* (2nd ed.). Jones and Bartlett Learning.

Barnard, C. (1938). *The functions of the executive.* Harvard University Press.

Bauman, Z. (1989). *Modernity and the Holocaust.* Cornell University Press.

Baumrind, D. (1964). Some thoughts on ethics of research: After reading Milgram's "Behavioral Study of Obedience". *American Psychologist, 19*(6), 421–423. https://doi.org/10.1037/h0040128

Baumrind, D. (1966). Effects of authoritative control on child behavior. *Child Development, 37*(4), 887–907.

Baumrind, D. (1979). IRBs and social science research: The costs of deception. *IRB: Ethics & Human Research, 1*(6), 1–4. https://doi.org/10.2307/3564243

Baumrind, D. (1985). Research using intentional deception: Ethical issues revisited. *American Psychologist, 40*(2), 165–174.

Baumrind, D. (2013). Is Milgram's deceptive research ethically acceptable? *Theoretical and Applied Ethics, 2*(2), 1–18.

Baumrind, D. (2015). When subjects become objects: The lies behind the Milgram legend. *Theory & Psychology, 25*(5), 690–696.

Beecher, H. K. (1966). Ethics and clinical research. *New England Journal of Medicine, 274*(24), 1354–1360. https://doi.org/10.1056/NEJM196606162742405

Beauvois, J. L. (2010). Obéissance, influence, pouvoir de la télévision, "Le jeu de la mort". Réponses à des interrogations légitimes qui m'ont été adressées. 4/6/2010 [Obedience, influence, power of television 4 "Game of Death". Responses to legitimate questions addressed to me]. Game show: Making the "participants" obey with Milgram [archive], on maniprop.com,

February 15, 2010. Accessed February 22, 2010. OR http://liberalisme-democraties-debat public.com/spip.php?article119. Both no longer available 21 Apr 2022.
Beauvais, J. L., Didier, C., & Oberlé, D. (2012). The prescriptive power of the television host. A transposition of Milgram's obedience paradigm to the context of TV game show. *European Review of Applied Psychology / Revue Européenne de Psychologie Appliquée, 62*(3), 111–119.
Burger, J. M. (2009). Replicating Milgram: Would people still obey today? *American Psychologist., 64*(1), 1–11. https://doi.org/10.1037/a0010932. PMID: 19209958.
Bierstedt, R. (1954). The problem of authority. In M. Berger, T. Abel, & C. H. Page (Eds.), *Freedom and control in modern society* (pp. 67–81). Van Nostrand Company.
Binet, A. (1900). *La suggestibility*. Schleicher.
Binet, A., & Henri, V. (1894). De la suggestibility naturelle chez les enfants [On natural suggestibility in children]. *Revue Philosophique de la France et de l'Etranger, 38*, 337–347.
Blass, T. (1999). The Milgram paradigm after 35 years: Some things we now know about obedience to authority. *Journal of Applied Social Psychology, 29*, 955–978.
Blass, T. (2004). *The man who shocked the world: The life and legacy of Stanley Milgram*. Basic Books.
Blau, P. M. (1964). *Exchange and power in social life*. Wiley.
Browning, C. R. (1992). *Ordinary men: Reserve Police Battalion 101 and the final solution in Poland*. HarperCollins.
Buss, A. (1961). *The psychology of aggression*. Wiley.
Cartwright, D. (Ed.). (1959). *Studies in social power*. University of Michigan Press.
Charcot, J. M. (1881). *Oeuvres Completes*. Bureaux du Progres Medical.
Citro, C. F., Ilgen, D. R., & Marrett, C. B. (Eds.). (2003). *Protecting participants and facilitating social and behavioral sciences research*. The National Academies Press.
Clarke, S. (1999). Justifying deception in social science research. *Journal of Applied Philosophy, 16*, 151–166.
Elms, A. C. (1982). Keeping deception honest: Justifying conditions for social scientific research stratagems. In T. L. Beauchamp, R. R. Faden, R. J. Wallace Jr., & L. Walters (Eds.), *Ethical issues in social science research* (pp. 232–245). Johns Hopkins University Press.
Frank, J. D. (1944). Experimental studies of personal pressure and resistance I: Experimental production of resistance. *Journal of General Psychology, 31*(1), 23–64.
Friedrich, C. J. (1958). *Authority*. Harvard University Press.
Funder, D. C. (2009). Persons, behaviors and situations: An agenda for personality psychology in the postwar era. *Journal of Research in Personality, 43*(2), 120–126.
Hofling, C. K., Brotzman, E., Dalrymple, S., Graves, N., & Pierce, C. M. (1966). An experimental study of nurse-physician relationships. *Journal of Nervous and Mental Disease, 141*, 171–180. https://doi.org/10.1097/00005053-196608000-00008
IMDB. (2017). *The weakest link (TV Series 2000–2017)*. Internet Movie Data Base. Accessed December 26, 2021, from https://www.imdb.com/title/tt0268862
Johnson, R., & Cureton, A. (2022). Kant's moral philosophy. In E. N. Zalta (Ed.), *The Stanford encyclopedia of philosophy* (Spring 2022 Edition). https://plato.stanford.edu/archives/spr2022/entries/kant-moral/
Katz, J. (1987). The regulation of human experimentation in the United States: A personal odyssey. *IRB: Ethics & Human Research, 9*(1), 1–6. https://doi.org/10.2307/3563644
Levine, B. E. (2018). *Vital ignored truths in Milgram's Obedience to Authority Studies*. Accessed January 27, 2023, from brucelevine.net
Milgram, S. (1963). Behavioral study of obedience. *The Journal of Abnormal and Social Psychology, 67*(4), 371–378. https://doi.org/10.1037/h0040525
Milgram, S. (1964a). Group pressure and action against a person. *Journal of Abnormal and Social Psychology, 69*(2), 137–143. https://doi.org/10.1037/h0047759
Milgram, S. (1964b). Issues in the study of obedience: A reply to Baumrind. *American Psychologist, 19*(11), 848–852.

Milgram, S. (1965). Some conditions of obedience and disobedience to authority. *Human Relations, 18*(1), 57–75. https://doi.org/10.1177/001872676501800105

Milgram, S. (1975). *Obedience to authority: An experimental view*. Harper and Row.

Milgram, S. (1979). Préface de la deuxième edition française Soumission à l'autorité: un point de vue expérimental. In A. G. Miller. (1995). Constructions of the obedience experiments: A focus upon domains of relevance (p.41). *Journal of Social Issues, 51*(3), 33–53. https://doi.org/10.1111/j.1540-4560.1995.tb01333.x

Miller, A. G. (1986). *The obedience experiments: A case study of controversy in social science*. Praeger.

Miller, A. G. (1995). Constructions of the obedience experiments: A focus upon domains of relevance. *Journal of Social Issues, 51*(3), 33–53.

Mischel, W. (2009). From *personality and assessment* (1968) to personality science, 2009. *Journal of Research in Personality, 43*(2), 282–290. https://doi.org/10.1016/j.jrp.2008.12.037

Oberlé, D., Beauvois, J., & Courbet, D. (2011). Une transposition du paradigme d'obéissance de Milgram à la télévision: enjeux, résultats et perspectives [Applying Milgram's obedience paradigm to television: issues, results and prospects]. *Connexions, 95*(1), 71.

O'Leary, C. J., Willis, F. N., & Tomich, E. (1970). Conformity under deceptive and non-deceptive techniques. *The Sociological Quarterly, 11*(1), 87–93.

Overmier, J. B., & Seligman, M. E. (1967). Effects of inescapable shock upon subsequent escape and avoidance responding. *Journal of Comparative and Physiological Psychology, 63*, 28.

Perry, G. (2013a). *Behind the shock machine: The untold story of the notorious Milgram psychology experiments* (Revised ed.). The New Press.

Perry, G. (2013b). Deception and illusion in Milgram's accounts of the obedience experiments. *Theoretical and Applied Ethics, 2*(2), 79–92.

Perry, G. (2021, April 16). Social psychology and reality TV. *Gina Perry*. Accessed December 9, 2021, from http://www.gina-perry.com/2021/04/16/social-psychology-and-reality-tv/

Perry, G., Brannigan, A., Wanner, R. A., & Henderikus, S. (2020). Credibility and incredulity in Milgram's obedience experiments: A reanalysis of an unpublished test. *Social Psychology Quarterly, 83*(1), 88–106. https://doi.org/10.1177/0190272519861952

Peterson, C., Maier, S., & Seligman, M. (1993). *Learned helplessness: A theory for the age of personal control*. Oxford University Press.

Reicher, S., & Haslam, S. A. (2006). Rethinking the psychology of tyranny: The BBC prison study. *British Journal of Social Psychology, 45*, 1–40.

Reiter, E. (1996). *Making fast food: From the frying pan into the fryer* (2nd ed.). McGill-Queen's University Press. ISBN: 9780773513877.

Rice, A. (1985). *The Vampire Lestat*. Random House Publishing Group.

Rokeach, M. (1961). Authority, authoritarianism, and conformity. In I. A. Berg & B. M. Bass (Eds.), *Conformity and deviation* (pp. 230–257). Harper.

Russell, N. (2011). Milgram's obedience to authority experiments: Origins and early evolution. *British Journal of Social Psychology*. https://doi.org/10.1348/014466610X492205

Santos, C. R. (1978). A theory of bureaucratic authority. *Canadian Public Administration, 21*(2), 243–267. https://doi.org/10.1111/j.1754-7121.1978.tb01764.x

Seligman, M. (2002). *Authentic happiness*. Free Press.

Simon, H. A. (1965). Administrative decision making. *Public Administration Review, 25*(1), 31–37. https://doi.org/10.2307/974005

Slater, L. (2004). *Opening Skinner's box: Great psychological experiments of the twentieth century*. W.W. Norton.

Slone, L., & Hull, J. (2006). Deception of research subjects. In E. A. Bankert & R. J. Amdur (Eds.), *Institutional review board: Management and function* (2nd ed., pp. 201–215). Jones and Bartlett Learning.

Snow, C. P. (1961). Either-or. *Progressive, 25*(2).

Sorkhabi, N., & Larzelere, R. L. (2019). Diana Blumberg Baumrind (1927-2018). *American Psychologist, 74*(7), 850. https://doi.org/10.1037/amp0000492

Steinle, F. (1997). Entering new fields: Exploratory uses of experimentation. *Philosophy of Science, 64*(4), S65–S74. https://doi.org/10.1086/392587

Steinle, F. (2002). Experiments in history and philosophy of science. *Perspectives on Science, 10*(4), 408–432. https://doi.org/10.1162/106361402322288048

Sullivan, W. (1963, October 26). 65% in test blindly obey order to inflict pain: Yale experiment shows many became distraught over cruelty but did not stop. *The New York Times, 10*.

Turowetz, J., & Hollander, M. H. (2018). From 'Ridiculous' to 'Glad to Have Helped': Debriefing news delivery and improved reactions to science in Milgram's 'Obedience' Experiments'. *Social Psychology Quarterly, 81*(1), 71–93. https://doi.org/10.1177/0190272518759968

Vande Kemp, H. (1999). Diana Baumrind: Researcher and critical humanist. In D. Moss (Ed.), *Humanistic and transpersonal psychology: A historical and biographical sourcebook* (pp. 249–259). Greenwood Publishing Group.

Weber, M. (1947). *The theory of social and economic organization*. Oxford University Press.

Wolfson, A. (2005, October 9). A hoax most cruel. *The Courier Journal* (Louisville, KY). http://www.courier-journal.com/apps/pbcs.dll/article?AID=/20051009/NEWS01/510090392

Zimbardo, P. G. (2007). *The Lucifer effect: Understanding how good people turn evil*. Random House.

Chapter 7
Tearoom Trade: The Ethics of Studying Social Problems

There are precious few at ease with moral ambiguities. So, we act as though they don't exist.
—Wicked *"Wonderful" Stephen Schwartz and Winnie Holzman.*

7.1 Introduction

This chapter explores the case of *Tearoom Trade*, a study conducted in the mid-1960s on the behavior and lifestyles of men who frequented public restrooms, known as tearooms, used by homosexuals for casual sexual encounters. The study was one of the first to document that many of the men who went to the tearooms were married, well-educated, relatively affluent and good community members. It was carried out before the 1974 Department of Health Education and Welfare regulations requiring the formation of what became known as IRBs to approve all research proposals before they could be submitted for funding consideration.

Tearoom Trade is frequently featured in human research protections tutorials and handbooks as a negative exemplar of what is wrong with social behavioral research. But it played a role in the development of current medical and social science research ethics including the *Belmont Report's* (1979) three basic principles to guide IRB reviews of proposed biomedical and social behavioral research.

7.2 Study Background and Description

Laud Humphreys earned a divinity degree at Seabury-Western Theological Seminary in Evanston, Illinois, in 1955 and then spent over 10 years as a minister in the Episcopal Church in Oklahoma, Colorado and Kansas before going to graduate school in sociology at Washington University in Saint Louis. As a minister, he counseled homosexuals but did not attempt to reform them (Galliher et al., 2004:24). In 1960, he married, and the couple eventually adopted two children.

H. Perlstadt, *Assessing Social Science Research Ethics and Integrity*, Clinical Sociology: Research and Practice, https://doi.org/10.1007/978-3-031-34538-8_7

Humphreys began his graduate work in 1965. One of his first graduate school professors, Helen Gouldner, suggested that he study the gay bars of Saint Louis as part of a proposed research project in which she encouraged students to get out of the ivory tower. When he had first decided to pursue graduate work in sociology, Humphreys learned about a recent sociology dissertation at the University of Missouri, Columbia, by Irma Bendel Mathes (1966) on adult male homosexuality and male–male parental role structure. She had contacted the Mattachine Society, a semisecret homosexual group that had been established in Los Angeles in 1950 and had then spread across the country. She asked that her survey be distributed to its members, who would then send her their completed questionnaires. In this way, she would not know who received or returned a survey, and if the survey did not contain specific identifiers, she would not be able to link respondents to their answers. But Humphreys thought that one needed to directly observe homosexuals rather than only relying on questionnaires (Galliher et al., 2004:18). Going to gay bars was the first step.

A year later, Humphreys learned about *The Boys of Boise: Furor, Vice and Folly in an American City* by John Gerassi (1966), an editor at *Time* magazine. In November 1955, police in Boise, Idaho, arrested three clients of an alleged organized underworld ring of male homosexual prostitutes aged 13–20. Other arrests followed and became national news though a *Time* article. The "crime wave" resulted in the firing of the police chief and a probation officer, the expulsion of the son of a city councilman from West Point and the conviction of a bank vice president. In addition, a homosexual delinquent prostitute murdered his father and received a 10-year sentence for manslaughter. As the Boise incidents suggest, the costs of being ousted included criminal conviction, loss of job and blackmail.

A review of *The Boys of Boise* appeared in the *Annals of the American Academy of Political and Social Science* by Joseph Bensman (1967), an associate professor of sociology at City College of the CUNY. Bensman acknowledged that Gerassi's journalistic treatment and ability to identify what is important and dramatic far exceeded that of most sociologists. But these strengths had biased his selection of data, theory and mode of analysis.

Political scientist Nelson Polsby thought that *The Boys of Boise* was somewhat hysterical in tone and displayed little analytical intelligence. He was also concerned that Gerassi had based his conclusions about the awareness of sexual deviance in the community on a sample size of 12. Polsby (1967:691) wrote, "The book falls short of professionally acceptable standards of rigor in the accumulation of data, the marshalling and interpretation of evidence, and in its interplay with relevant theory to disqualify it as a tool of higher education."

Both Humphreys and his major advisor, Lee Rainwater, were aware of Gerassi's book. Rainwater acknowledged the "thorough journalistic study of one community (Boise, Idaho) in which excessive public attention to the dangers of homosexuality proved destructive not only to the lives of individuals but to community more generally" (Humphreys, 1970a, 1970b:xv). Humphreys was clearly aware of it by the time he finished the dissertation, and it may have guided his sample selection methodology.

Compared to the *Boys of Boise*, *Tearoom Trade*, Humphreys' (1975) book about the findings of his study, has stood the test of time. In their defense of the study, Irving Louis Horowitz and Lee Rainwater contented that without it, "We would once again be thrown back on simple-minded, psychological explanations that are truly more voyeuristic than analytic" (Humphreys, 1970a, 1970b:189). Years later, *Tearoom Trade* was frequently mentioned in the 2007 reporting of the arrest of Senator Larry Craig (R-Idaho) for solicitation in a men's room in the Minneapolis airport (see Frankel, 2007; Mac Donald, 2007).

7.2.1 Study Design and Methods

Humphreys began observations for his dissertation research in April 1966. He followed ethnographic techniques for observing deviant groups, subcultures and activities in St. Louis. He worked his way into the homosexual scene by going to bars and parties. He then began conducting observation of tearooms in public parks. "Tea time" was the vernacular term used to describe when homosexuals gathered in public restrooms to engage in sex with other men. (The individuals Humphreys observed were performing fellatio, which at that time was as felony.) The restrooms were located in public parks near major thoroughfares and highways, away from other park facilities such as playgrounds, tennis courts and picnic areas, but with nearby parking.

When he began going to public restrooms in parks, Humphreys paced near the door as if waiting for a contact. He soon realized he was disrupting the action. While no conversations take place within the tearooms, Humphreys was able to approach and talk with some of the men outside them. He became acquainted with 12 of them, his "intensive dozen." Over some meals and drinks together, he disclosed his real purpose for visiting parks with established tearooms. All 12 agreed to be interviewed. Two agreed to be taped and the other interviews were reconstructed from notes.

These proved to be the richest source of data for the study (Humphreys, 1975:36–37). The "intensive dozen" also suggested that he take on the role of lookout or watch queen. A watch queen was often a voyeur who obtains sexual gratification from observing others engaged in sexual acts. The voyeur becomes a participant observer who does not attract undue attention or distort the behavior of the participants. The watch queen stands near the door or windows in order to see who is coming toward the restroom. He coughs when someone approaches. The cough would break the prevailing silence of the ongoing sexual encounters. He then nods if the coast is clear or the entering party is a regular (Humphreys, 1975:27).

According to the American Anthropology Association (2004), ethnographic research may include methods that Humphreys employed: unobtrusive direct observation, structured and unstructured interviewing, focused discussions with individuals and community members, and audio recordings. The Association notes that the process of obtaining informed consent may be continuous and incremental throughout the course of the research, and review of consent obtained may be periodic. At the Federal level, Section 46.116(d) of the 1991 Common Rule (*45 CFR 46*) authorizes IRBs to waive informed consent or approve a consent procedure that alters or eliminates some or all of the elements of informed consent if four conditions are met: (1) the research is of no more than minimal risk; (2) the change in consent procedures will not harm the respondents; (3) the research could not practicably be carried out without the waiver or alteration; and (4) whenever appropriate, additional information will be provided to subjects after participation.

Humphreys contended that his research was of minimal risk. He conducted his research before the 1971 AAA guidelines and the 1971 *HEW Institutional Guide on Protecting Human Subjects,* "the Yellow Book" (DHEW, 1971; Schrag, 2009). He took what today would be considered fair precautions by keeping names and addresses in a safe deposit box. It seems reasonable to assume that the agreement of Humphreys' "intensive dozen" to participate in the study may be a type of informal community consent, which is obtained from those whose interests would be affected by the proposed research (King et al. (2014). Although they agreed, the dozen could easily have alerted fellow tearoom visitors at any time and ended Humphreys' research efforts.

Humphreys' research design called for identifying a target population and interviewing them to gather basic demographic information on their occupations, race, area of residence and marital status. He realized that the dozen who were willing to talk with him early on were most likely atypical, because they were more overt, less defensive and better educated. He therefore sought to obtain a more representative sample that included more working-class men, but had no way of identifying or approaching them. Rainwater suggested tracing the license plates of cars parked near the tearooms to generate a sample of participants (Humphreys, 1975:37, 30, 41).

7.2.2 Creating Samples

Acting on Rainwater's suggestion, in September 1966, Humphreys began generating a systematic sample of cars parked near ten public restrooms in four different parks in the St. Louis metropolitan area. Like other participant observers, Humphreys kept field notes describing the setting, participants and activities in the tearooms on a portable tape recorder concealed under a box on the front seat of his automobile. His notes included the license numbers of as many cars during each half-hour break that equaled approximately 10% of the average volume of likely autos at that time on that day of the week. Although not a random sample, he found that the results were fairly representative on a time basis for the largest park which accounted for roughly half of the observed homosexual activities.

He told friendly policemen he was conducting market research and asked if they would give him access to license registers. The registers contained the names and addresses of the car owners as well as the brand name and year of the car. He then checked the cars against his field notes and rejected two cases. His final, nonrandom sample included 100 participants whose cars were found near ten public restrooms in four different parks in the metropolitan area (Humphreys, 1975:29, 31,33, 37). Today, of course, the Internet makes it easy to obtain this information.

With the addresses of the cars in his sample, he was able to drive by and record a description of the tearoom users' residences and neighborhoods. Since he did this at Christmastime, he was able to note the type of religious decorations in front of homes. He saw children's toys and bicycles and boats or trailers in the driveways. "For Rent" signs often had the number and types of rooms and in some cases, the price (Humphreys, 1975:38).

During his graduate school career, Humphreys also worked as a research assistant at the Medical Care Research Center in Saint Louis. At one point, he was asked to develop a questionnaire for a social health survey of men (Humphreys, 1975:41). He based his survey instrument on similar studies conducted in Michigan and New York. The items covered family background, socioeconomic factors, personal health and social history, religious and employment data, friendship networks, marital relationships and sexual practices. With the permission of the study director, Humphreys added a randomized subsample drawn from the license numbers of cars at the tearooms. Only Humphreys and a trusted graduate student working with him conducted interviews with this subsample. The subsample was asked the same questions as everyone else in the social health survey of men (Humphreys, 1975:42–43).

Humphreys and his graduate assistant were able to complete only 50 of 75 planned subsample interviews, because 10 of the tearoom respondents refused to do the survey, and another 15 did not complete the interview. When conducting these interviews, Humphreys changed his hairstyle and wore appropriate clothes compared with the disguise he used when he was acting as the watch queen. He also drove a different car when conducting the surveys, since the one he had used to visit the tearooms was recognizable.

Although Humphreys reported that he recognized each of the men he interviewed from observing them at the tearoom, it is not known if any of the respondents recognized him and then refused to start or complete the interviews for that reason (Humphreys, 1975:42). It appears he honored all requests not to participate in or complete the survey.

As would be expected, the men who completed the interviews were slightly over-representative of the middle and upper classes. They were suburbanites and more highly educated. From preinterview information, some men had moved and left no forwarding address. Others were in manual jobs, and those who refused to take the survey tended to live in Italian and working-class German neighborhoods.

He created a comparison group by randomly selecting a sample of potential respondents in the men's health survey. He found 50 who matched the 50 men in his tearoom subsample on occupation, race, residential area and marital status. He trained two other graduate students, and they conducted interviews. If a man declined to be interviewed, he was replaced with the next name on the list (Humphreys, 1975:42–43).

Humphreys had noticed that the majority of out-of-state license plates had stickers from nearby military installations (Humphreys, 1975:39). These military men were more likely to be involved in homosexual activity than military men in the control group (Galliher et al., 2004:34). Men in the subsample and the comparison sample from the main health survey were not informed that they had been chosen specifically to obtain more personal information that would be part of his dissertation research on homosexuals (Warwick, 1973:32–33).

As noted above, Humphreys took what today would be considered reasonable precautions to protect the identity of those interviewed through safeguarding the names and addresses of his subjects. The master list was kept in a safe deposit box, and each interview card kept under lock and key (Galliher et al., 2004:31). He concealed all identifiers in his dissertation and publications. He conceded that a respondent from the tearoom might still be able to identify himself in the book but most would not be able to do so.

7.3 The Ethics Controversy

Humphreys passed his dissertation defense on May 16, 1968. Two days later, Washington University Chancellor Thomas H. Eliot (Galliher et al., 2004:27) wrote to Humphreys stating that it appeared he had failed to follow university regulations and federal law regarding the protection of human subjects when he conducted his dissertation research. The chancellor added that Humphreys may have violated Missouri criminal law by failing to report felonious behavior or even by aiding and abetting criminal sexual acts. The chancellor concluded that the degree might have to be revoked. In addition, Humphreys was charged with violating the terms of his predoctoral research fellowship from the NIMH (Glazer, 1972:110). The Chancellor then informed the NIMH of these concerns and asked that it investigate, as well as suspend a pending grant to Humphreys' advisor, Lee Rainwater.

Washington University apparently had some sort of human subjects review process in place when Humphreys defended his dissertation, but it is uncertain what policy, if any, was active when he began his research in the spring of 1966. This was 5 years before HEW issued its 1971 guide on protecting human subjects. The required paperwork for dissertations carried out at that time was post hoc, affirming that the rights and welfare of the subjects had been protected, that appropriate informed consent was obtained and that the risks and benefits had been assessed. In response to the Chancellor's request, the NIMH sent a team to investigate the dissertation research and Rainwater's pending grant.

A NIMH memo of July 31, 1968, noted that with respect to Humphreys' research, "sodomists are rarely if ever prosecuted for this felony, and lookouts or watch queens probably never" (Glazer, 1972:110; Galliher et al., 2004:21, 42). It went on to state that Humphreys' research purpose and the absence of felonious intent would have most likely resulted in acquittal. But the Chancellor decided that Humphreys, who had been a lecturer in sociology during the 1967–1968 academic year, would no longer be employed at the university or allowed to work on Rainwater's grant.

In a letter to Executive Vice Chancellor George Pake dated June 21 of that year, the secretary of the sociology department (Galliher et al., 2004:27) took responsibility for failing to submit the proper human subjects' forms for Humphreys' dissertation. This satisfied the Chancellor, who notified Humphreys that he had been cleared of all charges, and the degree would be awarded (Galliher et al., 2004:27).

However, on July 18, 1968, the *St. Louis Post Dispatch* (see Galliher et al., 2004:27) published a story about the controversy between the sociology department and the administration at Washington University that included references to Humphreys' dissertation. Several of the 12 cooperating respondents who knew that Humphreys had been studying them as part of his dissertation research called him to ask if they were in jeopardy (Glazer, 1972:110). He assured them that they were not in danger. They seemed satisfied, and he asked them to pass the word around the local tearooms. Humphreys then got in touch with the other cooperative correspondents.

Humphreys and Horowitz intended to publish the dissertation as a book. It was originally submitted to Oxford University Press, which turned it down despite excellent reviews. It was then sent to Aldine Publishing Company. According to Horowitz (2010:140–141), the dissertation was accepted at the University only on the condition that it would not be published or its contents revealed to a wider public for 2 years. An excerpt from the dissertation was published 18 months later in *Society* (Humphreys, 1970a). The book, *Tearoom Trade* (Humphreys, 1970b) came out that same month and went on to win the 1970 C. Wright Mills Award from the Society for the Study of Social Problems, which acknowledges books that critically address an issue of contemporary public importance and advance the social scientific understanding of the topic.

After the publication of Humphreys' book in 1970, a few other men came to realize they had been included in the study and contacted him. It appears, however, that they were untouched by the publicity surrounding *Tearoom Trade*. To protect the participants, Humphreys proceeded to burn tapes, delete passages from transcripts and shred other material. Later, when Humphreys feared he might get subpoenaed, he gave his friend James Henslin the master list to take from Missouri to Illinois, where Henslin later burned it in his backyard (Galliher et al., 2004:45; Henslin, 2001:144). Humphreys came out of the closet at the 1974 meeting of the American Sociological Association (ASA) during an emotional exchange with Edward Sagarin, a professor of sociology and criminology at the CUNY, who strongly believed that gay men and lesbians, as members of a large, unrecognized minority, deserved civil rights. Humphreys' coming out as a gay man also ended his marriage (Humphreys, 2009).

It is difficult to assess the state of human research protections between 1966 and 1968, when Humphreys was conducting his fieldwork. In 1962, the Ethics and Standards Committee of the American Association for Public Opinion Research

(AAPOR) reported that legislative action at the state and local level was making it difficult for researchers doing surveys of public opinion, marketing and social science to meet their responsibilities to the public and governmental units. It concluded that unless actions were taken by the AAPOR, regulations will be imposed upon public opinion and other researchers. Two years later, field interviewers reported that some 250 communities in 34 states had requirements ranging from interviewers registering with the local police chief to an automatic $50 fine for any house-to-house surveys (Arnold, 1964).

In the early 1960s, officials at the NIH began questioning the agency's tradition of relying exclusively on the moral character of investigators to safeguard human subjects and its lack of systematic monitoring of researcher conduct (Williams, 2005:71–72). In February 1966, the Surgeon General issued a policy, "Clinical Investigations Using Human Subjects," which required institutions receiving PHS grants to have a committee conduct a prior review of proposed research with human subjects to assess the rights and welfare of the research subjects, the appropriateness of the informed consent method and the balance of risks and benefits. This was revised in 1971 and became a federal regulation in 1974 (*21 CFR 310.102(f)*). Although the policy addressed self-regulation, it did not adequately define key terms such as "rights and welfare of potential subjects," "informed consent," and "risks and potential benefits." This lack of definitions confused committees and led to arbitrary application of the policy (Williams, 2005:71–73).

7.3.1 The Moralizers

The excerpt from Humphreys' dissertation proved to be a lightning rod. Journalist Nicholas von Hoffman (1970a) wrote a column in *The Washington Post* expressing strong disapproval of Humphreys' study. He argued that regardless of Humphreys' precautions or his intent to obtain reliable data, Humphreys had collected information without the knowledge of the people involved, which could potentially have been used for blackmail, extortion and the worst kind of mischief. His column begins:

> We're so preoccupied with defending our privacy against insurance investigators, dope sleuths, counterespionage men, divorce detectives and credit checkers, that we overlook the social scientists behind the hunting blinds who're also peeping into what we thought were our most private and secret lives. But there they are, studying us, taking notes, getting to know us as indifferent as everybody else to the feeling that to be a complete human involves having an aspect of ourselves that's unknown (von Hoffman 1970a: B1, B5).

The Trans-Action/*Society* article (von Hoffman 1970b) noted that 54% of the men were married and living with their wives, and that the door-to-door survey revealed no evidence that these unions are particularly unstable, nor that any of the wives were aware of their husbands' secret sexual activities. Though measures were taken, as detailed above, to remove identifying details, Humphreys did include several in-depth composite descriptions of the men who frequented the tearooms. One such composite was the subject "George," a second-generation German raised as a Lutheran. He served in the army during the Korean War and was a truck driver like his father. He weighed over 200 pounds and had tattoos on both forearms. At the time of the study, he had been married 14 years and had seven children.

Humphreys did not put quotation marks around the name "George," and it was only toward the end of the article that he explained that George was a composite of several men. An inattentive reader might easily have assumed that George was a real person, and it is understandable why critics concluded that some of the men would recognize themselves. Humphreys walked a very fine line between portraying his subjects as real people, rather than stereotypes, and protecting their identities.

He wrote, "I have tried to make it impossible for any close associate to recognize the real people behind the disguised composites portrayed in this article. But I have worked equally hard to enable a number of tearoom players to see themselves in the portrait of George" (Humphreys, 1970a, 1970b:25). He succeeded on both counts: while some men did recognize themselves in the study, no one was blackmailed or extorted as a result of its publication.

In their defense of Humphreys, Horowitz and Rainwater (1970), identified a dispute between journalists and social scientists over undercover reporting and confidentiality of sources. They noted that the *Washington Post* columnist von Hoffman applied a standard of investigative conduct for sociologists to which few journalists could measure up, and that journalists themselves collect information that could be used for blackmail or extortion. Journalists may claim to be protected by the First Amendment, but courts do hold journalists in contempt if they do not cooperate with grand juries by surrendering their notes or identifying contacts. While social scientists who do not cooperate with grand juries could be held in contempt, today they must first receive IRB approval before they can begin observing and collecting data.

This dispute goes back to Robert E. Park, one of the founders of the Chicago School of Sociology in the 1920s and 1930s. Park was a reporter for several major city newspapers before studying sociology. He thought of the sociologist as a kind of super reporter who focused on what was actually going on rather than what seemed to be happening. Using his journalistic background in first-hand reporting, he encouraged the development of participant observation as an objective methodology for studying the city and its problems (Burnet, 1964). With respect to the *Tearoom Trade* study, the journalist/social scientist tension found expression in the pages of the journal that first published Humphreys' lightning rod piece. Von Hoffman's (1970b) column was reprinted in the May issue of *Society*, along with a response by Humphreys' major advisor, Horowitz and Rainwater (1970:12–13).

One example of a journalist whose reportage on a social problem is widely used in social science courses is Barbara Ehrenreich (Dingwall, 2006). Ehrenreich, who holds a PhD in cellular biology from The Rockefeller University, became a political activist and wrote about the US health care system and the sexual politics of sickness, among other topics relating to social problems. Between 1991 and 1997, she was a regular columnist for *Time* magazine.

In 1997, shortly after welfare reform was enacted, she met with Lewis Lapham of *Harper's Magazine* and suggested that the magazine have a reporter investigate the effects of welfare reform on the working poor. Ehrenreich, who had never gone "under cover," would spend 3 months working as a waitress in Florida, a house cleaner and nursing home aide in Maine and a Walmart retail associate in Minnesota. She created fake job resumes and references to conceal her identity as a journalist and social investigator, fashioning herself as a homemaker returning to the workforce with little relevant experience (Liebenthal, 2014).

Based on these work experiences, Ehrenreich then went on to write *Nickel and Dimed: On (Not) Getting by in America* (Ehrenreich, 2001), which made the *New York Times* best-seller list. During one of her early bookstore appearances in Key West, she was approached by a woman who said she was working at the restaurant when Ehrenreich was being interview for the job. The woman told Ehrenreich that her first impression was that she was hiding something. Ehrenreich was afraid the woman would say she thought she was a highly educated, sophisticated sort of person, that is, a journalist or social scientist, but the woman said, "I thought you were just out of jail or a shelter" (Liebenthal, R. 2014).

Dingwall (2006) pointed out that her work is held up as an example of the sort of investigation that sociologists ought to do, but that would not pass an IRB review because of the lack of consent among the parties, although most names and identifying details were changed. In addition, if Ehrenreich were an academic researcher, her use of deception would undoubtedly have raised ethical issues and required justification.

Two years after von Hoffman's condemnation, Donald P. Warwick presented a more academic and ethically based assessment of *Tearoom Trade*. At the time, Warwick was Chair of the sociology department at York University in Toronto. His article appeared in the first volume of *The Hastings Center Studies*. The Center is a research institute dedicated to the discussion of ethical questions posed by the life sciences and more generally to analyzing contemporary moral dilemmas in medicine and science. Warwick (1973:29) found only a few existing, well developed and generally acceptable standards for evaluating research from an ethical perspective. Such standards would come 6 years later, with the publication of the Belmont Report (1979), with its identification of the three ethical principles necessary to the protection of human subjects, beneficence, justice and respect for persons.

But Warwick had a much broader concept of research ethics, which included not just the individual research participant/subject, but also the researcher, the larger society and the researcher's profession (Warwick, 1973:30). He presents a list of Humphreys' misrepresentations and disguises, which "must surely hold the world record for field research" (Warwick, 1973:30). Humphreys served as watch queen, hid a tape recorder in his car, told the police he was doing market research to get information from license plates, changed his appearance and car when conducting the health survey, informed those in the survey that they were part of a random anonymous survey and distorted the survey by blending the homosexual subsample into the total sample, and all justified on the grounds of situation ethics (Warwick, 1973:31–32).

Like von Hoffman, Warwick discussed the possible consequences of Humphreys' misuse of information. The data could have been use for blackmail or criminal prosecution. Once the study made headlines, some of the men, including those who were aware that they were being studied, were anxious and fearful of being identifiable. Warwick asserted that any conscientious professional person must be concerned about the anxiety he creates in people as a result of his work, especially when a researcher imposes himself on others for his own ends, without their knowledge. The men in the tearoom did not, after all, ask to be studied (Warwick, 1973:34).

Although Warwick (1973:36) was not opposed to studying controversial topics like homosexuality, he was concerned that Humphreys set himself above considerations of appearances and how the public might view sociologists such as himself and the field more generally.

A final concern addressed in Warwick's article was the balance between the freedom of the individual researcher and her or his fellow researchers in various allied professions. Warwick (1973:35) claimed that offensive behaviors such as illegal activities, deception and misrepresentation on the part of researchers were likely to have a negative effect on the research environment. He noted that "in some circles ... social scientists are sly tricksters who are not to be trusted" (Warwick, 1973:37). He thought that *Tearoom Trade* was one of a few social scientific studies that would have lent itself directly to a grand jury investigation. In his opinion, the government ought to have stepped in and prevented the most flagrant abuses of social research, including public deception.

Humphreys hoped to improve the lot of homosexuals in American society. Warwick (1973:37) acknowledged that Humphrey's concern for their vulnerability was admirable, but pointed out that Humphreys does not present any factual basis for assuming that *Tearoom Trade* would bring about a positive change. But Warwick himself only states an impression that a widespread reading by the larger public might well produce negative effects. This highlights the problematic nature of social science models designed to identify the likelihood of intended and unintended consequences.

7.3.2 *Humphreys' Postscript*

Aware of the growing controversy around his work, Humphreys (1975:167–174) added a postscript to the enlarged second edition entitled, "A Question of Ethics." In it, he discusses an essay by Kai T. Erikson that was published when Humphreys was completing his systematic field observations. Erikson's starting point was an article published 10 years earlier by Becker and Greer (1957), which suggested that a participant observer may collect data openly in the role of researcher, or covertly in some disguised role. Borrowing the symbol of masks from Erving Goffman's (1959) *Presentation of Self in Everyday Life*, Erikson (1967:367) asserted that the practice of using masks in social research compromises both the people who wear them and the people for whom they are worn.

Humphreys argued that research in tearooms required a disguise to gain entrance into social situations that would otherwise be closed to outsiders and that tearooms were in fact public restrooms in a public park and not a private domain. It was the police, the press and other agents of social control who made the tearooms a public issue. With respect to the survey portion of the study, he admitted that he'd given subjects a less-than-full presentation of what he was doing. He argued, essentially, that the research could not reasonably have been done without some level of deception and disguise.

He asserted that the ethics of social science are those of situation ethics. Situation ethics is a Christian ethical theory principally developed in the 1960s by, among others, Joseph Fletcher, an Episcopal priest. Fletcher wrote that "even a transient sex liaison, if it has the elements of caring, of tenderness and selfless concern, is better than a mechanical, egocentric exercise of conjugal rights between two uncaring or antagonistic marriage partners" (Fletcher, 1966).

Humphreys also raised the larger issue of whether socially sensitive topics such as sex, religion or suicide should be studied, given that studying them might endanger the ethical integrity of the researcher or the profession/discipline. He argued that concern about possible harm to fellow professionals should take a secondary place to concern for those who might benefit from the research, and that preventing harm to participants/respondents should be the primary interest of the researcher. Several years before the *Belmont Report*, Humphreys wrote, "Those who engage in the study of deviant behavior . . . must become accustomed to the process of weighing possible social benefits against possible costs in human discomfort" (Humphreys, 1975:170).

Humphreys reported that earlier in his career, he had administered examinations in Christian ethics to candidates for the Episcopal priesthood. He learned that questions about means or ways of doing things were always relative. Later, he applied this insight to social science methods and concluded that specific methods are not "good" or "bad," but only "better" or "worse" than others.

7.4 Related Participant Observation Studies of the Period

In the early 1970s, sociologist Carol A.B. Warren (1974) did her dissertation on a middle-class, white male gay community in San Diego. Like Humphreys, her work grew out of a class paper. She had friends in the male gay world and several of them agreed to be interviewed. Her mentor, Jack Douglas, liked the paper and encouraged her to do her dissertation on the gay community. She was considered to be an attractive young "fag hag," a term from the period that could be used affectionately to describe a woman who is best or good friends with one or more gay men and whose presence was accepted and unquestioned. The sociable world of the male gay community also involved both lesbian and heterosexual women (Warren, 2003:502). Warren did not have to take on the role or disguise herself.

Looking back 30 years later, Warren (2003:500) wrote, "I began to write field notes as I socialized, unrestrained by IRBs or more than perfunctory notions of confidentiality, harms and benefits, or informed consent." She was aware that the gay males kept their homosexuality secrets from most family and work associates if they were in business or professional occupations and feared stigmatization (Warren, 1976:160). In contrast to Washington University, the University of San Diego had a typical set of guidelines for conducting research.

Warren thought that stigma affected both the deviants and the researchers who studied them. In contrast to Humphreys, who observed actual sex acts, Warren and others studied sexual subcultures rather than sex acts. Humphreys' work became controversial and widely known because he observed and studied sex acts. In the 1960s and 1970s, stigma was prevalent in the world of gay research. Those who studied homosexuality either publicly identified as heterosexual or said nothing about their own sexual interests.

A few years later, Barbara Ponse, a student at the University of Southern California, wrote her dissertation the lesbian community. She spent 3 years doing participant observation in lesbian communities along with in-depth interviews with women living in those communities. Ponse (1978:14) left her first academic position at Washington University in St. Louis partly because she had been pressured to declare herself a lesbian even though it was not her self-identity. She left academia and started a successful practice as a psychotherapist.

7.4.1 Personal and Professional Ethics

In his commentary on disguised observation in sociology, Erikson (1967) distinguished between personal ethics and professional ethics. "Personal ethics" refers to the way an individual conducts him or herself, while "professional ethics" reflects the way a group of colleagues define their special responsibility to one another and to the social groups, communities and organizations in which they conduct research. Sociologist Arlene Kaplan Daniels (Glazer, 1972:115) expressed very grave doubts about relying on a researcher's personal sense of honor, ethics or professional discretion, no matter how well-developed these may be in that individual. She suggested that since research involves professional ethics, the professional associations should develop a control structure that eliminates the necessity of depending primarily upon the integrity of individuals.

The solution that emerged to ensure the integrity of research on human subjects, however, was to give control to IRBs at institutions that held fiduciary responsibility for federal research grants-rather than to social science professional associations, which had no direct control over the research and, at the time, had rudimentary codes of ethics.

7.4.2 Ethics of Journalism and Social Sciences

Professors of business law Levin and Roline (2002) provide a basis for comparing the ethics of journalism and social sciences. They discuss the 1992 case of *Food Lion vs Capital Cities/ABC, Inc.* Prime Time Live, an ABC network news show, learned that the US Department of Labor was investigating complaints about employees working off the clock and being fired before they would qualify for the Food Lion profit sharing plan. In addition, the Government Accountability Project was looking into unsanitary food-handling practices. ABC News Management gave their prior approval for the reporters to disguise their identities. The reporters taped other Food Lion employees relabeling old food with new freshness dates (Levin & Roline, 2002:575–576).

The case went to trial and on appeal, the two reporters were found guilty of breach of their duty of loyalty to the company and of trespass on Food Lion's property in conducting their undercover investigation. Food Lion was awarded $1.00 for each offence (Levin & Roline, 2002:595–596). These nominal damages were a symbolic slap on the wrist to the reporters and ABC, Inc. The reader should compare this to the sanctions against social science researchers who could face loss of funding and obstructions to publishing their findings in scientific journals.

In their analysis of the *Food Lion* case, Levin and Roline (2002) raised several questions: How candid must journalists be about who they are? Can society adequately protect public health and welfare without undercover journalism? If undercover journalism is necessary, how far should a journalist be able to go in investigating alleged wrongdoing? At the time of the Food Lion case, the Society of Professional Journalists 1987 code of ethics did not address the issue of undercover reporting. The 2014 code states that "journalists should avoid undercover or other surreptitious methods of gathering information except when traditional open methods will not yield information vital to the public" (Levin & Roline, 2002:590–591).

In contrast, sociologists, ethnographers and students of social problems are expected to meet scientific guidelines for methods and ethical treatment of the subjects. Once again, this means obtaining IRB approval before they can begin observing and collecting data. In contrast, journalists follow a professional code that is far more capacious, and may observe people who have not consented.

In his discussion of disguised observations in sociology, Erikson (1967:372–373) recognized that sociologists may take jobs or become members of groups and then subsequently find themselves in places or situations where they become aware of the possibility of conducting research. Sociologists cannot always introduce themselves as researchers or announce that their interactions may be providing ideas for future research. Erikson argued that while it may or may not be ethical for a journalist not to reveal his identity or purpose in the course of gathering information, it did not follow that a sociologist could do the same. Sociologists have a different relationship to the community, are collecting data for a different purpose and have a set of different professional and scientific interests to protect.

Along these lines, philosopher Chris Herrera (2003:359) wrote "Some attempt must be made to adjust our standards so that science remains good in the dual sense of being epistemically robust and considerate of the people who, after all, are not given the choice of whether to participate in the social scientist's project."

The current codes of ethics of the ASA (2018) and the APA state that:

> Informed consent may be dispensed with only where research cannot reasonably be assumed to create distress or harm or is conducted in public places.
>
> Confidentiality is not required with respect to observations made in public places and activities conducted in public or other settings where no rules of privacy are provided by law or custom (ASA, 2018:10.5(c); APA, 2002: 803.1).
>
> Confidentiality must be observed when disclosure of responses could place participants at risk of criminal or civil liability or damage their financial standing, employability, or reputation. (ASA, 2018:10.5(c); APA, 2002:805.1(b)).

7.5 Humphreys' Impact on Ethics

As readers will recall, the publication of the *Belmont Report* in 1979 marked a turning point in research ethics. It was the end product of the National Commission for the Protection of Human Subjects created by the National Research Act of 1974. The Commission drew upon a variety of resources, many of which were included in a two-volume appendix. The Report identified the three basic ethical principles of Respect for Persons, Beneficence and Justice. It also contained guidelines to assure that future biomedical and behavioral research includes informed consent, assessment of risks and benefits, and fair procedures to select research subjects.

Two years later the US Department of Health and Human Services and the Food and Drug Administration agreed upon statutory regulations governing existing research involving human subjects. In 1991, these were revised and codified in the regulations of 15 Federal departments and agencies, as *45 CFR 46*, referred to as the "Common Rule." Since then, the Common Rule has been periodically updated and revised.

Experimentation with Human Beings (Katz, 1972) was one of the first major works on research ethics and served as a primary resource for the *Belmont Report,* revisions in the federal regulations 45 CFR 46 and IRB tutorials. Katz was a physician and professor at Yale Law School and was a member of the US Public Health Service Tuskegee Syphilis Study Ad Hoc Advisory Panel to the Assistant Secretary for Health and Scientific Affairs of the Department of Health, Education and Welfare (HEW).

The book contained numerous case studies from medicine, biology, psychology, sociology and law, including Humphreys' *Tearoom Trade*. In "What Constitutes Harm?," Katz asked his readers: how should the authority of the investigator be affected by the following, and what difference does it make if the subject accepts the harm:

a) Degree, e.g., slight to severe
b) Type, e.g. to body, emotions, conduct character, personal and social values, dignity, anonymity or reputation
c) Explanation of harm e.g., disclosure or nondisclosure about being a participant or about specific aspects of the design
d) Balancing of harm, e.g., against benefits to subject, science or society
e) Recipients of harm, e.g., subjects who are considered worthy, inferior, normal or deviant
f) Awareness of harm, e.g., the ability to know, predict, and comprehend consequences (Katz, 1972:324–325)

Katz (1972:326–329) then inserted reprints of Humphreys' 1970 article, "Tearoom Trade: Impersonal Sex in Public Places," as well as von Hoffman's "The Sociological Snoopers" and the response by Horowitz and Rainwater, "Journalistic Moralizers." The expectation was that the reader would answer the questions raised in Katz's study after reading and comparing the reprints.

Robert J. Levine, a professor of Medicine at Yale, wrote several papers for Appendix I of the *Belmont Report.* These were written to assist the Commission in considering the basic ethical principles that should underlie the conduct of research involving human subjects. In his paper "The Role of Assessment of Risk Benefit Criteria in the Determination of the Appropriateness of Research Involving Human Subjects," Levine (1976a:2-25, 26, 27) considers the social risks where truly informed consent cannot be secured prior to initiating the research. His example is *Tearoom Trade*, where the experimental subjects are not even aware of the unseen observer. He pointed out that the study illustrated two types of risk to society that may occur as a consequence of conducting social research.

The first was that: individuals who learned they had been identified through their license plates might develop a distrust of social institutions, e.g., the Department of Motor Vehicles. He considered this to be a societal cost when assurances of confidentiality and privacy are breached. The second was that if Humphreys was known to be studying homosexuals and was seen spending time at public restrooms, it may be assumed by anyone who saw him that homosexuals frequented those restrooms. This could draw police attention to the restrooms (Levine, 1976a:2-26, 2-27). In fact, when Humphreys first started going to restrooms, a man, who was possibly a plain clothes park patrolman, told him not to hang around here because "we're clamping down on this park … so, try the john at the north east corner of (Reagan) Park" (Humphreys, 1975:6–7). It appears that law enforcement was willing to tolerate homosexual activities in the park restrooms as long as it did not lead to filing complaints.

Readers will recall that regulars at the tearoom ultimately vetted Humphreys and suggested that he take on the role of watch queen. In another Levine paper relevant to *Tearoom Trade*, "Appropriate Guidelines for the Selection of Human Subjects for Participation in Biomedical and Behavioral Research," Levine (1976b:4-18) defines community consultation as the process of meeting with the community in which the research is planned. The purpose is to learn from the prospective subjects how to better conduct negotiations for informed consent with individuals in the community. In addition, the researcher may learn whether those consulted perceive the potential benefits as being worthy of taking on the risks of research, if the risks are only experienced by a small proportion of the community.

As distinct from Levine's papers that appeared in the *Belmont Report*'s Appendix, the *Report*'s principles focused solely on individuals and ensuring that each would benefit from the research, be respected and chosen fairly. Over the years, some IRBs would waive documented informed consent for observational studies while others would not. Thirty-six years later, Levine (2012) asked whether the *Belmont Report* provided guidance for community research, something he had addressed in the original publication. His conclusion was no.

But that did not mean that the *Report* did not provide resources for planning and conducting ethical research involving the community. Levine suggested that community consultation in socially sensitive research would increase the subjects' perception of justice in the research and give them a feeling of control that humanizes the relationship between the researchers and the participants, thereby promoting respect for persons.

One example of such an approach is the University of Kansas's Community Tool Box (2022). The Tool Box is designed to help people evaluate community initiatives but can be applied to biomedical and social science research protocols. It calls for collaborative planning between researchers and community members from diverse backgrounds to clarify the research objectives and strategies as well as to identify community concerns and available resources to support the research effort.

The notion of community consultation was similarly supported by Friesen et al. (2017:15, 19, 20), when the Common Rule was revised in 2017 to address the concerns of social and behavioral researchers. In their article, they explore some significant criticisms of the *Belmont Report*. They argue that the relationship between the three *Belmont* principles and their applications should not be deductive, since this would result in focusing on narrow aspects of the research process. They propose that the principles ought to apply broadly to all aspects of research involving human subjects.

For example, respect for persons should no longer be thought of as a principle that is captured merely by the process of informed consent, but as one that guides the entire research process. In some cases, informed consent can be forgone in favor of "broad consent." Levine (1976b:4-8) thought this could include consulting with the community or group that would be potential subjects of proposed research. Again, we see how this could be applied to *Tearoom Trade*, where Humphreys was vetted by the regulars at the tearoom, which enabled him to continue to collect observations.

7.5.1 Interpreting and Implementing Research Ethics

Training materials in social science research ethics often present case studies, such as *Tearoom Trade*, in which the principles of human research protections have been either deliberately violated or not observed. These materials include online tutorials for investigators, handbooks for IRB members and staff and sections in student textbooks and anthologies on biomedical and social science ethics. The most questionable are those that summarize the studies in a paragraph or two, followed by a statement listing one or two key ethical issues of concern. As philosopher Hilde Lindemann Nelson (2004) pointed out, these are like Aesop's fables with just enough of a narrative to lead to the inevitable moral or ethical conclusions.

This approach to ethics often fails to raise more complex issues that should be examined, and, while the summary may be factual, it may not be complete or accurate. Similarly, Griffin (1993) maintained that while historical narratives may appear to be merely descriptive, they actually are an artful blend of explanation and interpretation that reflect a specific set of values. A narrative may present facts that are not verified, as the rhetorical intent is to correct and prevent exploitation of innocent participants in research. Some authors may be moral entrepreneurs (Becker, 1963) whose intent is to crusade for a rule that would right what they perceive to be a social evil. The approach of the author of this chapter may be found in the preface.

The Institution Review Board Member Handbook, now in its fourth edition (Amdur & Bankert, 2022), provides IRB members with valuable information on the structure and processes involved in carrying out their responsibilities to ensure that appropriate steps are taken to protect the rights and welfare of humans participating as subjects in biomedical and social behavioral research. The *Handbook* begins with a brief history of the IRB system. Unfortunately, its cursory assessments of the *Tearoom* Trade study contain several factual errors. The following has appeared unchanged in all four editions beginning with the first in 2003.

> In the early 1970s social scientist Laud Humphries [*sic*] conducted a study of homosexual behavior in public restrooms. Dr. Humphries was able to function as a watch queen outside public restrooms where people gathered to engage in anonymous homosexual activity. Humphries recorded the license plates and other identifying information from the people who came from these kinds of interactions and used this information to obtain names and addresses. He went to the homes of his study subjects and presented himself as an interviewer to collect information about the subject's background and family life. Many of the subjects were living with their family in a situation where it would have been devastating to reveal information about homosexual activity. At no time did the subjects understand that they were participating in research. In published reports of this study, the level of detail revealed the identity of some of the subjects (Amdur & Bankert, 2022:14).

As this chapter has shown, Humphreys originally paced outside or just inside the restrooms, but once he became a watch queen, he was positioned inside the restroom near a window or door so he could see who was approaching. Inside, his cough served as an alarm and his nod served to communicate all clear. At least a dozen subjects knew they were participating in research specifically on their community and agreed to be interviewed. They also appear to have spread the word that

Humphreys was not a threat at the tearooms, though without mentioning he was doing observation research on them and their activities. In some cases, this can be considered a type of community informed consent.

While some of the participants may have recognized themselves in Humphreys' book and articles, as opposed to published newspaper and other accounts, they were worried enough to contact Humphreys and learned that their identities were not revealed. As mentioned earlier, he had kept the master list and each interview card under lock and key.

7.6 Discussion and Conclusion

Tearoom Trade raises relevant questions concerning research ethics and human research protections, and it continues to be presented as a cautionary tale of unethical social behavioral research. As this chapter has shown, some ethical issues surround ing the study are well worth considering, but commentaries should not be summarized at the cost of reliability, validity and accuracy in an effort to encourage researchers to choose the most ethically appropriate protocols for their proposed studies. For example, despite the best efforts of the authors, editor and publisher, Humphreys' name is misspelled in all four editions of the *Institutional Review Board Member Handbook* (Amdur, 2003:17; Amdur & Bankert, 2007:15, 2011:14, 2022:14).

Timothy F. Murphy, a Chicago-based writer educated in both philosophy and literature, made a valid observation on applying today's research ethics to studies conducted long ago and researchers long dead. He wrote:

> One point to keep in mind, when looking at the past, is the distinction between wrong doing and blameworthiness. It can be tempting to condemn all researches in the past as blameworthy because their work failed in some way to meet standards now in place. . . .Some of them may be judged less harshly because of mitigating factors, such as factual ignorance, cultural ignorance, evolution in moral understanding and organizational indeterminacy. . . .Moral understanding refers to changes in the way we interpret morality. . . .Organizational indeterminacy refers to unclear responsibility within an organization or group . . . (that is) failures of their organizations as a whole (Murphy, 2004:5).

In Humphreys' case, as has been discussed, he obtained facts though deception and taking advantage of opportunities to access names and addresses from license plates and then added a subsample of men to a men's health survey. He certainly did not have cultural ignorance or bias with respect to the homosexual community at that time. In the late 1960s, he encountered organizational indeterminacy in a poorly formed and implemented review process for dissertation research at Washington University.

In 1971, 3 years before the 1974 Department of Health Education and Welfare (HEW) regulations required the formation of (IRBs) to approve all research proposals before they could be submitted for funding consideration, the American Anthropological Association (AAA) published a formal code of ethics for anthropological research. The 1998 AAA version stated in part that "anthropological researchers must be open about the purpose(s), potential impacts and source(s) of support for research projects with funders, colleagues, persons studied or providing information, and with relevant parties affected by the research" (Biswas, 2015:251).

In my opinion, the ethical issues raised by *Tearoom Trade* are real and present problems for ethnographers whose research involves gaining access to a group or subculture and then scientifically studying its beliefs, social structure and behaviors. This requires that some preliminary observations be made in order to develop hypotheses and decide what aspects of the group or subculture to study. Over time, the observational study may be supplemented by data collection instruments such as unstructured or semistructured interviews and questionnaires, as the ethnographer learns more about the participants, their values and their social interactions.

Furthermore, ethnographers want to observe people behaving spontaneously in natural settings. They seek to minimize the tendency of people to change their behavior when they know or become aware that they are being studied or cameras are rolling. To do so, the ethnographer may dress like those being observed—that is, take on a disguise—and not request documented informed consent prior to or during the observations and data collection phases of research.

Until the 2018 revisions to the Common Rule, sociologists, ethnographers and students of social problems were subject to IRB approval before they could begin observing and collecting data. Under the revision, observations of public behavior when sensitive information may be collected would be classified as exempt research without requiring any administrative or IRB review, provided that data security and information privacy protections policies are followed (NPRM, 2015).

Deception is unnecessary in the medical clinical model, except for using placebos. But some degree of deception may be necessary in social science and ethnographic research when totally naïve participants are required. As a result, ethnographers and some social psychologists must develop protocols for studies involving multifaceted situations that do not provide any hard and fast answers to the complex ethical dilemmas they will encounter (Ferdinand et al., 2007; Wainwright & Sambrook, 2010). The resulting inconsistency across IRBs and the ability of journalists to conduct similar observations without ethical approval has been a sore point for social scientists and ethnographers.

Journalists and many social scientists see themselves as serving the public good. The question is how to balance privacy and protections against this good. Humphreys' study was groundbreaking in presenting a clear description of certain homosexual behaviors and lifestyles, and it contributed to the public good by challenging stereotypes of and repression against homosexuals.

References

AAA. (2004, June 4). *AAA Executive Board Statement on Ethnography and Institutional Review Boards*. American Anthropology Association.

Amdur, R. J. (2003). *Institutional Review Board: Member Handbook*. Jones and Bartlett Publishers.
Amdur, R. J., & Bankert, E. A. (2007). *Institutional Review Board: Member Handbook* (2nd ed.). Jones and Bartlett.
Amdur, R. J., & Bankert, E. A. (2011). *Institutional Review Board: Member Handbook* (3rd ed.). Jones and Bartlett.
Amdur, R. J., & Bankert, E. A. (2022). *Institutional Review Board: Member Handbook* (4th ed.). Jones and Bartlett.
APA. (2002). *Ethical principles of psychologists and code of conduct*. American Psychological Association. Accessed September 28, 2021, from https://www.apa.org/ethics/code/ethics-code-2017.pdf
Arnold, R. G. (1964). The interview in jeopardy: A problem in public relations. *Public Opinion Quarterly, 28*(1), 119–123. https://doi.org/10.1086/267227
ASA. (2018). *Code of ethics*. American Sociological Association. Accessed September 28, 2021, from https://www.asanet.org/sites/default/files/asa_code_of_ethics-june2018.pdf
Becker, H. S. (1963). *Outsiders: Studies in the sociology of deviance*. Free Press.
Becker, H. S., & Geer, B. (1957). Participant observation and interviewing: A comparison. *Human Organization, 16*(3), 28–32. https://doi.org/10.17730/humo.16.3.k687822132323013
Belmont Report. (1979). *The Belmont Report: Ethical principles and guidelines for the protection of human subjects of research*. Accessed October 4, 2021, from https://www.hhs.gov/ohrp/regulations-and-policy/belmont-report/read-the-belmont-report/index.html
Bensman, J. (1967). Review of The boys of Boise: Furor, vice, and folly in an American City, by J. Gerassi. *The Annals of the American Academy of Political and Social Science, 373*, 284–285. http://www.jstor.org/stable/1037424
Biswas, S. (2015). Ethics in anthropological research: Responsibilities to the participants. *Human Biology Review, 4*(3), 250–263.
Burnet, J. (1964). Robert E. Park and the Chicago School of Sociology: A centennial tribute. *Canadian Review of Sociology/Revue Canadienne de Sociologie, 1*(3), 156–164. https://doi.org/10.1111/j.1755-618X.1964.tb00747.x
DHEW. (1971). *The Institutional Guide to HEW Policy on Protection of Human Subjects*. "The Yellow Book". Department of Health Education and Welfare. Accessed January 2, 2023, from http://ia601308.us.archive.org/0/items/institutionalgui00nati/institutionalgui00nati.pdf
Dingwall, R. (2006). Confronting the anti-democrats: The unethical nature of ethical regulation in social science. *Medical Sociology Online, 1*(1), 51–58. Accessed October 4, 2021, from https://www.academia.edu/1184594/Confronting_the_anti_democrats_The_unethical_nature_of_ethical_regulation_in_social_science
Ehrenreich, B. (2001). *Nickel and dimed: On (not) getting by in America*. Henry Holt & Co.
Erikson, K. T. (1967). A comment on disguised observation in sociology. *Social Problems, 14*(4), 366–373. https://doi.org/10.2307/798850
Ferdinand, J., Pearson, G., Rowe, M., & Worthington, F. (2007). A different kind of ethics. *Ethnography, 8*(4), 519–543. https://doi.org/10.1177/1466138107083566
Fletcher, J. (1966, January 21). Theology: Situation ethics: Between law & love. *TIME Magazine, 87*(3):55. Accessed April 22, 2022, from https://content.time.com/time/magazine/article/0,9171,835076,00.html
Food Lion, Inc. v. Capital Cities/ABC, Inc. - 194 F.3d 505.
Frankel, T. C. (2007, August 31). In Forest Park, the roots of Sen. Craig's misadventure. *St. Louis Post-Dispatch*.
Friesen, P., Kearns, L., Redman, B., & Caplan, A. L. (2017). Rethinking the *Belmont Report*? *The American Journal of Bioethics, 17*(7), 15–21. https://doi.org/10.1080/15265161.2017.1329482
Galliher, J. F., Brekhus, W. H., & Keys, D. P. (2004). *Laud Humphreys: Prophet of homosexuality and sociology*. University of Wisconsin Press.
Gerassi, J. (1966). *The boys of Boise: Furor, vice and folly in an American city*. Columbia Northwest Classics.
Glazer, M. (1972). *The research adventure: Promise and problems of field work*. Random House.

Goffman, E. (1959). *The presentation of self in everyday life*. Anchor Books.

Griffin, L. J. (1993). Narrative, event-structure analysis, and causal interpretation in historical sociology. *American Journal of Sociology, 98*(5), 1094–1133. https://doi.org/10.1086/230140

Henslin, J. M. (2001). *Sociology: A down-to-earth approach* (5th ed.). Allyn & Bacon.

Herrera, C. D. (2003). A clash of methodology and ethics in 'undercover' social science. *Philosophy of the Social Sciences, 33*(3), 351–362. https://doi.org/10.1177/0048393103252782

Horowitz, I. L. (2010). Publishing as a vocation: The necessity of independent scholarly media. *Journal of Scholarly Publishing, 41*(2), 131–144. https://doi.org/10.1353/scp.0.0077

Horowitz, I. L., & Rainwater, L. (1970). Journalistic moralizers. *Society, 7*, 12–13. Reprinted in Denzin, Norman K. (1973) *The Values of Social Science*, 2nd edition. New Brunswick, NJ: Trans-Action Books. Pp 151–164.

Humphreys, L. (1970a). Tearoom trade: Impersonal sex in public places. *Society, 7*(3), 10–25.

Humphreys, L. (1970b). *Impersonal sex in public places*. Aldine Publishing.

Humphreys, L. (1975). *Tearoom trade: Impersonal sex in public places enlarged edition with a retrospective on ethical issues*. Aldine Publishing.

Humphreys, L. (2009). Rev. Dr. Laud Humphreys | Profile. *LGBTQ Religious Archives Network*. Accessed April 22, 2022, from https://lgbtqreligiousarchives.org/profiles/laud-humphreys

Katz, J. (1972). *Experimentation with human beings: The authority of the investigator, subject, professions, and state in the human experimentation process*. Russell Sage Foundation.

King, K. F., Kolopack, P., Merritt, M. W., & Lavery, J. V. (2014, December 13). Community engagement and the human infrastructure of global health research. *BMC Medical Ethics, 15*, 84. https://doi.org/10.1186/1472-6939-15-84

Levin, D. A., & Roline, A. C. (2002). Undercover reporters, tort law, and the First Amendment: Food Lion v. ABC and the future of surreptitious newsgathering. *The Kansas Journal of Law and Public Policy, 11*(3), 575–628. https://doi.org/10.2139/ssrn.323060

Levine, R. J. (1976a). *The Belmont Report: Ethical principles and guidelines for the protection of human subjects of research* (pp. 2-1–2-59). The National Commission for the Protection of Human Subjects of Biomedical and Behavioral Research. https://videocast.nih.gov/pdf/ohrp_appendix_belmont_report_vol_1.pdf

Levine, R. J. (1976b). *The Belmont Report: Ethical principles and guidelines for the protection of human subjects of research* (pp. 4-1–4-103). The National Commission for the Protection of Human Subjects of Biomedical and Behavioral Research. https://videocast.nih.gov/pdf/ohrp_appendix_belmont_report_vol_1.pdf

Levine, R. J. (2012). BELMONT REPORT*: Guidance for community research* [PowerPoint slides]. Accessed October 4, 2021, from https://www.niehs.nih.gov/news/assets/docs_a_e/belmont_report_guidance_for_communit y_research_508.pdf

Liebenthal, R. (2014, March 5). Living with a wild god: A conversation with Barbara Ehrenreich. *Harper's Magazine*. Accessed October 4, 2021, from https://harpers.org/2014/03/living-with-a-wild-god-a-conversation-with-barbara-ehrenreich

Mathes, I. B. (1966). *Adult male homosexuality and perception of instrumentality, expressiveness and coalition in parental role structure*. Doctoral dissertation, Missouri University-Columbia (as cited in Galliher, J. F., Brekhus, W. H., & Keys, D. P. (2004). *Laud Humphreys: Prophet of homosexuality and sociology*. Madison, WI: University of Wisconsin Press).

Mac Donald, L. M. (2007, September 2). America's toe-Tapping menace. *The New York Times*. Accessed October 4, 2021, from https://www.nytimes.com/2007/09/02/opinion/02macdonald.html?ei=5087%0A&em=&en=543db0d43dfd6f76&ex=1188964800&pagewanted=print

Murphy, T. F. (2004). *Case studies in biomedical research*. MIT Press.

Nelson, H. L. (2004). Four narrative approaches to bioethics. In G. Khushf (Ed.), *Handbook of Bioethics. Philosophy and Medicine* (Vol. 78, pp. 167–182). Kluwer Academic Publishers.

NPRM. (2015). *Summary*. Notice of Proposed Rulemaking. Accessed October 28, 2021, from https://www.hhs.gov/ohrp/regulations-and-policy/regulations/nprm-2015-summary/index.html

Polsby, N. W. (1967). Review of *The boys of Boise: Furor, vice and folly in an American City*, by J. Gerassi. *American Journal of Sociology, 72*(6), 691.

Ponse, B. (1978). *Identities in the lesbian world.* Greenwood Press.
Schrag, Z. M. (2009). How talking became human subjects research: The federal regulation of the social sciences, 1965–1991. *Journal of Policy History, 21*(1), 3–37.
University of Kansas Community Tool Box. (2022). *Section 5. Our Evaluation Model.* Accessed January 29, 2023, from https://ctb.ku.edu/en/table-of-contents/overview/model-for-community-change-and-improvement/evaluation-model/main
von Hoffman, N. (1970a, January 30). Sociological snoopers. *The Washington Post*, p. B1.
von Hoffman, N. (1970b). Sociological snoopers and journalistic moralizers. *Society, 7*(7), 4–8.
Wainwright, D., & Sambrook, S. (2010). The ethics of data collection: Unintended consequences? *Journal of Health Organization and Management, 24*(3), 277–287. https://doi.org/10.1108/14777261011054617
Warren, C. A. B. (1974). *Identity and community in the gay world.* Wiley.
Warren, C. A. B. (1976). Women among men: Females in the male homosexual community. *Archives of Sexual Behavior, 5*(2), 157–169. https://doi.org/10.1007/bf01541872
Warren, C. A. B. (2003). Sex and gender in the 1970s. *Qualitative Sociology, 26*(4), 499–513. https://doi.org/10.1023/b:quas.0000005054.79173.08
Warwick, D. P. (1973). Tearoom trade: Means & ends in social research. *The Hastings Center Studies, 1*(1), 27–38. https://doi.org/10.2307/3527471
Williams, E. D. (2005). *Federal protection for human research subjects: An analysis of the Common Rule and its interactions with FDA regulations and the HIPAA Privacy Rule.* The Library of Congress. Accessed September 10, 2021, from http://www.fas.org/sgp/crs/misc/RL32909.pdf

Chapter 8
The Stanford Prison Experiment: The Power of the Situation

The degree of civilization in a society can be judged by entering its prisons.
— *attributed to Fyodor Dostoevsky,* The House of the Dead

8.1 Introduction

Philip Zimbardo is best known for his 1971 Stanford Prison Experiment (SPE). Early in his career, he conducted experiments in the psychology of deindividualization, in which a person in a group or crowd no longer acts as a responsible individual but is swept along and participates in antisocial actions. After moving to Stanford University, he began to focus on institutional power over the individual in group settings, such as long-term care facilities for the elderly and prisons. His research proposal for a simulated prison was approved by the Stanford University Human Subjects Research Review Committee in July 1971. He built a mock prison in the basement of the University's psychology building and recruited college-aged male subjects to play prisoners and guards. The study began on Sunday, August 8th, and was to run for 2 weeks but ended on Friday morning August 13th. In less than a week, several of the mock guards hazed and brutalized the mock prisoners, some of whom found ways of coping, while others exhibited symptoms of mental breakdown.

Incidentally, on Saturday, August 21st, three prisoners were killed trying to escape from San Quentin State Prison on Alcatraz Island in San Francisco Bay. This was followed 3 weeks later by a prison riot at Attica Prison in upstate New York (Sawyer, 2021). Zimbardo immediately became an expert on prison riots and prisoner abuse. He testified before a US House Judiciary subcommittee in October 1971. His special knowledge continued to be recognized decades later. In 2004, he served as an expert defense witness in the court martial of a guard at Abu Ghraib, the US military prison in Iraq.

In 2007, Zimbardo (2008: vi, vii, xi) published *The Lucifer Effect: Understanding How Good People Turn Evil*, a detailed account of the SPE. He wanted to challenge the traditional focus on individual personality and characteristics as the major explanation for people committing evil deeds, and instead emphasize the

H. Perlstadt, *Assessing Social Science Research Ethics and Integrity*, Clinical Sociology: Research and Practice, https://doi.org/10.1007/978-3-031-34538-8_8

organizational and group situations that enable them to do so. As an individuated person himself, Zimbardo readily accepted responsibility for his personal ethical and administrative mistakes during the SPE.

8.2 Preliminary Experiments

Zimbardo conducted a set of rather complex experiments that enabled him to conceive, design and carryout the SPE. As noted above, he was interested in the psychology of deindividuation, first proposed by Festinger et al. (1952); according to Zimbardo (1970: 249–250), deindividuation occurs when members are submerged in a group and not given special attention by others. They experience a reduction of their inner constraints and are more likely to express hostility toward parents or people in authority who they may have felt shaped those constraints.

Deindividuation happens when a person becomes part of a larger group and takes on the beliefs and attitudes of the group. The person is caught up in the crowd or mob and may do things they ordinarily would not do. Zimbardo's three deindividuation studies were elaborated in his undergraduate senior seminar at New York University, his research at Stanford on hypnosis and his Social Psychology in Action class.

8.2.1 The NYU Deindividualization Experiment

During the 1966–1967 school year, Zimbardo and students in his undergraduate senior seminar at New York University's campus in the Bronx conducted what would become Zimbardo's first complex experiment on deindividualization, anonymity and aggression (Zimbardo, 1969:265–269; 2008:299–300). Like the Milgram experiments (see Chap. 6), it involved administering electric shocks. Specifically, female subjects from an introductory psychology class at New York University's campus in the Bronx were to deliver electric shocks to a female confederate victim.

Eight subjects were randomly assigned to the deindividualized group (I) or individualized group (D). Each was given a very large lab coat (size 44) and an open-faced hoodie to wear over her head. Group (I) was given large name tags to wear while group (D) could not readily identify individuals in their group. In order to void experimenter bias, all instructions were given via tape recordings. The subjects in the individualized group were always addressed by the names on their name tags, while the deindividualized group subjects were addressed en masse. The students in each group were told that two of them would administer the shock while the other two would merely observe. If the two were pressing the key at the same time, the intensity of the shock would not be increased. An obedient subject would be free to administer a shock without doubling the intensity of the shock. Each subject was given a sample typical shock the victim would receive.

In addition to deindividualizing the subjects, Zimbardo portrayed one victim as nice and the other as obnoxious. The first was described on the instructions tape as a sweet girl who wanted to work with developmentally disabled children and earn some money for her fiancé who was in medical school. The other was described as a transfer student who was making money by modeling to pay for trips to Ivy League schools for dates because she couldn't stand the Jewish students at the NYU Bronx campus.

The subjects were placed in separate cubicles facing a one-way mirror. Lights were turned off for the (D) group but only dimmed for the (I) group. The victim-subject could be seen through the one-way mirror talking with the experimenter who appeared to be giving her a test. When the victim gave an incorrect answer, a signal light came on and the subjects were to immediately press the shock key. Each time the victim was supposedly shocked, she reacted as if she had extreme pain. After the tenth trial, she reacted so strongly that her hand came out of the electrode strap, but the experimenter quickly strapped her back in. The testing continued for another ten trials.

The measures of aggression were whether a shock was administered and for what duration. The subjects could administer shocks for up to 2.50 s. The mean duration for the deindividualized group was 0.90 s, twice as long as the 0.47 mean for the individualized group; this difference was significant. Zimbardo (1970:270) found that over the trials, the individualized group shocked the purportedly nice victim less and less, but the purportedly obnoxious victim more and more, but the deindividualized group increasingly shocked both victims. He noted that his findings agreed with Milgram's remotest proximity (no feedback) condition between the teacher/aggressor and learner/victim (see Chap. 6). Remoteness reduced inhibitions about the victim, as well as not being embarrassed in front of other group members.

In his subsequent Stanford experiment, Zimbardo would individualize the prisoners and deindividualized the guards. The prisoners wore a smock-like dress with a prisoner number on the front and back to individualize them. They also wore a woman's nylon stocking to cover their hair (a substitute for head shaving), and rubber clogs. A heavy chain was bolted onto their right ankle, which could be attached to the ankle of another prisoner, forming a chain gang. The deindividualized guards wore uniforms from a local army surplus store. They wore reflective sunglasses and had no name tags. This may have contributed to increasingly aggressive interactions between the two groups.

8.2.2 Research on Liberating Behavior Through Hypnosis

In 1971, Zimbardo moved from NYU to Stanford, where he held positions as both a tenured professor and fellow at the Center for Advanced Studies in Behavioral Sciences. During this time, he was continuing to develop his ideas about individuation and deindividuation. He held that an individuated person's actions were reasonable and orderly, while a deindividualized person's actions were impulsive and chaotic (1970). Most people's lives are ordered by a daily schedule or clock time—when to wake up and go to bed, when to eat meals, when to go to or return home from school or work. It occurred to him that an individual's time perspective could be altered by hypnosis, when subjects are instructed in such a way that they feel like time is passing very slowly, that is, expanding the present (Zimbardo et al., 1971:307; 1972:282).

Zimbardo received a grant from the Office of Naval Research (ONR) to conduct an experiment on hypnosis and mind control. He recruited 30 Stanford undergraduates from an introductory psychology course who were high scorers on a hypnotic susceptibility scale. The 15 males and females were randomly assigned to one of four groups. Twelve subjects were trained by a hypnotist, starting in small groups of eight and finally in groups of two. In addition, each subject was exposed to one of the three researchers acting as hypnotists. The training included giving the subjects suggestions to allow the present to expand and the past and future to become distanced and insignificant.

The other subjects were assigned to one of three groups. Two of the three groups received the same expanded present, time distortion instructions. Six were hypnotic simulators who were told to imagine how hypnotized subjects would respond, and to act as if they were hypnotized throughout the study. Another six subjects were in the present expanded control group, which received the time distortion instructions, but without any mention of hypnosis. The last six subjects were in the normal time control group. They were asked to think of their own conception of time and describe it as a metaphor, e.g., time is money (Zimbardo et al., 1971:305).

Subjects were tested in pairs within the same condition, although on most tasks they were isolated in separate cubicles. The hypnotic subjects were given a 5-min relaxation induction at the start of the experimental sessions, which were designed to increase suggestibility and suspend critical faculties. The simulators were given the same period of time to prepare themselves to be good hypnotic simulators. One task was to expose the subjects to an ambiguous situation that could be considered humorous or repulsive. All subjects heard an outtake of a radio commercial for the 1953 movie *The Caddy* starring Dean Martin and Jerry Lewis. It was ultimately not broadcast because it contained bloopers, with the comedians becoming more obscene and vulgar, and the recording engineers could be heard laughing in the background.

Two judges observed the overt reactions of the subjects through a one-way mirror, after which the subjects reported their reactions on a questionnaire. The next task required the subjects to make something in 5 min out of a large, two-pound mound of clay. The subjects left their cubicles, entered the room with the clay on the floor and worked with it separately or together. After 5 min, the experimenter told the subjects to finish up and return to their cubical to complete a questionnaire on this task.

A major finding was that the hypnotized subjects were most likely to have altered their temporal perspective and boundaries between present and future than the other subjects. They laughed aloud more and were more preoccupied with physically messing around with the clay, rather than making something with it. No differences were found between female and male subjects. Another finding was that the hypnotic subjects were more likely to display social emotional contagion. When one hypnotized subject began laughing the others quickly joined in the laughter. One hypnotized subject who could not find a name in a phone book became angry and began to tear pages out. When the other two subjects in his group were given phone books, they also started ripping out pages. The experimenters had to return the subjects to a state of deep relaxation (Zimbardo et al., 1971:318–320).

One takeaway from the hypnosis experiments was that a person's time sense could be manipulated from clock time to subjective time. The hypnotized subjects were uninhibited in that they were not task oriented. They were wasting time, laughing and messing around; they were not on the clock. Zimbardo (1970:161–162) would build on his findings from these experiments, applying them to his prison experiment. He realized that if the mock prisoners were deprived of sleep as a group, their daily time sense could be altered and they, like the hypnotized students, could become uninhibited, deindividuated and exhibit inappropriate behavior.

8.2.3 The Stanford Student Project

Like Milgram's experiments, Zimbardo's most well-known experiment grew out of a student project. In the spring of 1971, he asked students in his Social Psychology in Action class to choose from among a set of projects that would investigate the changes an individual undergoes in the process of adapting to a new environment and role. Options included the elderly entering homes for the aged, people joining cults and new convicts being jailed or imprisoned. Several students ran a mock prison in their dormitory over a weekend. While Zimbardo was aware this had taken place, he did not know what had actually happened until the students gave their in-class report in May. The students expressed intense feelings of anger, frustration, shame and confusion about their behavior during the project. Zimbardo held a debriefing with all of them. He realized that only a controlled experiment, with random assignment of the roles of guards and prisoners, could separate the dispositional factors of behavior, which are based primarily on participants' attitudes and personalities, from the situational factors of behavior, which emerge from the environment, institutional rules and role expectations (Zimbardo, 2008:32, 494–495).

Zimbardo (2008:26, 493–494) was also interested in the antiwar confrontations between students and police units and the National Guard that broke out in May 1970, following the invasion of Cambodia. These confrontations had spread across the country, from Kent State, where four students were killed, to Stanford, where the administration building was effectively closed down and shots were fired at the home of the commander of the Stanford University Reserve Officers Training Corps (ROTC), a program to train commissioned officers for the US Armed Forces.

In the spring of 1971, Zimbardo began conversations with the new chief of police of the City of Palo Alto about depolarizing the situation by holding reciprocal visits and tours between police officers and college students. The chief of police became interested in how men and women became socialized to the role of police officers, and how a rookie became a good cop. Zimbardo told the police chief that he could set up an experiment in which rookie cops and college students would be both mock guards and prisoners.

As noted above, Zimbardo had a contract with the ONR which funded a number of studies at Stanford: hypnosis and mind control (Maslach et al., 1972; Zimbardo et al., 1971; Zimbardo et al., 1973); false confessions (Maslach, 1971) and individuation and interpersonal aggression (Zimbardo, 1970; Maslach, 1974). The US Navy and Marine Corps were concerned about conflicts between guards and prisoners in naval prisons. Zimbardo wanted to demonstrate that the conditions of the prisons were not a result of the type of individuals working and incarcerated in them, but rather emerged from the prison environment, rules and role expectations. If successful, he hoped to help the Navy develop training that would eliminate the deplorable conditions in the prisons (Haney et al., 1973). The ONR agreed to a no-cost extension to pay for the SPE (Zimbardo, 2008).

8.3 From Application Through Prisoner Rebellion

On Sunday, July 31, Zimbardo (1971a) completed his application to the Stanford University Human Subjects Research Review Committee for approval of the study "Role Playing in a Simulated Prison." The review committee quickly approved the application and the experiment began exactly 2 weeks later, on Sunday, August 14, 1971. Zimbardo noted that neither the researchers nor the committee knew in advance exactly what would happen or when. It was an exploratory study to document as completely as possible the emergence of a prison environment with respect to roles and behavior.

Rather than developing research hypotheses, his application had identified a few basic parameters for the study and then proposed to observe and document how they evolved. Ideally, Zimbardo hoped the study would yield insights into what occurs in real prisons. Notably, 3 years later, the Department of Health, Education and Welfare (HEW) published regulations for the use of Human Subjects that required the formation of IRBs.

Zimbardo's application specified that he would recruit participants through newspaper advertisements for volunteers to participate in a psychology study of imprisonment. All volunteers would be given an information sheet, which was attached to the application. On the application, Zimbardo wrote:

> There may be some potential emotional stress created by this temporary loss of freedom among the prisoners and by the need for surveillance and control among the guards. We will maintain careful observation of both groups, with professional staff living in [rooms] adjacent to the experimental prison cells. Subjects will be notified of the potential

> stressfulness of the experience and during a preliminary interview will be encouraged not to participate if they are at all anxious (Zimbardo, 1971a:1).

In addition, the project would require physical activity, including exercise and cleaning rooms and halls. It would also require number counts.

On his Stanford Research Review application, Zimbardo answered "No" to the questions, "Is deception to be used at any point?" and "Does deception affect the informed consent?" The application asked if the participants would be submitted to humiliation, harassment, irritation or public or private embarrassment. Zimbardo answered "Yes":

> Prison subjects' privacy will be minimized. Prison subjects will have to wear prison uniforms. Prison subjects will have to follow orders and rules. Prison subjects will be discouraged from quitting. These negative effects are among the major anticipated side effects of being in a prison and form an essential possible outcome of this study (Zimbardo, 1971a, 2).

Zimbardo also indicated that a background questionnaire and personality inventory would probably be used in the selection of participants to exclude extreme responders, since he wanted the guards and prisoners to be as homogeneous and normal as possible. He anticipated that participants might be retested at the end of the study to note any transient changes in their self-reports. With respect to confidentiality, Zimbardo promised that all information would be coded, with a master list available only to the PIs.

The participants were given a written information sheet about the study (Zimbardo, 1971b). They were to be paid $15 a day and would be randomly assigned to play the roles of either prisoners or guards for the duration of the study. The length of the study would vary from about 5 days to 2 weeks, depending on several factors, such as the prisoner's sentence or the work effectiveness of the guards.

The prisoners would be provided food and accommodations, which met minimal standard nutrition, health and sanitation requirements. Medical and psychiatric facilities would be accessible should any of the participants desire or require such services.

Participants also agreed to have their behavior observed, to be interviewed and perhaps to take psychological tests. Films of parts of the study would be taken and participants would agree to allow them to be shown, assuming their content had scientific value. The informed consent form clearly stated that participation in the research project would involve a loss of privacy. Zimbardo promised that when the experiment ended, he would debrief each participant individually, as well as the group as a whole.

Finally, the participants were told that the study would explore the development of norms that govern behavior in a novel situation, and the differential perceptions of being in a prison from people who are initially comparable, but then arbitrarily assigned to play different roles. Unstated in the informed consent form were underlying research questions about how powerfully the labels of prisoner and guard might be in influencing behavior, and how long it might take for the simulating prisoners and guards to behave in a manner similar to prisoners and guards in real-life prisons.

Zimbardo had indicated that the prisoners would be discouraged from voluntarily leaving the study. Notably absent was any explicit wording on the information sheet informing participants they were free to withdraw from the study at any time without penalty or loss of the promised or pro-rated compensation to which they were entitled. Zimbardo's justification was presumably that, like real prisoners, those in the SPE ought not to have been given an easy way out. The participants were to enter a contractual agreement, promising to participate for the full duration of the study. No prisoner could leave once jailed, except through established procedures.

8.3.1 Constructing the Mock Prison

With the Research Review Committee's approval, Zimbardo moved quickly. He constructed a mock prison in the basement of the Stanford Psychology Building with three cells; a small closet repurposed as a solitary confinement space for disobedient prisoners; and a hallway repurposed as the prison yard where meals were served, meetings were held and visitors could meet prisoners. He set up a hidden observation point and videotaping facilities and bugged the prisoner's cells. The cells were close enough to each other that the prisoners could communicate with each other by shouting. Zimbardo ordered food for the prisoners from the student union. Additionally, he contacted the Stanford University's health, legal, fire and police departments to notify them about the experiment.

Zimbardo's (1970) research on deindividualization suggested, as noted above, that sleep deprivation and unusual time schedules could lower the threshold of behavioral constraint. He proceeded to set up three 8-h shifts for the guards. The day shift ran from 10 a.m. to 6 p.m.; the evening shift, from 6 p.m. to 2 a.m.; and the morning shift, from 2 a.m. to 10 a.m. (Zimbardo, 2008:56). These shift names and hours differed by 3 h from many standard 8-h work shifts (7:00 a.m. to 3:00 p.m., 3:00 p.m. to 11:00 p.m., and 11:00 p.m. to 7:00 a.m., though not 9:00 a.m. to 5:00 p.m.) The prisoners were strategically sleep deprived. They were awakened around 2:30 a.m. by the incoming morning shift and ordered to stand outside their cells to be counted. They had less than 4 h of sleep until the 6 a.m. wakeup call and count.

Potential subjects were asked to complete a questionnaire and were then interviewed in depth by two psychology graduate student researchers. In the end, the 24 applicants selected were judged to be the most physically and mentally stable, most mature and least involved in antisocial behaviors (Haney et al., 1973). Ranging in age from 18 to 24, the finalists included young men who ranged from recent high school graduates to those with bachelor's and master's degrees. The participants did not know each other, save for two brothers who became guards but were assigned to different shifts. As planned, the 24 finalists were randomly assigned to be either prisoners or guards. Zimbardo noted that none of the volunteers wanted to be a guard—all preferred to take the prisoner's role. The nine initial prisoners were then randomly assigned to one of three cells.

Zimbardo based his experimental set-up in part on what he had learned about prisons from Carlo Prescott, who had recently been released from San Quentin State Prison. One of the students in the spring social psychology class had invited Prescott to talk to the class about his experiences (Zimbardo et al., 2000). Prescott described prisoners having bags placed over their heads, inmates being bound together with chains and buckets being used in place of toilets in cells (Prescott, 2005).

Zimbardo subsequently asked Prescott to coteach a new summer school course in 1971 on the psychology of imprisonment. Prescott invited other men and women who had been imprisoned, as well as prison guards and lawyers, to talk to the summer school class. With this special course and Prescott's mentoring, Zimbardo was able to bring a situational savvy to his experiment (2008, 68).

8.3.2 *Creating a Total Institution*

Sociologist Erving Goffman (1961) wrote that total institutions control and regiment the daily activities of members, such as eating, sleeping, working and recreation, which are carried out in the immediate presence of many others. Privacy is at a minimum. Everyone is treated alike and expected to follow a set of explicit formal house rules enforced by the staff. Examples of total institutions in Goffman's research included prisons, concentration and prisoner of war (POW) camps, psychiatric hospitals, boarding schools, military barracks and monasteries.

Prisoner of War (POWs) are soldiers who are captured by their enemy during a war. The prisoners are then transported to a prisoner of war (POW) camp. In these camps, prisoners are forced to work, and attempts are made to induce them to reject their political or social beliefs and accept those of their captors. Camps put rebellious prisoners in solitary confinement.

Zimbardo had the formidable task of creating a total institution de novo. In some ways, the start-up of the Stanford County Jail resembled a prisoner of war camp where captured soldiers and military police were brought together for the first time, as compared to an ongoing civilian prison with its guards and inmate community into which new prisoners and guards must adjust (Zimbardo, 2008:46).

On Saturday, August 13, Zimbardo held an orientation meeting with the guards where he discussed the purpose of the experiment, gave them their assignments and suggested means of keeping the prisoners under control without using physical punishment. Zimbardo (2008:54–55) explained that he wanted to understand the psychological barriers that prisons create between people. The guards were told that the prisoners knew there were limits on what could happen to them in the experimental setting, unlike in real prisons, where prisoners can be beaten. The guards could not physically abuse the prisoners in any way but could create some degree of fear. The guards, however, could act arbitrarily and would be totally in control. The prisoners were to always be called by the prison number on their uniforms. Once during each of the three shifts, the guards could line up the prisoners for a "count," using their prison ID number to establish that all prisoners were present and to test them on their knowledge of prison rules (Haney et al., 1973).

The experiment's research questions were as follows: what will the prisoners do to try to gain power in the prison, even total power, and will they work against the guards to regain some of their freedom? Three guards would be assigned to each of three shifts based on their preferences. Zimbardo said that the night shift might be the easiest because the prisoners would be sleeping about half the time. The guards would have relatively little to do but would have to stay awake in case the prisoners attempted to plan something. This subtly suggested that that the prisoners might revolt.

The guards then met with "Warden" David Jaffe, the undergraduate student who had led the prison project in the social psychology class that spring. As part of their project, the class had developed a set of rules and procedures for the guards. Jaffe and the guards settled on a list of 17 rules that the prisoners in the Stanford County Jail would follow. These rules covered five major characteristics of a total institution: regulation of daily activities, respect for property, privileges controlled by the guards and staff, respect for authority and taboo or forbidden words.

The rules governing daily activities at the Stanford County Jail included that all prisoners must remain silent during rest periods, after lights out, during meals and when they were outside their cells in the prison "yard" (a long, narrow basement corridor). They must participate in all prison activities and keep their cells clean at all times, with beds made, personal effects neat and orderly and floors spotless. The prisoners were not to move, tamper with, deface or damage walls, ceilings, doors or other prison property and were never to operate ceiling lights. In addition, prisoners had to address each other by number, the guards as "Mr. Correctional Officer," and the warden as "Mr. Chief Correctional Officer." They were to stand whenever the warden, the prison superintendent (Zimbardo) or any visitor arrived and wait for orders to be seated or to resume activities (Zimbardo, 2008:44–45).

Privileges controlled by the guards, warden and superintendent included lavatory visitations, which were limited to 5 min, and smoking after meals or at the discretion of the guards. As in real-world jails and prisoner-of-war camps, mail would be inspected and censored. The guards could listen in on the conversations between a prisoner and his visitors and limit the visit to 5 min. The prisoners were aware that if they said anything negative about the prison they could suffer later (Zimbardo 94–95). Failure to obey any of the above rules could result in punishment. Finally, prisoners must never refer to their condition as an experiment or simulation. They are imprisoned until paroled.

8.3.3 The Prisoners Rebel

On Monday morning, Prisoner 5704, who had been denied his after dinner smoke the night before, got Prisoners 819 and 7258 to tear the numbers off their uniforms in protest against the unacceptable living conditions. Readers will recall that prisoners were required to wear a smock-like dress identified with a prisoner number. The guards stripped the rebellious prisoners naked and would not allow them to redress until they had replaced their numbers. After that incident, Prisoner 5704, the ringleader of the revolt, convinced his two cellmates (Prisoners 7258 and 3401) to do something more, whereupon 3401, who had supported prisoners considering a hunger strike during breakfast, now suggested they push their beds against the door of Cell 1, cover the door opening with blankets and shut off the lights—a clear violation of Rule #6 against operating the ceiling lights.

When the guards could not break into Cell 1, they suddenly rushed into Cell 2 that had, in Zimbardo's opinion, "the top-of-the-line trouble makers" (Prisoners 819, 8612 and 1037). The guards grabbed the three cots and hauled them out into the Yard (hallway). A struggle ensued, with much pushing, shoving and shouting. Prisoner 819 screamed "No, no, no! This is an *experiment*. Leave me alone!" His cellmate 8612 added, "A fucking simulation. It's a fucking simulated experiment. It's no prison."

In the melee that followed, Prisoner 8612 ended up naked. He thrust his hands between the bars in the door of Cell 2, with his palms upward in a pleading gesture (Zimbardo, 2008:61). One of the guards smacked his club against the bars near 8612's hands, and a few minutes later, another guard shot bursts of cold fire extinguisher foam into the cell.

8.4 Who's Who in the SPE

The SPE was like a stage production consisting of a cast of volunteer subjects playing prisoners, guards and prison administrators, as well as two from central casting, an ex-convict and prison chaplain playing themselves, and cameo walk-on appearances by prisoner's parents on visiting night, followed by a department colleague and his wife who showed up after the visitors left. In addition, playing a supporting role was Christina Maslach, who had been Zimbardo's teaching assistant and collaborator on the hypnosis study. This chapter will discuss these groups and individuals to better analyze and understand their actions and their impacts on the evolution of the SPE simulation, bringing in relevant theoretical perspectives and empirical findings.

8.4.1 The Prisoners

SPE prisoners, readers will recall, were Stanford male undergraduates who volunteered to participate in a study and were randomly assigned to play the role of prisoner or guard. Zimbardo (2008:504) did not present a set of hypotheses in advance of conducting the experiment, but he would later categorize the behavior of several prisoners in terms of Erving Goffman's (1961:61–64) four types of inmate adaptation to total institutions. They are:

1. Withdrawal where the inmate drastically curtails his involvement and interactions with both staff and fellow inmates,

2. Intransigence when the inmate refuses to cooperate with the staff in any way which, in a prison, could including rebelling or rioting,
3. Colonization where the inmate creates a personal niche within the institution and may mess up just prior to their slated discharge to increase the likelihood of remaining incarcerated; and
4. Conversion when the inmate assists staff in dealing with fellow inmates and exhibits a highly disciplined, moralistic approach to issues which are considered in an all or nothing context.

Goffman thought that most inmates adapt an opportunistic combination of the four types to maximize their chance to avoid physical and psychological harm. Zimbardo (2008:51, 62, 69, 71, 72) explicitly labeled prisoner 8612 as the rebel/intransigent, and he provided sufficient information on three other inmates to be able to classify them: Prisoner 819 for withdrawal, 3401 for colonization and 2093 for conversion.

8.4.1.1 Prisoner 819: Withdrawal

It was hard to withdraw from the SPE, where the prisoners were subject to headcounts and cell inspections in addition to communal meals and occasional meetings with prison officials and visitors. 819 thought the first counts on Sunday and Monday were just a joke. When he laughed, he did 20 push-ups without complaining. Similarly, prisoners 819 and 5486 found it funny to be ordered to sing their prison numbers; after laughing they were ordered to jumping jacks as punishment. 819 was commanded to sing a solo tune repeatedly but couldn't satisfy the guards (Zimbardo, 2008:47–50).

On Monday morning, the prisoners were told about toilet privileges, which involved being blindfolded and led outside the prison entrance as a chain gang on a circuitous route to the toilet. They would be given a short time and must remain silent. The guards noticed that 819 smiled and found it funny. A little later 819 quit doing exercises and refused to continue. The other prisoners stopped to show their solidarity, but 819 decided to continue for their sake. 819 was then sent to the solitary confinement space, "the Hole," with a defiant swagger. He was joined by 8612 and both missed breakfast (Zimbardo, 2008:58).

Prisoner 819 was back in Cell 2 when the guards rushed in after they couldn't get into Cell 1, where the prisoners had barricaded themselves. This started a prison rebellion. As the guards dragged the cots into the hallway, 819, readers will recall, screamed "No, no, no! This is an experiment!" adding, "Leave me alone! . . . You're not going to take our fucking beds!" (Zimbardo, 2008:61).

Over the rest of that day, 819 was reluctant to participate. At the afternoon count, one of the "good" guards, Geoff Landry, had the prisoners sing their numbers up a scale, in the fashion of "do-re- mi." All the prisoners except 819 sang. He refused to join the other prisoners, shouting out, "Thank you, Mr. Correction Officer, for a fine day!" Many hours later, when it was time for the Tuesday 2:30 a.m. count, 819 had to be dragged out of bed. Much of the prisoners' experience is nicely summed up in a letter 819 wrote to his friend, in which he stated that he sleeps, shouts his number and get hassled (Zimbardo, 2008:65, 70, 82, 91).

Prisoner 819's parents, brother and sister visited him on Tuesday night. Two of the guards hung around close enough so that 819 was aware that if he said anything negative about the prison he would suffer. After his parents left, he told his brother and sister about "the Hole," but when he pointed to it, one of the guards said not to talk about it. His sister asked him about the numbers on his smock and what the prisoners do all day. He explained the numbers and told her what they do all day. But when he talked about the problems he had with the guards on the night shift, the nearby guard stopped him again. He managed to say that the guards get them up early in the morning. "Some guards are really good but they all have clubs" (Zimbardo, 2008:94–95).

Father McDermott, the actual prison chaplain, showed up on Wednesday and offered to meet with those prisoners who wanted to talk with him as well as some who requested that religious services be held on the weekend. After meeting with seven prisoners, he asked about the one reluctant prisoner who said he was sick and wanted more sleep. Zimbardo had told him that earlier that day, 819 had torn open pillows and scattered feathers all over his cell. He was put in the "Hole" and his two cellmates had to clean up the mess. Zimbardo had one of the guards encourage 819 to talk with the priest in the hopes he might feel better. When they met, Father McDermott asked 819 about his visit with his family the night before. He then wanted to know how 819 was feeling, to which he replied that he had a headache and felt kind of drained and nervous. Then he broke down and started crying. The priest alerted Zimbardo, who asked 819 if he wanted to be released. But 819 wanted to continue and agreed to behave himself (Zimbardo, 2008:101–105).

Zimbardo took 819 to the staff R&R room. A while later, one of the guards had the prisoners chanting that 819 was being punished because he messed up the cells. Zimbardo went back to the R&R room and found 819 having an emotional breakdown. Zimbardo told him that he was a psychologist and not a prison superintendent and that it was time for 819 to go home. 819 left the experiment because of a severe preexisting medical condition.

8.4.1.2 Prisoner 8612: Intransigence/Rebellion

Prisoner 8612, one of the top trouble makers, was so intransigent that he was released from prison within 36 h of starting the experiment. His problems began when he was arrested on Sunday morning by a Palo Alto police officer, "Officer Bob." The officer somewhat apologetically said that he was taking 8612 downtown for booking on suspicion of burglary. Prisoner 8612 told the officer he knew his rights and asked to see the warrant for his arrest. While Officer Bob was considering a response, it dawned on 8612 that it was Sunday and that he had been told to wait for the experiment to begin that day. He dropped his interest in the warrant when he remembered he had signed up for it, not for the money, but to see how he'd feel being oppressed as a political prisoner (Zimbardo, 2008:36–37).

On Monday morning, Guard Vandy claimed that he did not like the way 8612 made his bed. He threw the blankets and sheets on the floor and ordered 8612 to remake the bed. 8612 lunged at the guard and was sent to the Hole, which already held 819. Both prisoners missed breakfast. Later, 8612 was back in Cell 2 when the guards suddenly broke in frustration because they could not get into Cell 1, where the prisoners had barricaded themselves. The guards pulled the three cots into the yard as 8612 furiously resisted, starting the rebellion. He shouted "It's a fucking simulated experiment. It's no prison. And fuck Dr. Zimbardo!" He ended up naked and moaned, "They took our clothes, and they took our beds! This is unbelievable!" (Zimbardo, 2008:58–61). As the guards moved on to Cell 3, 8612 and his cellmate 1037 called out to Cell 3 to barricade themselves. Guard Landry came at them with a fire extinguisher and shot bursts of skin-chilling carbon dioxide into Cell 2, ordering them to shut up and stay away from the door. The morning shift of three guards was attempting to control nine prisoners.

Around 6 p.m. on Monday, when the night shift was arriving, 8192 picked the lock on his cell and attempted to escape. He was shoved back into his cell where he again screamed obscenities. He had taken off his stocking cap and was told to put it back on, to which he responded:

> I can't put it on my head, it's too tight. I'll get a headache. What? I know that's really weird. That's why I'm trying to get out of here... they keep saying 'No, you won't get a headache,' but I know I will get a headache. (Zimbardo, 2008:72)

After his attempted escape, he was again sent to solitary confinement in the Hole. When he was released from confinement at lights out, he screamed that he was burning up inside. He met with Warden Jaffe who talked with Craig Haney, a graduate research assistant. Haney spoke with 8612 and thought that he might be play acting, given his antiwar activities at the university the year before. 8612 had broken Rule 9, which stated that prisoners must never refer to their condition as an experiment or simulation, which threatened the deception essential to the experiment and the roles of the participants.

Without consulting Zimbardo, who was out to dinner, Haney contacted 8612's girlfriend, who quickly came and took him away. Craig told them they might want to go to Student Health in the morning where staff were available to provide help if needed (Zimbardo, 2008:77–78). Not just Haney, but the whole of the research team suspected he had faked his symptoms (Banuazizi & Movahedi 1975; Zimbardo et al., 1972). It is possible that some of the other prisoners followed suit.

Regardless, half the prisoners would be released early (Zimbardo, 2008, 186) because of emotional and cognitive disorders.

Zimbardo (2008:496) later noted that 8612's utterance that the SPE was an experiment or simulation was a key event in the study. Everyone had to impose communal self-censorship, allowing everyone to know it is just an experiment, but acting and speaking as if it were a real prison. 8612 then claimed that in real prisons they don't take your clothes and bed away. Suddenly everything stopped in a moment of dead silence. Someone replied but they do. After that, everyone—prisoners, guards and staff—accepted the self-imposed limit on expressing the obvious truth.

8.4.1.3 Prisoner 3401: Colonization

Prisoner 3401 was the only Asian-American participant, and the shortest, at 5 feet, 2 inches in height. He seems to have wanted to fit in. Zimbardo (2008:136) described him as usually quite serious and polite when he was dealing with the guards. During breakfast on Monday morning, as noted above, he had shown solidarity with prisoners considering a hunger strike. A few hours later he agreed with 5704 that it was time to resist. 3401 suggested that his fellow Cell 1 prisoners push their beds against the cell door (Zimbardo, 2008:60, 63). He became a colonizer only when he learned that Prisoner 8612, the defiant inmate, returned from his Monday evening meeting with Zimbardo and Carlo Prescott. 8612 told the other prisoners that "I could not get out! They wouldn't let me out! "You can't get out of here!" (Zimbardo, 2008:67 70).

The other prisoners came to believe that if this rebellious leader couldn't get out, they, too, were stuck in jail for the duration of the experiment. Zimbardo commented that had a real impact on the prisoners and transformed the SPE into the Stanford Prison. This change came from the prisoners themselves, who accepted the reality of the SPE. They considered themselves unable to quit the experiment on demand and walk out at will (Zimbardo, 2008, 70–71).

This is an example of how a subordinate group legitimizes the authority and rules of an organization and supports those with power over them. Max Weber (1947, 324) noted that voluntary submission is a basic criterion of authority. Peter Blau (1964, 200) elaborated on this, explaining that authority rests on the acceptance of social norms that are enforced by a collectivity of subordinates on its individual members. That is, social constraints compel individuals to comply. The failure of the prisoner rebellion and the capitulation of its leader sent a powerful message to the other study participants that resistance was futile, and it was in their best interest to recognize the legitimacy of the prison guards.

Prisoner 3401 had a parole board hearing on Wednesday. He informed the board that he deserved parole because he believed his conduct had been beyond reproach and that his full rehabilitation can be assured. The guards, however, reported that 3401 has been a two-bit trouble maker and meekly mimicked bad behavior. Craig Haney asked what his role was in the prisoner uprising, to which 3401 honestly replied that he didn't stop it and in fact had encouraged it. Prescott said that he would not parole 3401 if he were the last man in the prison (Zimbardo, 2008: 134–135).

This would seem to have sealed 3401's fate for the rest of the experiment. Goffman (1961:61–64) held that colonizers may take actions to remain incarcerated. It turned out that 3401 did not want parole, if it meant that he would forfeit his compensation, which he really needed (Zimbardo, 2008:140). That evening 3401 developed a full body rash and had to be released. Again, a medical condition justified a prisoner-participant getting released from jail. He received appropriate medication from Student Health Services and was sent home (Zimbardo, 2008:143).

8.4.1.4 Prisoner 2093: Conversion

According to Goffman (1961:61–64), the convert has a more disciplined and moralistic approach to life. He identifies with and assists the staff when dealing with fellow inmates and displays enthusiasm for the institution. Prisoner 2093, however, identified with an ideal prison guard, insisting that the SPE guards demonstrate moral responsibility. When he was interviewed for the experiment, he replied that 10 years from now he would like to improve efficiency in unorganized and inefficient areas of our government.

He told the two Palo Alto police officers who arrested him on Sunday that he was prepared to be arrested without any resistance. 2093 was 5 feet, 8 inches tall, with 170 pounds of solid muscle.

One of the officers, Officer Bob, thought that 2093 might be some kind of "nut case" who wanted to prove something with his karate lessons. Officer Joe, later told Zimbardo that 2093 was like a military drill officer or a sergeant in the army. The other prisoners nicknamed him "Sarge" because of his militaristic style of obediently following orders. 2093 had strong values that would eventually come into conflict with those of the guards (Zimbardo, 2008:38–39, 47).

After breakfast on Monday, when two prisoners refused to return to their cell, three guards pushed them into their cell. Just then, 2093 called out that he was willing to volunteer to clean the dishes, perhaps in an attempt to ease the rising tensions that would go on to lead to the prisoner uprising. After lunch, the guards lined up the prisoners and ordered them to state their numbers, starting with the prisoner at the end. 2093 started it off in a fast, loud response which the other prisoners picked up with some variations (Zimbardo, 2008:59, 64).

Tuesday evening was visiting night. The prisoners were served a hot meal with seconds and double desserts. Guard Helmann was sitting at the head of the table and asked 2093 if he never had it so good and whether his mother ever gave him seconds? 2093 answered "No" to both, whereupon Helmann picked some food off 2093's plate and walked away. 2093's father showed up at visiting night. 2093 bragged that he had memorized all 17 rules that must be obeyed. His father asked what right does the research team have to enforce that, and mentioned civil rights. Helmann, who was hovering nearby, interjected that people in prison have no civil rights. 2093's father wanted more privacy to speak with his son but Guard Helmann told him that was not allowed. 2093's father appeared upset but accepted this limit. 2093 told his father about the counts, exercises, chores and lights-out. 2093 added that he expected it to be worse. His father asked how, and Helmann explained that two of the original prisoners are no longer in prison and two were in maximum security (Zimbardo, 2008:93, 118).

During the Wednesday night count, Guard Helmann suddenly asked 2093, "Why are you such an ass-licker? Why do you try to be obedient so much?" 2093 retorted that "it's in my nature to be obedient" (Zimbardo, 2008:120). A few minutes later, Helmann opened the door to the Hole. Inside was 416, who had replaced 8612, the intransigent rebel who was released on Monday night. 416 was holding a sausage in each hand because he didn't eat them at dinner. Helmann announced that none of them would have blankets tonight. Helmann ordered 2093 to tell 416 that "you're going to kick his ass if he doesn't eat the sausages." 2093 asserted that he would not use a profane word toward another human being and that he was willing not to have a bed tonight. Guard Landry suggested that 2093 say, "you're going to kick him in the rear end." 2093 walked over to 416, repeating the exact same words to him, explaining that he did so because he was ordered to. Zimbardo (2008:121–124) wrote that this was a power struggle between Helmann, the most controlling, power-hungry guard and the totally obedient prisoner, who was a man of principle.

Prisoner 2093 appeared before the Parole Board on Thursday. He told them that he had followed all the rules from day one and would not give up his pay in exchange for parole. He had spent summer quarter at Stanford living in the back of his car and had a little trouble sleeping the first night because the prison bed was too soft. He had been eating better in prison and had more time to relax than the previous 2 months. He also explained that he did not apply for parole on Wednesday because he didn't want to get ahead of other prisoners who were having a harder time than he was.

8.4.2 Prison Guards

While prisoners have been the focus of research ethics, fewer studies have been done on prison guards. In their review of the literature on stress and burnout among correctional officers, Schaufeli and Peeters (2000) found that correctional officers are expected to both guard prisoners and facilitate rehabilitation. Guards in the SPE, however, were only expected to be tough and maintain order and discipline. The purpose of the SPE was not to reform prisoners but to learn how prisons change people when they are faced with all-powerful guards (Zimbardo, 2008:65).

8.4.2.1 A Study of Guards at State Correctional Institutions

Criminologist Mary Ann Farkus (2000) conducted in-depth interviews with 79 officers at two medium-security state correctional institutions. She identified five types of prison guards. The most common were "Rule enforcers" (43%), who followed the rules, were inflexible in discipline and expected deference to their authority and obedience from the inmates. They observed distinctions in rank and obeyed their orders that came down the chain of command. They tended to work the second and third shifts when the warden and associate wardens were usually not at the prison. "Hard liners" were a subtype of Rule enforcers and accounted for approximately 14% of those interviewed. They held more militaristic values of being a guard, and were abusive and aggressive toward inmates. Like the Rule enforcers, they worked the later shifts.

One-fifth (21.5%) were "People workers," who modified the formal rules by creating their own informal reward and punishment system. They were seen as professionals trying to do their very best. They developed a comfortable style of working with inmates. They were most likely to work the first or day shift, and least likely to work the third or graveyard shift. "Synthetic officers" occupied a niche between the Rule enforcers and People workers. They closely followed the rules and identified with official goals, but tried to take circumstances into account. However, they were more likely than the People Workers to distrust the inmates. The Synthetic officers preferred the day shift and composed approximately 14% of the interviewees.

About 7.5% of those interviewed were classified as "Loners." They tended to be female and Black officers between the ages of 26 and 36. They closely followed the rules to validate their authority to the inmates and coworkers and avoided making mistakes.

8.4.2.2 The Stanford Prison Guards

On Friday when the SPE ended, all participants were invited to a debriefing session (Zimbardo, 2008:182–183). The former inmates named three guards who, like Farkus's Hard liners, had been creatively abusive or specifically singled them out for abuse. The SPE prisoners identified two guards who resembled Farkus's People workers and had done small favors for them or had distanced themselves from the more abusive guards, Other SPE guards had done their job and gone by the book, similar to Farkus's Rule enforcers.

Zimbardo (2008:202–203) analyzed hours of video tapes and found 25 incidents of prisoner–guard interactions. Two independent raters scored the interactions on Asking Questions, Giving Commands, Offering Information, Using Individuating (positive) or Deindividuating (negative) References, Making Threats, Giving Resistance, Helping Others and Exhibiting Aggression. Overall, negative hostile interactions outnumbered positive interactions between guards and prisoners. Guards were more likely than prisoners to be assertive.

The number counts were times when abuse was most likely to occur and guards had increased their harassment of prisoners over time. No deindividuating reference occurred during the very first two count interactions, compared with an average of 5.4 such references in the very last two counts just before SPE ended. The guards averaged 0.3 depreciating insults during the first two counts but averaged 5.7 times on the last counts. The night shift was headed by Hellmann, nicknamed "John Wayne," because he was the hardest on the prisoners. His shift issued an average of 9.3 commands versus 4.0 for the other two shifts, and he made twice as many deprecating insults (5.2 versus 2.3).

This supports Farkas (2000), who found that Hard liners and Rule enforcers were more likely to work the second and third shifts, while corrections officers, who were

People workers, were more likely to work the first shift and less likely to work the third. It also suggests that Zimbardo's attempts to set unusual hours for the shifts may have contributed to a time disorientation that lowered social inhibitions for the SPE guards on the morning shift, which started at 2 a.m., when few if any members of the research team were around.

8.4.3 Father McDermott

After the Monday rebellion, Zimbardo created the Grievance Committee of prisoners who were elected by their comrades. The committee demanded that glasses be returned, that there be less physical and verbal abuse and that religious services be provided for prisoners who wished to attend them. Zimbardo contacted a Catholic priest he knew to play prison chaplain. As it turned out, Father McDermott (not his real name) had actually served in this role in Washington, DC. He agreed to talk with some of the prisoners on Wednesday and then give Zimbardo his honest evaluation of how realistic the prison experience seemed (2008, 101).

He met with the prisoners in chairs against the wall between Cells 2 and 3, with Zimbardo in a chair next to the priest. The conversations started with brief introductions followed by questions about the prisoner's life, his family, how he was being treated, how he was feeling and whether he had any complaints. As prison chaplain, he asked if he could offer any assistance.

Father McDermott asked several of the prisoners whether they or their family had sought legal counsel because the prisoners did not have much pull in their present situation. Zimbardo (2008:102–105) was pleased that the priest had been drawn into the simulation, but wary when McDermott promised to contact 7358's mother so she could arrange for legal help from his cousin who worked in the local public defender's office. He called and told her that her son needed legal representation if he wanted to get out of the Stanford County Jail. She then called her nephew in the public defender's office, who in turn called Zimbardo. A meeting was scheduled for Friday morning.

8.4.4 Carlo Prescott

Readers will recall that Prescott, the former inmate of San Quentin State Prison, had been invited by a student in Zimbardo's social psychology class to talk about his experiences. Afterward Zimbardo asked Prescott to coteach a new summer school course in 1971 and kept him on as an SPE advisor. When Father McDermott told Zimbardo that he was going to follow up concerning legal counsel for Prisoner 7258, Zimbardo quickly improvised a parole process. Parole was not part of the original information or instructions given to the prisoners. Zimbardo then asked Prescott to chair the parole committee.

Chairing the Parole Board would be a role reversal for Prescott, whose own petitions for parole had been denied many times (Zimbardo, 2008: 54, 57–58, 68, 100). He began the first SPE Parole Board meeting by telling the other three members—research assistant Craig Hanney, a male graduate student, and a female secretary, both of whom knew little about the study—that parole boards had turned down ideal candidates for arbitrary and/or biased reasons, e.g., because a candidate was raised in a low-income neighborhood or because they didn't like the prisoner's face. In short, prisons are a big business and need prisoners (Zimbardo, 2008:131, 498). Prescott dealt with the student prisoners in much the same way he had been dealt with by real parole boards.

The first parole candidate was Prisoner 4325 from Cell 3 who said he was charged with assault with a deadly weapon but wished to plead not guilty. Prescott cynically asked if he is implying that the arresting officers, who have had a number of years of experience, just happened to pick him up out of all of Palo Alto? He went on to ask about 4325's criminal history that had put him in a situation to be arrested, then asked if he had shot or stabbed someone. Haney, Zimbardo's graduate student research assistant, and other board members tried to shift the questioning to how 4325 had been adjusting to prison life. Prescott, however, wanted to know what the prisoner would do if he were to be released. 4325 said he was going to UC Berkeley to study physics. Prescott's follow-up asked him about his religious beliefs and why he has not taken advantage of the prison's programs of group or vocational therapy.

Prescott had been asked these types of questions at his parole hearings, although Prescott knew that the SPE did not offer therapy programs (Zimbardo, 2008:132–133). It is not clear how well the research staff prepared 4325 to answer detailed questions about his crime.

When Prisoner 3401 was brought into the board meeting with a paper bag over his head, Prescott wanted it removed so he could see his face. 3401 is revealed to be Asian American. Prescott played the race card. "While Oriental people are likely to be good citizens, very few are in prisons" (Zimbardo, 2008:135). Prescott told 3401 that after hearing his previous answers, he considered him to be a constant trouble-maker who derided the simulated prison. "I wouldn't parole you if you were the last man in the prison. I think you're the least likely prospect to parole Zimbardo, 2008:135). 3401 really needed his money and was unwilling to forfeit it for early release. In that sense, he was a colonizer who wanted to remain in prison.

Zimbardo (2008:142–143) was taken aback by Prescott's transformation from someone he had worked with developing the project to his performance as Parole Board Chair. This blurred the line between the simulation and reality of the parole process. Zimbardo knew that Prescott had nightmares before his Parole Board hearings, in which he had only a few minutes to present his case to board members who were not really listening to him.

8.4.5 A Psychology Department Colleague and Wife

Gordon Bower was Zimbardo's colleague in the psychology department, a very serious scholar and former graduate school roommate. But Zimbardo (2008:98) considered him a "bleeding-heart liberal." On Tuesday evening, Bower and his wife happened to be in the psychology building and saw the prisoners on the fifth floor where they had been temporarily moved, to avoid a rumored raid on the prison. Bower and his wife went out and bought the prisoners some doughnuts. Later they went down to the basement, found the door open and saw Zimbardo. Bower asked Zimbardo what was going on, and Zimbardo briefly described the research. Bower wondered what the independent variable was, at which point Zimbardo got angry and asked him to leave.

Bower's question was not irrelevant, though it did not take into account the fact that the SPE was more of a simulation than an experiment. Although participants were randomly assigned to the roles of guard and prisoner, the study did indeed lack explicit, independent and dependent variables. A simulation is designed and carried out when an investigator wants to understand the natural dynamics and relationships in a social situation but it is not feasible to conduct the study in a real-world setting. Good simulations are interactive, and researchers (or game players) often adjust the ongoing scenario.

Unlike many social psychological laboratory experiments, in which the experimenter manipulates the situation according to a predetermined research design, Zimbardo let the simulation evolve and had to improvise adjustments: the Grievance Committee which he created on Monday after the rebellion, agreeing to let prisoners leave the experiment due to health or medical conditions, bringing in a prison chaplain, establishing the Parole Board and ending the SPE early. He knew he had no control group but envisioned conducting group comparisons in the future (Zimbardo, 2008:197).

8.4.6 Prisoner 1037's Parents

Prisoner 1037 started out being rebellious, but after that, he slowly withdrew while remaining minimally cooperative. During the Monday morning rebellion, he joined his cellmate, 8612, in urging the occupants of Cell 3 to barricade themselves in and to fight the guards, for the time had come for violent revolution. A bit later, when Prisoner 1037 refused to come out of his cell, three guards threw him to the ground, handcuffed his ankles and dragged him by his feet out into the hallway. With his feet chained together, they dragged him into the Hole.

Prisoner 1037 was subsequently elected to sit on the Grievance Committee representing Cell 2. The committee met with Zimbardo and presented its demands: return glasses, administer less physical and verbal abuse and offer religious services. Zimbardo told them he would meet with the staff that night and make some changes.

But later that evening, when Prisoner 1037 learned from his cellmate, 8612, that no one could quit, he felt he was really a prisoner and was totally helpless.

On Tuesday evening, Prisoner 1037's parents came to see him. His mother was worried about his appearance. On her way out, she brought this up with Zimbardo. She said her son looked haggard and had not been sleeping through the night, because the guards woke them up for something called counts. Zimbardo explained what counts were. He then asked the father if his son could take it, to which the father replied, "Sure he can, he's a real leader" (Zimbardo, 2008:97). But the mother was not deterred.

That night, she wrote a letter to Zimbardo in which she repeated her concerns, adding that neither she nor her son had expected anything as severe as what she had seen and heard. She reported that her son at first had been sorry that he had volunteered but had gone through several different moods and was more resigned now. She closed with the thought that this would be the hardest money he would ever earn in his life.

At the Wednesday parole board hearing, Prescott noted that 1037 seemed rather depressed. 1037 told the parole board that on Monday he rebelled, thinking he was being treated unjustly, but that evening he finally realized that he was unworthy of better treatment. After that, he did his best to cooperate. Zimbardo (2008:138) noted that this statement resembled the same of kind declarations made by American POWs who were the subjects of mind-control experiments during the Korean War. During his hearing, 1037 told the board that he would consider parole even if it meant forfeiting his salary. On Thursday, Zimbardo told Prisoner 1037 that he would be immediately paroled and would get full pay for the entire experiment after the study and final surveys were completed. His parents picked him up during visiting hours on Thursday evening.

8.4.7 Christina Maslach

Christina Maslach had been Zimbardo's teaching assistant and had collaborated with him on other research projects, as well as serving as an informal editor of several of his books. She had just completed her Ph.D. at Stanford and was about to join the psychology department at UC Berkeley as an assistant professor. She was also romantically involved with Zimbardo—they would be married a year after the prison study ended. She was not closely involved in the ongoing simulation because she was part of a team that was scheduled to do a thorough evaluation of staff, prisoners and guards on Friday.

On Thursday, she unexpectedly became directly involved when she was asked to serve on the Parole Board as a replacement for Haney, who had a family emergency. She apparently did not participate very much in the hearing. That evening, she came down to the prison to meet Zimbardo for a late dinner. On her way in, she stopped to talk with one of the guards, who she described as being very pleasant, polite and friendly. Later on, she was told by one of the research staff that she should take a look at the meanest, toughest guard, Hellmann "John Wayne," who had just come on duty. When she looked through the observation point, she was stunned to discover it was the same guard she had chatted with earlier, who now moved and talked differently, cursing with a southern accent and swinging his club (Zimbardo, 2008:169).

When she was in the superintendent's office with Zimbardo, he told her to look at the prisoners chained together by their ankles with paper bags over their heads on their way to the toilet. She said that she had already seen it and averted her gaze. She began to cry and told Zimbardo that she was leaving and to forget about dinner. He ran after her and told her no one else had reacted as she just had. The others who had failed to convince Zimbardo to release specific prisoners to end the experiment early lacked legitimate or expert power over Zimbardo (2008:237, 457–458). However, as Zimbardo's romantic partner, Maslach possessed personal referent power, which involves a threat of rejection from a person who is highly valued or loved by another (French and Raven, 1959:154–155). Maslach replied that she did not care if everyone in the world thought that what was going on was okay, she thought it was simply wrong, and that Zimbardo was personally responsible for the prisoners' suffering. The argument was intense, unlike any they had had before. He acknowledged his responsibility and decided he would end the experiment on Friday morning (Zimbardo, 2008:170–171).

8.5 Discussion and Conclusion

The SPE proved to be highly controversial. Like Milgram's study, Zimbardo's evolving experimental design and findings challenged how people might act in a situation requiring obedience to an authority, whether a researcher or prison guard. The SPE raised ethical issues on informed consent and protecting vulnerable subjects. Also, like Milgram's study, it was replicated both scientifically and on television and became part of larger discussions about prison riots, abuses and penal reform.

8.5.1 Ethical Issues

Two ethical issues raised by the SPE are the ability of subjects to withdraw from a research study at any time, and the failure to minimize harm and end the study when abusive behavior escalates. Regarding the matter of withdrawing, according to the Participant Information Sheet, "It is obviously essential that no prisoner can leave once jailed, except through established procedures" (Zimbardo, 1971b:1). The first procedure to be established was at the Saturday orientation meeting for the guards. Prison Warden Jaffe, the undergraduate who had led the student class project, and the guards created the list of 17 rules that the prisoners would have to follow.

Readers will recall that Rule 9 stated that prisoners must never refer to their condition as an experiment or simulation, which threatened the deception essential to the experiment and the roles of the participants. Prisoner 8612 had shouted that it was a "simulated experiment" and been sent to the Hole. However, the official reason, which became the second procedure to be established, was that he appeared to exhibit extreme psychological distress (Zimbardo, 2008:222). He was sent home on Monday evening after only 36 h in jail. The third procedure was following the SPE Parole Board's recommendations for releasing specific prisoners.

When he submitted his application to the Stanford Review Committee, Zimbardo (2008:120, 235) thought that neither he nor the members of the research committee imagined in advance that any oversight was necessary in an experiment in which college students technically had the freedom to stay or to go, if at any time the going became rougher than they could handle. The Review Committee application asked many of the same questions that would subsequently become required criteria by the Common Rule (*45 CFR46.111(a)(6)*, including the criterion that "when appropriate, the research plan makes adequate provision for monitoring the data collected to ensure the safety of subjects."

Today, an IRB could require the creation of a Clinical Study Oversight Committee (CSOC) or a Data and Safety Monitoring Board (DSMB). Both are an independent group of experts that advises study investigators on adverse events and unanticipated problems involving risks to or safety of the subjects.

Depending on the scope and risks involved, the DSMP may assign the responsibility for data and safety monitoring to the principal investigator (PI), the sponsoring entity, or a data safety monitoring committee or board. Committees oversee projects with greater than minimal risk, while boards are usually reserved for studies that may have major risks for research participants (Amdur, 2006).

The DSMP includes the schedule for reviewing the data and progress of the study, the reporting of adverse events, and rules outlining under what circumstances individual participants should be stopped from continuing their participation in the study and under what conditions the study as a whole should be terminated (NHLBI, 2008).

However, if the research is not a clinical trial, but does involve greater than minimal risks to participants, IRB approval of a data safety monitoring plan is required and a Data and Safety Monitoring Board (DSMB) or Observational Study Monitoring Board (OSMB) may be required (NHLBI, 2008).

In hindsight, an independent monitoring board should have been in place.

When the SPE ended, Zimbardo (2008:189, 234–235) admitted that he had a serious conflict of interest as PI and prison superintendent. He thought that if someone else had been acting as superintendent, he would have been able to assess the situation more objectively and would likely have ended the experiment earlier. But, more to the point, he also acknowledged that the experiment required oversight and that someone should have had authority over him to end it.

8.5.2 Should the Prison Experiment Be Replicated?

Scott Plous, a former student of Zimbardo's and a professor at Wesleyan University who maintained the Stanford Experiment Website (n.d.), contended that the standards for using human participants in research would not permit such an experiment today and that it is thus unlikely to ever be replicated (Alexander, 2001).

In 2004, David Frohnmayer, president of the University of Oregon, stated that Zimbardo's work has never been replicated; the fact that it cannot be repeated because of the ethical restrictions of human subjects committees is validation to some extent of the power of the experiment. Social psychologists do, however, continue to produce evidence that situational factors can have powerful influences over the behavior of individuals (Frohnmayer, 2004).

Zimbardo maintained that the participants suffered no long-term harm, even though some had symptoms of mental breakdown during the experiment (Alexander, 2001). He claimed that most subsequent research on prison roles has been limited to paper-and-pencil tests, asking people things like, "Imagine you were a guard, how would you behave?" (O'Toole, 1997).

One simulation-based study was conducted in 1979 at the University of New South Wales, Australia (Lovibond et al., 1979; Gross, 2008; Zimbardo, 2008:251). It involved three variations on prisons as total institutions. The Standard Custodial baseline experiment placed nonconvict volunteers in a situation closely resembling a medium-to-high-security prison. The prison officers addressed the prisoners by their numbers and the prisoners were required to address the officers as Sir or Mr., followed by their surname. The second experiment, Individualized Custody, differed from the baseline by emphasizing the need to keep the prisoners securely in custody while allowing inmates to retain their self-respect. In the third experiment, Participatory, the guards were trained to encourage and reinforce social and responsible prisoner behavior without an emphasis on keeping them securely in custody. Six prisoners and four guards spent 4 days in the experimental prison.

Not surprisingly, the Standard Custodial variation exhibited the most harassment by prison officers, while a few prisoners worked out ways to outsmart, belittle and frustrate the officers. The Participatory had the least hostility and developed relations of mutual tolerance and cooperation. The Individualized Custodial variation featured social distancing between the officers and the prisoners, resulting in very few incidents occurring. The researchers concluded that the observed hostile and confrontational behavior was the result of the social context, rather than the psychological characteristics of the participants. Morgan et al. (1979) argued that the experiment would more accurately match that of a school or hospital.

8.5.3 Research on Evil Practices

Zimbardo has spent a good deal of his career since 1971 studying the psychology of evil, pointing out what has been gained from the SPE and how it can help improve the prison system. The SPE demonstrated that the behaviors of guards and prisoners were not a result of their personality types but rather of values, norms and behavior generated by the prison environment, rules and role expectations. Individuals will vary in their role adaptations to specific situations. The focus, then, should be on the group, and not on particular individual psychological characteristics.

Zimbardo, like Milgram, contended that the intense psychological reactions experienced by participants during the experiment were transient and did not seriously or negatively affect the lives of the participants. Zimbardo administered a number of psychological tests before the experiment, while it was ongoing and immediately after it ended. He noted that the mood of those who were released early was, as expected, negative during the experiment, but the posttest revealed a great increase in positivity and a corresponding decrease in negativity among the prisoners. Interestingly, the guards also experienced an increase in positivity and a decrease in negativity between their intermediate and final test scores. He claimed that at the end of the study, both groups had returned to their initial baselines, suggesting that the changes were situation-specific and the result of the roles participants played (Zimbardo, 2008, 201).

Here, we can turn to an illustrative point of comparison, Abu Ghraib, the Iraq prison used by American forces in Iraq to hold prisoners of war. In 2003, it was the site of a scandal in which American military personnel tortured and abused inmates. Around midnight on October 25, 2003, three Iraqi detainees were dragged from their cells, made to crawl on the floor naked, chained together and forced into simulated sexual acts (358). The Schlesinger Report (2004) on the atrocities at Abu Ghraib prison during the war in Iraq identified a failure of command involving a lack of adequate procedures for the processing, interrogating and releasing of prisoners. Commanders had to improvise the organizational and command relationships, resulting in poor oversight of lower-level personnel. These are exactly the same issues that enabled the Stanford guards to abuse and humiliate their prisoners.

Zimbardo (2008, 331,347, 358–359) was asked to testify on behalf of Staff Sargent Ivan Fredrick, who was in charge of the night shift at Abu Ghraib. Since Frederick had pleaded guilty, Zimbardo's testimony focused on the situational and systemic factors that facilitated the torture and abuse. He drew parallels between the SPE and Abu Ghraib. Most incidents occurred at night, when high ranking prison officials were not likely to be around. He compared SPE guard "John Wayne" with a reserve corporal in Iraq as a catalyst for making things happen.

8.5.4 Conclusion

The SPE is perhaps one of the two or three best known social behavioral science research studies. It is discussed in many introductory psychology text books as a model for the power of the situation, as well as topics in other social science methodology and research ethics courses. It has generated comments, criticisms and implications for the real world of prisons. This chapter has shown how Zimbardo's previous work influenced his ideas and research design for the SPE. In contrast to many accounts, which are organized chronologically over the 6 days of the experiment, the focus here has been on how the prisoners, the guards, Carlo Prescott, the ex-convict who advised Zimbardo and served as head of the SPE Parole Board, and Father McDermott, the SPE prison chaplain, forced Zimbardo to take a more hands on approach to the experiment and create new procedures and entities to address their concerns. Fortunately, he relied on and followed their advice. Finally, as noted above, he listened to Christina Maslach, who successfully persuaded him to end the experiment early.

Acknowledgments I wish to thank Chris Herrera, Jonathan K. Rosen, David Segal and Ruth Spivak for their comments on this chapter.

References

Alexander, M. (2001, August 22). Thirty years later, Stanford Prison Experiment lives on. *Stanford Report*. Accessed April 22, 2022, from https://news.stanford.edu/news/2001/august22/prison2-822.html?msclkid=7d17df2ec26f11ec8086da6bf715d359

Amdur, R. J. (2006). Provisions for data monitoring. In E. A. Bankert, & J. R. Amdur (Eds.), *Institutional review board: Management and function*. 2nd edition (pp. 160–165). Jones & Bartlet

Banuazizi, A., & Movahedi, S. (1975). Interpersonal dynamics in a simulated prison: A methodological analysis. *American Psychologist, 30*, 152–160.

Blau, P. M. (1964). *Exchange and power in social life*. Wiley.

Farkas, M. A. (2000). A typology of correctional officers. *International Journal of Offender Therapy and Comparative Criminology, 44*(4), 431–449. https://doi.org/10.1177/0306624X00444003

Festinger, L., Pepitone, A., & Newcombe, T. (1952). Some consequences of deindividuation in a group. *Journal of Abnormal and Social Psychology, 47*, 382–389.

French, J. R. P., & Raven, B. (1959). The bases of social power. In D. Cartwright (Ed.), *Studies in social power* (pp. 150–167). Institute for Social Research.

Frohnmayer, D. (2004, November 30). *"Situational ethics, social deception, and lessons of machiavelli" Judge learned hand award Luncheon Oregon chapter of the American Jewish Committee Tuesday*. http://president.uoregon.edu/speeches/situationalethics.shtml

Goffman, E. (1961). *Asylums. Essays on the social situation of mental patients and other inmates*. Doubleday Anchor. http://www.diligio.com/goffman.htm

Gross, B. (2008, Winter/December). Prison violence: Does brutality come with the badge? *The Forensic Examiner*. http://www.theforensicexaminer.com/archive/winter08/6/

Haney, C., Banks, C., & Zimbardo, P. G. (1973). A study of prisoners and guards in a simulated prison. *Naval Research Review, 30*, 4–17.

Lovibond, S. H., Mithiran, & Adams, W. G. (1979). Effects of three experimental prison environments on the behaviour of non-convict volunteer subjects. *Australian Psychologist, 14*(3), 273–285.

Maslach, C. (1971). The "truth" about false confessions. *The Journal of Personality and Social Psychology, 20*(2), 141–146. https://doi.org/10.1037/h0031675

Maslach, C. (1974). Social and personal bases of individuation. *Journal of Personality and Social Psychology, 29*(3), 411–425. https://doi.org/10.1037/h0036031

Maslach, C., Marshall, G., & Zimbardo, P. G. (1972). Hypnotic control of peripheral skin temperature: A case report. *Psychophysiology, 9*(6), 600–605. https://doi.org/10.1111/j.1469-8986.1972.tb00769.x

Morgan, A. H., Lovibond, S. H., & Adams, W. G. (1979). Comments on S. H. Lovibond, Mithiran, & W. G. Adams: "The effects of three experimental prison environments on the behaviour of non-convict volunteer subjects". *Australian Psychologist, 14*(3), 273–287.

NHLBI. (2008). National Heart Lung and Blood Institute. *Data and safety monitoring policy*. http://www.nhlbi.nih.gov/funding/policies/dsmpolicy.htm

O'Toole, K. (1997, January 8). *The Stanford prison experiment: Still powerful after all these years. Stanford report*. Stanford University News Service. http://www.stanford.edu/news/gif/snewshd.gif

Prescott, C. (2005, April 28). The lie of the Stanford prison experiment. *The Stanford Daily*.

Sawyer, K. D. (2021). *George Jackson, 50 years later*. Accessed January 18, 2022, from https://sfbayview.com/2021/08/george-jackson-50-years-later/?msclkid=4afbd2c7c26b11eca875b013aedf20b3

Schaufeli, W. B., & Peeters, M. C. W. (2000). Job stress and burnout among correctional officers: A literature review. *International Journal of Stress Management, 7*(1), 19–48. https://doi.org/10.1023/A:1009514731657

Schlesinger Report. (2004). *Final report of the independent panel to review Department of Defense Detention Operations*. http://news.bbc.co.uk/nol/shared/bsp/hi/pdfs/24_08_04_abughraibreport.pdf

SPE Website. (n.d.). Stanford Prison Experiment Website. *The story: An overview of the experiment*. Accessed February 28, 2022, from https://www.prisonexp.org/the-story

Weber, M. (1947). *The theory of social and economic organization*. Oxford University Press.

Zimbardo, P. (1969). The human choice: Individuation, reason and order versus deindividuation, impulse, and chaos. In W. J. Arnold & D. Levine (Eds.), *Nebraska Symposium on Motivation* (Vol. 17, pp. 237–307). University of Nebraska Press.

Zimbardo, P. G. (1970). The human choice: Individuation, reason, and order versus deindividuation, impulse, and chaos. In W. J. Arnold & D. Levine (Eds.), *1969 Nebraska symposium on motivation* (pp. 237–307). University of Nebraska Press. Accessed January 19, 2022, from https://stacks.stanford.edu/file/gk002bt7757/gk002bt7757.pdf

Zimbardo, P. G. (1971a). *Application for institutional approval of research involving human subjects*. August, 1971. Available at: http://www.prisonexp.org/pdf/humansubjects.pdf. Accessed December 1, 2023.

Zimbardo, P. G. (1971b). *Prison life study: General information sheet*. August, 1971. Available at: http://www.prisonexp.org/pdf/geninfo.pdf. Accessed December 1, 2023.

Zimbardo, P. G. (2008). *The lucifer effect: Understanding how good people turn evil*. Random House.

Zimbardo, P. G., Haney, C., Banks, W. C., & Jaffe, D. (1972). *Stanford prison experiment*. Philip G. Zimbardo, Inc. (Tape recording).

Zimbardo, P. G., Haney, C., Banks, W. C., & Jaffe, D. (1972, April 8). The mind is a formidable jailer: A Pirandellian prison. *New York Times Magazine,* Section 6, 36, ff.

Zimbardo, P. G., Marshall, G., & Maslach, C. (1971). Liberating behavior from time-bound control: Expanding the present through hypnosis. *Journal of Applied Social Psychology, 1*(4), 305–323. https://doi.org/10.1111/j.1559-1816.1971.tb00369.x

Zimbardo, P. G., Marshall, C., White, G., & Maslach, C. (1973). Objective assessment of hypnotically induced time distortion. *Science, 181*(4096), 282–284.

Zimbardo, P. G., Maslach, C., & Haney, C. (2000). Chapter 11: Reflections on the Stanford prison experiment: Genesis, transformations, consequences. In T. Blass (Ed.), *Obedience to authority: Current perspectives on the milgram paradigm* (pp. 193–237). Lawrence Erlbaum Associates.

Chapter 9
The Yanomami: A Case of Retrospective Ethics

> *O brave new world, that has such people in 't!*
> *Shakespeare,* The Tempest *Act 5 Scene 1*

9.1 Introduction

Social scientists, and anthropologists in particular, have been recognized as important players in disaster and disease outbreak response because of their ability to assess social, economic and political factors in local contexts and positively shape the course of health interventions (Paul Farmer, 1996; Stellmach et al., 2018).

During the large-scale outbreak of Ebola Virus between 2013 and 2016, individuals and communities hid infected patients and their interments. For example, in Guinea, Liberia and Sierra Leone, relatives wiped, massaged, kissed and embraced sick relatives. At funerals, mourners touched the body, as did those who wrapped the body, laid it in a coffin and buried it. Alain Epelboin, an anthropologist helping the World Health Organization, talked with families and explained the reasons for changes to burial traditions. The family was only allowed to look at the deceased when the body was enveloped in disinfectant, before it was sealed in a plastic body bag. The funeral procession and burial, including prayer and speeches, were still permitted with a burial team in protective gear (Epatko, 2014).

Anthropologists study kinship to learn about people's everyday social relations and rituals. This can shed light on, among other things, the subsistence strategy of families and communities in hunter gatherer societies. Anthropologist Napoleon Chagnon had developed genealogies of Yanomami, who live in about 300 villages in the watershed between the Oronoco and Amazon rivers in Southern Venezuela and Northern Brazil. He had recently received his Ph.D. at the University of Michigan when he was asked by Michigan biogeneticist and physician James V. Neel to join an expedition to study genetic variations among the Yanomami. Chagnon's (1968) ethnography, *Yanomamö: The Fierce People*, was widely used in introductory anthropology classes.

The Yanomami live in forests by cutting and burning to clear areas for planting as well as hunting and gathering. They existed in relative isolation from the outside

H. Perlstadt, *Assessing Social Science Research Ethics and Integrity*, Clinical Sociology: Research and Practice, https://doi.org/10.1007/978-3-031-34538-8_9

world until the 1950s, when the first missionaries arrived (Neel et al., 1970:419). One of the earliest contacts was with the Mucajai River Yanomami. In 1957, a group of Americans and Canadians arrived in the Amazon under the auspices of the Unevangelized Fields Mission (UFM), later called Missão Evangélica da Amazônia (MEVA). In 1957 and 1958, they flew over the Mucajai, dropping cans containing fishhooks, knives, scissors and beads. In 1959, MEVA (2023) became a nonprofit, private law institution of a philanthropic nature, which has been working with the traditional peoples of Mazônia to facilitate the emergence of indigenous Christian churches. They also built a small, permanent mission station with an airfield (Peters, 1998:32–33).

Neel learned of measles outbreaks in Brazil and Venezuela in mid-December 1967. He quickly found a measles vaccine which he brought with him. When he and his team arrived, measles had already spread to the Yanomami. Neel and his colleagues dropped their research project and, in a humanitarian effort, vaccinated Yanomami in numerous villages.

In his book *Darkness in Eldorado: How Scientists and Journalists Devastated the Amazon*, Patrick Tierney (2000b), an investigative journalist, falsely accused Neel of making the measles epidemic "the worst epidemic in Yanomami history" by giving them a faulty measles vaccine that killed thousands of villagers who contracted the disease as a result of the vaccine. Tierney implied that Neel gave the vaccine not to save Yanomamo lives but to see how they would react to it. He called it "an exercise in preventive medicine" and asserted that the results were disastrous. Tierney also claimed that Chagnon exaggerated the level of violence in Yanomami society (Tobin, n.d.).

The book sparked an acrimonious debate within the AAA, which was finally resolved in 2005 with a vote by association members to rescind its acceptance of a 2002 final report on the book. The AAA Executive Board established a six-member Task Force to assess the issues raised by the book and recommend ways to improve anthropological field practices. The Task Force final report was critical of Chagnon for prioritizing his own research over the well-being of the Yanomami and questioned his claim that the Yanomami needed warfare to survive. The 2005 resolution also affirmed that the AAA would follow its own policies prohibiting ethics adjudications (Glenn, 2006).

This raises ethical questions about retrospectively imposing current ethical standards on health research and interventions conducted earlier. For example, by taking blood samples with or without consent, did Neel and Chagnon violate a Yanomami taboo against providing blood because the Yanomami believed it gives the recipient power over them? (Mann, 2001:421). Did Chagnon circumvent breaking a taboo when he asked people in one village about their ancestors in a different village? If so, the Yanomami cleverly nicknamed him s*haki*, the pesky bee.

Were the measles vaccinations a humanitarian effort to prevent an epidemic or a controlled experiment? Was informed consent obtained from individuals and/or communities, and more generally, what are the best ways to explain such a project to people unfamiliar with its purposes and methods? What types of inducements or compensations should be offered to people living in indigenous communities or societies? Finally, to what extent should professional social science associations develop and enforce codes of ethics covering practice and research in such settings?

This suggests that ethicists must consider the implications of a research intervention proposal on the wishes, risks and benefits for a specific community (Weijer & Emanuel, 2000). Patrick Taylor (2009:481), the Deputy General Counsel and Chief Counsel for Research Affairs at Children's Hospital Boston, thought that community relates to the historic view that retroactivity violates fundamental interests of free societies and by extension indigenous communities. He asked when does it become fair for a government (or a professional association) to charge individuals with retroactive obedience through regulations?

We need to ask why we differentiate between protecting individuals who volunteer to participate in research and communities which are the subject of the research? (Kahn, 2005:919). As we have seen, the Yanomami, as a community, received benefits and/or risks when labeled "the Fierce People" or as the combatants in the film "The Axe Fight." It is unclear whether an IRB would accept a leader or council to assure informed consent for the community. One solution is a partnership between researchers and the people in the communities. In a partnership, the communities would participate in protocol development, recruitment and sampling activities, approving information disclosure and deidentification of participants, reimbursing community members who help conduct the research, and how and when to disseminate reports and publications (Weijer & Emanuel, 2000; Kahn, 2005).

9.1.1 James Neel

James Neel, Ph.D., M.D., was a pioneer in of the field of human genetics and a founder of the American Society for Human Genetics. He established the Department of Human Genetics at the University of Michigan, one of the first departments in the United States. He served in the Army Medical Corp and was among the first physician-geneticists to visit Hiroshima and Nagasaki after World War II to advise the National Academy of Medicine on the genetic effects of exposure to radiation in the children of survivors of the atomic explosions. He played a significant role in organizing the Atomic Bomb Casualty Commission (ABCC) and its successor, the Radiation Effects Research Foundation (Michigan News, 2000).

In 1951, the Atomic Energy Commission (AEC) planned to stop funding for the ABCC's work in Japan. However, Neel appealed, and the AEC decided to continue to fund work on the genetic risks of radiation exposure. Over the next several years, the AEC would fund the research of Neel and W.J. Schull at the University of Michigan. This included continuing their population work in Japan, computer simulation studies, development of biochemical techniques to identify genetic variants, immunological studies and the Yanomami studies (American Society of Human Genetics, 2002). AEC funding was based on a peer-review system that mirrored that of the NSF, the NIH and other nonmilitary agencies (Santos et al., 2014).

9.1.2 The Genetics of Primitive Societies

Neel's primary research interest was to study the genetics and genealogies of people currently living in hunter-gather societies. Neel thought that genetic evolution, as evidenced in gene frequency changes, could occur more rapidly in societies that often split into new communities because of disagreements or territorial shifts. Polygynous marriages would maximize the genetic variance of a male's children, with headmen who had more wives having more children (Santos et al., 2014). Polygyny would also limit the supply of marriageable women unless unmarried men abducted women from another village.

In addition, Neel (1970:818–819) thought that preagricultural societies had developed immunity to the pathogens in their surroundings and could help geneticists explain the origins and nature of human diseases (Weiss & Ward, 2000). This required data on inbreeding, effective population size, differential fertility, age pyramids and survival curves as well as an accurate assessment of health and disease in the population under study. Such studies would need to be carried out by cross-disciplinary teams of anthropologists, linguists and geneticists.

Neel's 1962 field work was with approximately 100 Xavante people in Mato-Grosso, Brazil (Lindee, 2001:273–274). Neel and Brazilian geneticist Francisco M. Salzano collected detailed demographic data, reproductive histories, anthropometric measurements, medical examinations and biological samples (blood and saliva) for immunological and genetic tests (Salzano, 2000).

Neel continued to draw blood samples on his 1966 and 1967 expeditions to the Yanomami and found that eight of ten tested Yanomami villages had almost no measles antibodies. A measles outbreak could have resulted in a 20–30% death rate (Mann, 2001:419).

9.1.3 The Measles Outbreak

In preparation for his 1968 expedition, Neel was joined by Napoleon Chagnon, who was part of the 1966 and 1967 Michigan expeditions. In December 1967, Neel learned of a measles outbreak among the Yanomami in Brazil, which had spread along the Orinoco River. Neel quickly acquired the Edmonston B vaccine, which he had obtained gratis from Lederle Laboratories and Parke-Davis for humanitarian purposes. Edmonston B was being replaced by the Schwarz vaccine, which had fewer side effects but did not give as long-lasting immunity (Mann, 2001:417).

Neel developed a vaccination strategy. He planned a public-health campaign of prophylactic vaccination among those Yanomami communities most likely to face early exposure to measles (AAA, 2002). He would vaccinate villages at the periphery of Yanomami territory that had already been studied and were not to be visited as part of his 1968 expedition. He would give half of the vaccine to Salesians, a Catholic missionary group serving the Yanomami, to inoculate the people in those villages. He hoped to vaccinate half the village at once and the other half 2 weeks later, to avoid having all villagers suffer a reaction at the same time (American Society of Human Genetics, 2002:4). But as is often the case, an epidemic outpaces medical science and public health initiatives, so Neel improvised.

Measles had reached Yanomami territory before Neel's small advance party arrived at the Ocamo River mission station on January 22nd. The next day 40 individuals were vaccinated with Edmonston B alone. The rest of the measles vaccine, plus gamma globulin, which increases protection, were with the main party investigating Yanomami and Ye'cuana villages on the Erebato River. Neel reported outbreaks of wild measles, which we would now attribute to untraceable community spread. He spent at least 2 weeks vaccinating with gamma globulin and giving medical care as needed. Neel's party administered 1000 doses and gave the rest to missionaries and medical auxiliaries of the Venezuelan government (Michigan News, 2000; Cantor, 2001). However, very few Venezuelan officials followed the trajectory of the epidemic (Hurtado & Salzano, 2004:7).

In the late 1990s, Neel received a note from Chagnon who had learned about the book the investigative journalist Tierney was writing on the Yanomami. Neel promptly made photocopies of relevant field notes and related materials that would document what happened in 1968. He put them all in a file marked YANOMAMA 1968 Insurance and placed the file in the archives of the American Philosophical Society in Philadelphia. In 2000, historian and sociologist of science Susan Lindee found the file and used it to counter Tierney's claims (Dreger, 2015:48).

9.2 Napoleon Chagnon

Napoleon Chagnon began ethnographic field work with the Yanomami in 1964. He intended to study a recently contacted tribe in Brazil but shifted his focus to the Yanomami after a military coup took place in Brazil. His dissertation research was funded by the NIMH (Iannone, 2013:258). He planned to collect data on Yanomami genealogy and lineages through participant observation, interviews and surveys. But unlike most anthropologists who settle into one village for the duration of their study, Chagnon collected his data from several villages, traveling in 1966 to help Neel in his efforts (Borofsky, 2005:42). The data on genealogy and lineages would then be compared with their genetic ancestry as revealed in their blood samples.

The Yanomami were known as a very warlike people who had at times dominated several weaker tribes, and whose raiding parties included the abduction of women (Cantor, 2001). In 1966, Chagnon completed his dissertation *Yanomamö Warfare, Social Organization and Marriage Alliances* (Borofsky, 2005). In 1968, Chagnon published *Yanomamö, The Fierce People*, based on his dissertation. The Yanomami refer to themselves as "*waitiri*," the fierce and valiant, and Chagnon adopted it for the title of his book (Cantor, 2001). The book, along with an accompanying film by anthropologist Timothy Asch, was included in introductory anthropology classes for many years. The 1975 film *The Ax Fight* shows a long-standing lineage conflict flaring into a confrontation and violence in a Yanomami village (Nichols, 1996:9).

Anthropology is a scholarly enterprise that lacks an objective measure of excellence and is subject to disagreements and doubts (Walsh & Lehmann, 2021:32). Some of Chagnon's critics were anthropologists who worked in the Amazon Basin with similar peoples. At first, Chagnon considered some to be expressions of professional jealousy, but a few became increasingly political in tone, especially from political activists who claimed his publications were causing harm to the people he studied. Over the course of his career, Chagnon became both an outlier in anthropology "who rubs people the wrong way" (Iannone, 2013, 259–260), and a public anthropologist who addresses social issues beyond the discipline and encourages broad, public conversations with the explicit goal of fostering social change (Borofsky, 2004).

9.2.1 Chagnon, Anthropology Outcast

Over the years, Chagnon compiled careful accounts of the births, deaths and family trees for every person in a Yanomami village. He developed techniques for calculating genetic relatedness between two genealogically related people to measure their degree of kinship and used his growing genealogical records to examine how participation in intervillage violence might affect reproductive success (Borofsky, 2005:7–8; Kellman, 1982). His work challenged the romantic notion that the natural state of the human an altruistic and peace-loving noble savage; this "made Chagnon an outcast among anthropologists" (Hammer, 2013).

In an article in *Science*, Chagnon (1988) proposed a theory of tribal violence linking homicide, revenge, kinship obligations and warfare. His findings on the Yanomami revealed that men who have killed have more wives and offspring than men who have not killed. This generated much controversy among cultural anthropologists and made Chagnon unpopular among social scientists who believed that culture alone shapes human behavior (Wong, 2001). According to anthropologist Marshall Sahlins (2000), Chagnon's arguments in *Science* "may have had the shortest half-life of any study ever published in that august journal."

Critics pointed out that Chagnon overestimated the number of Yanomami who kill by misinterpreting the term *unokai*. While it generally refers to those who kill others it can include those with a reputation to have caused deaths by witchcraft. So actual killers are hard to distinguish from those who have symbolically killed (Monaghan, 1994).

According to Chagnon (2014:6), the Yanomami were a large tribe facing unexpected attacks from neighboring tribes. A village would stand and fight or flee to settle in a safer area some distance away. He held an evolutionary perspective on the biological basis of human behavior. He coedited *Evolutionary Biology and Human Social Behavior: An Anthropological Perspective* (Chagnon & Irons, 1979). Its chapters explore human social behavior from a Darwinian perspective. In one chapter, Chagnon described how male Yanomami manipulated kinship rules. This drew the attention of Edward O. Wilson (1975), who had written *Sociobiology: The New Synthesis* to explain the evolutionary mechanics behind social behavior. Sociobiology is "the extension of population biology and evolutionary theory to social organization" (Wilson, 1978: xx). Wilson thought that the Yanomami might provide the clearest view of the conditions under which the human mind evolved in earliest history (Mann, 2001).

Ultimately, the dispute was over the merits of sociobiology in anthropology. Chagnon's opponents argued that the violence he claimed was inherent in Yanomami society was neo-Darwinian and placed them in a Hobbesian state of nature, that is, "a war of every man against every man" for everything, regardless of the interests of others. Critics consider sociobiology to be a simplistic explanation for complex human behaviors. When anthropologists find biological factors, they assume causality and recast their own interpretations as scientific fact. Chagnon, however, saw himself as opposing those who have a fixed belief that human beings are no more or less than a product of culture (Monaghan, 1994).

Franz Boas, a founder of American anthropology, believed that no single perspective could encompass the diversity of human cultures and societies. The Michigan Department of Anthropology, where Chignon earned all his degrees and worked for several years, was one of the earliest departments to encompass both the humanities and natural sciences.

However, in 1998, Stanford University disbanded its department of anthropology and created two new entities. The Department of Cultural and Social Anthropology (CASA) featured tracks in culture and society, and in archaeology, while the Department of Anthropological Sciences covered culture, social relations and language, archaeology and evolutionary studies, population and environment, and medical anthropology and genetics. At the time, the CASA website instructed "students interested in biological and evolutionary approaches to anthropology are urged to consult the Department of Anthropological Sciences" (Tooby, 2000). Although influenced by philosophical differences, the split also involved personality conflicts and intradepartmental politics (Leslie, 2000).

9.2.2 *The Gold Rush*

Gold was discovered in Yanomami territory in the early 1970s, and within a few years, small groups of independent gold-diggers (*garimpeiros*) had become a threat to the environment and the Yanomami. This led to the establishment in 1978 of the Commission for the Creation of a Yanomami Park (CCPY), a Brazilian nongovernmental nonprofit organization working to defend the territorial, cultural, civil and political rights of the Yanomami.

The next year, Survival International asked its supporters to lobby the Brazilian government for Yanomami land rights. Survival International, a charitable nonprofit based in London with offices in six countries, supports tribal peoples' desires to keep their ancestral lands. After the government revealed plans to divide the Yanomami land into 19 separate pockets, it coordinated demonstrations at Brazilian embassies in 20 countries. In 1992, the Yanomami indigenous land was approved and registered. This ensured that indigenous people had the constitutional right to the exclusive use of an area in the Brazilian states of Roraima and Amazonas, equivalent to the area of the state of Indiana (CCPY, n.d.).

Three years earlier, Survival International was to receive the 1989 Right Livelihood Award that honors and supports courageous people solving global problems. It invited Davi Kopenawa, a shaman and chief spokesperson for the Yanomami in Brazil, to accept the award on its behalf at a ceremony held in the Swedish Parliament. In 1991, Davi would travel to New York to meet with the Secretaries General of the United Nations and the Organization of American States, as well as with high officials of the World Bank (Golden, 1991: B1). However, Chagnon and his supporters dismissed Davi as a parrot of human rights groups and said he does not speak for the tribe (Monaghan, 1994: A19).

During this time period, Chagnon could not acquire research permits to study the Yanomami. In 1975, Venezuela began requiring foreign scholars, who wanted to work in border areas such as Amazonas, to be affiliated with a Venezuelan institution. As a result, Chagnon was unable to enter the region from 1976 to 1983. He returned in 1984 as part of a 3-year study of rural and indigenous housing through the Central University of Venezuela. In 1989, he secured a research permit to make a documentary film for FUDECI, the research, education and technological transference program of the Academy of Physics, Mathematics and Natural Sciences. The program supports scientific research on the conservation and sustainable management of the Amazon rainforests (Task Force, 2002a:41, 44). Between August 1990 and March 1991, Chagnon and Brewer-Carías shot 11 h of film for a documentary on Yanomami groups that "had never been contacted by any person," as well as 12 other groups, for research purposes (Task Force, 2002a:43).

However, the Director of Indigenous Affairs received requests from CONIVE, the national indigenous organization and SUYAO, the Yanomami cooperative founded with the help of Salesian missionaries, that the research permit for the film be suspended. After the permit was suspended, the director wrote Chagnon requesting he consult with CONIVE, SUYAO and the Salesians before the permit could be restored. Chagnon refused, saying it was a campaign against him by "a sham organization organized by leftist anthropologists in league with the missionaries" (Task Force, 2002a:42).

The only way Chagnon could get research permits was through Charles Brewer Carías, a Venezuelan explorer and naturalist. In the early 1960s, Brewer Carías had suggested that Neel and Chagnon study the Yanomami. Trained as a dentist, he served as such on the 1968 Neel expedition. Later he would photograph mesas around Angel Falls in Venezuela, lecture for the New York Botanical Garden and invent the Brewer Explorer Survival Knife (Stoll, 2001). With the help of Brewer Carías, Chagnon was able to affiliate with *Fundación para la Ayuda de la Familia Campesina e Indígena* (FUNDAFACI), the Foundation to Aid Peasant and Indigenous Families.

The foundation, established in 1989 to protect indigenous and peasant families, had political clout under the leadership of Cecilia Matos, a key mediator between Venezuelan President Pérez and many questionable business associates. The inclusion of Chagnon in the research program of the Foundation sought to give it respectability (Task Force, 2002a:41). Together, Chagnon and Brewer Carías made eight expeditions between August 1990 and March 1991, taking 3000 photographs and 11 h of film.

Chagnon was directly involved in attempts by Brewer Carías and Matos to create a Yanomami reserve and scientific biosphere in 6000 square miles (a little larger than Connecticut) in the remote Siapa Highlands. It was to be directed by Brewer Carías and Chagnon and subsidized by FUNDAFACI (Sahlins, 2000). Both the film project and reserve biosphere plan came to an abrupt end in 1993 when President Pérez was impeached and removed from office and Matos fled the country (Task Force, 2002a:43–44). The Venezuelan Congress then elected Ramón José Velásquez President in early June.

In July 1993, a series of raids and counter raids by independent gold diggers and Yanomami culminated in the massacre of Yanomami Indians from the village of Hamuxi. Between 14 and 19 Yanomami women and children were killed. At least two communal huts were later burned (Chagnon, 1993; Amnesty International, 1993). Venezuelan President Velásquez appointed Chagnon to an investigative commission headed by Brewer-Carías, who owned a mine in Bolivar state to the north that critics claimed was illegal.

The appointments were highly controversial. In September, Indians at a church gathering proceeded to march through the capital of Amazonas state in southern Venezuela carrying placards that read: "Brewer-Carías and Chagnon out of Yanomami Territory" (Brooke, 1993). The government was forced to name a second commission that included the Salesian bishop of the state of Amazonia and one of his priests. When it arrived with a military escort, it ordered the Brewer-Carías and Chagnon-led group to leave, which it did the next day (Monaghan, 1994: A19; Chagnon, 1993; D'Antonio, 2000).

Chagnon (1993) was furious. In his view, the Salesians were demanding that his commission be abolished and a second commission appointed. He claimed that until 1991 the missionaries had attracted converts by offering shotguns, which in turn had contributed to the growing violence. In 1992, Amazonia became a full Venezuelan state and this would weaken the secular authority of the Salesians. Finally, Jorge Britton, one of their supporters who presented himself as a defender of indigenous people, sent formal denunciations to US grant making agencies and Chagnon's university, citing native opposition to his work. The lines were drawn and future confrontations were inevitable.

9.3 The Acrimonious Debate

The 1993 meeting of the AAA was scheduled for mid-November in Washington, D.C. A few weeks earlier, supporters of the Salesians anonymously mailed packets to anthropologists intended to defame Chagnon. Packets were also placed on a free literature table in the Washington Hilton and Towers. Frank Salamone, chair of sociology and anthropology at Iona College, invited Chagnon and Father Jose Bortoli of the Salesian missions to speak at sessions that were put on the program at the last minute. They had previously traded charges that the other was manipulating the Yanomami for their own ends. But they were old friends, shook hands and declared a truce. Salamone noted that Chagnon sought truth through empirical methods and Bortoli through a metaphysical method (Cantor, 2001; *Michigan News*, 2000:part 3).

Chagnon thought that the single most important issue facing the Yanomami was their health.

Bortoli likewise urged anthropologists to focus on health, and on developing the Alto Orinoco-Casiquiare Biosphere Reserve, a national park set up for the Yanomami by the Venezuelan government and protecting human rights (Winkler, 1994).

9.3.1 Getting to El Dorado

The legend of El Dorado, Spanish for "the gilded one," stems from an initiation ceremony for the new leader of the Música people of central Columbia. Accompanied by four high priests, the new leader would be taken out on a raft. He would be naked except for a covering of gold dust and would make offerings to the gods by throwing gold objects and emeralds into the lake (Cooper, 2013). El Dorado appeared in Voltaire's satirical novella *Candide* (1759) as a hidden utopian kingdom where poverty is nonexistent because gold is so plentiful that it is looked upon as common pebbles. In Joseph Conrad's novel *Heart of Darkness* (1899), the Eldorado Exploring Expedition was a group of five white treasure hunters on the Congo River in Africa who were willing to kill natives and damage the environment.

With the publication of *Darkness in El Dorado*, the title of which drew on the legend's cultural meaning, Tierney (2000b) exposed the festering, acrimonious debate within anthropology. Tierney had a special interest in South America. In his 1989 book *The Highest Altar: The Story of Human Sacrifice*, he described modern day shamans who allegedly still practiced human sacrifice in Peru and Chile. Tierney decided to study the Yanomami, first in Brazil, where the Amazon gold rush had brought epidemics, guns, alcohol and prostitution, and then in Venezuela, along the Orinoco and in the mountains. Over the next 10 years, he made six trips to the Amazon-Orinoco region, spending 15 months in the field and visiting 30 of the villages that Chagnon had studied. What he found was sharply at odds with what Chagnon described (Tierney, 2000a:50).

When researching the impact of the Amazon gold rush, Tierney asked Chagnon for contacts and other information. Tierney accompanied a group of independent gold diggers through swamps and mountains to learn about their graft and corruption. He thought of the miners as one of the last tribes of El Dorado with their own mythology, ritual combats and closed circle of bloodletting (Publishers Weekly, 1997).

Sometime during 1995 Tierney sent drafts of *Last Tribes of El Dorado: The Gold Wars in the Amazon Rain Forest* (Tierney, 1997) to University of Chicago anthropologist Terence Turner, who worked with indigenous peoples of the Brazilian Amazon. Turner was interested in the political struggles of the indigenous peoples and associated ecological, cultural and rights issues. He was also involved in advocacy and human rights work. Turner had gone to Brazil in March 1991 as head of a Special Commission of the AAA and interviewed Davi Kopenawa (Special Commission, 1991). The Commission was to investigate the situation and recommend actions that might be taken by the Association in support of the Yanomami. The Commission denounced the National Indian Foundation of Brazil (FUNAI) for refusing access by anthropologists and other scientific investigators as well as medical personnel to the Yanomami area. Tierney then met Turner at the Pittsburgh International Airport (Srikameswaran, 2000).

Tierney also sent drafts to University of Hawaii anthropologist Leslie E. Sponsel, who had studied the ecology of foraging among various indigenous groups in the Venezuelan Amazon and who was a founding member and Chair of the AAA Commission for Human Rights from 1992 to 1995. Sponsel recalled that Tierney had sent him some chapters and thought that Tierney was going to focus on mining and its impact on the indigenous people and their environment. But Tierney expanded a chapter cleverly called "Napoleonic Wars" into a new book, with a focus on Chagnon. Sponsel didn't approve of the focus or the pun because he believed that the gold mining business was worse than whatever Chagnon did (Brown, 2000:5).

9.3.2 *The Controversy over* El Dorado

W.W. Norton scheduled the release of *Darkness in El Dorado* for November 15, 2000, to coincide with the opening of the AAA annual meeting in San Francisco. In late July or early August 2000, Sponsel and Turner, who by then was at Cornell University, received page proofs of *Darkness in El Dorado*. Both had been leaders on the AAA human rights and ethics committees. They were aware that *The New Yorker* planned to publish a piece by Tierney (2000a) entitled "The Fierce Anthropologist" before the November AAA meeting.

On August 31, they sent what they considered to be confidential emails to Louise Lamphere, President, and Don Brenneis, President-elect of the AAA, with the subject line "Imminent Anthropological Scandal" (Turner & Sponsel, 2000). They wrote that the focus of the scandal was the long-term study of the Yanomami of

Venezuela by geneticist Neel, Chagnon and other anthropologists. Citing their uncorrected proofs of *Darkness in El Dorado*, Turner and Sponsel said that in 1968, Neel—assisted by Chagnon—had given an unsafe measles vaccine to many Yanomamo and thus had "greatly exacerbated, and probably started, the epidemic of measles that killed 'hundreds, perhaps thousands'. . .of Yanomami." (Sponsel and Turner used that spelling of Yanomamo; even this tiny difference was code for which side of the fight an anthropologist was on (Tobin. n.d.).)

They wanted Lamphere and Brenneis to be prepared to deal with the book because the AAA would be called upon by its own membership and the general media to take collective stands on the issues, as well as to make appropriate apologies to counteract what may turn out to be a public relations disaster. Because the book would contain sensational revelations about anthropology, they believed it would be widely read both inside and outside the profession.

Turner and Sponsel then informed Lamphere and Brenneis of steps they had already taken. They had contacted Barbara Johnston, the chair of the Committee for Human Rights asking her to devote the committee's Open Forum at the annual meeting to the book. With Johnston's consent, they invited Tierney to participate in the Forum, and he accepted. They agreed with Johnston that the committee should draft a press release that Lamphere and/or Brenneis, perhaps with the approval of the AAA Executive Board, could circulate to the media. In addition, they thought that the AAA's Ethics Committee, the Society for Latin American Anthropology and the Association for Latina and Latino Anthropology should be notified and involved. Given the number of people and organizations mentioned, it should not have been surprising when the confidential email went viral on academic email lists and beyond.

On September 20, the *Chronicle of Higher Education* reported that the book's claims would taint the entire discipline, and a few days later, *The Guardian* ran a front page headline reading, "Scientist Killed Amazon Indians to Test Race Theory" (Miller, 2001). The article was virtually unedited from the Turner–Sponsel email (Sponsel, 2002:151). The story subsequently appeared in *Time Magazine*, *The New York Times* and on National Public Radio (NPR). The book's credibility rested on the fact-checking of *The New Yorker* (Dreger, 2011) and that the book was one of five finalists for the 2000 National Book Award in nonfiction. (Srikameswaran, 2000). Although Tierney revised parts of the book before it was ready for printing, both he and W. W. Norton no longer printed or distributed page proofs as part of their marketing strategy.

In late October, Anthropologist John Tooby (2000) asked "Did two US scientists start a genocidal epidemic in the Amazon or was *The New Yorker* duped?" Tooby argued that the book should have been in the fiction category since many of its sources are demonstrability false on many points that are central to its most sensational claims. The excerpt in the *New Yorker* was a collection of anecdotes and accusations purporting to show, among many charges, that Chagnon's depictions of Yanomamo violence were "greatly exaggerated," that his data was error-ridden, that he stirred up conflict among the tribesmen by trading steel tools for the data he needed, and that the Yanomamo feared and hated him (Tobin, n.d.).

Three days later the editors of *The New Yorker* (2000) published a rebuttal. They noted that Tierney raised questions about the choice of vaccines that Neel and Chagnon used, but in *The New Yorker* article Tierney did not claim that the vaccine spread the virus and noted that Neel stated the vaccination was an exercise in preventive medicine.

Tierney never asserted that Chagnon was the sole cause of violence among the Yanomami. He wrote that the missionaries had been giving machetes to the Yanomami since the 1950s. In contrast, Chagnon gave machetes in exchange for names of dead relatives, which violated taboos, and for obtaining blood samples in different villages, which may have resulted in discord among them. In a separate release, the editors said that Chagnon originally agreed to be interviewed but then backed out and threatened to sue (Geertz, 2001).

9.3.3 The 2000 AAA Annual Meeting

The Association held two extraordinary sessions at its 2000 annual meeting in San Francisco on the rapidly evolving controversy. The first was a seven-member panel on Thursday evening followed by an open comment session on Friday evening where members could present their views on the book. Tierney sat at one end of a long panel table and at the other end sat Northwestern University anthropologist William Irons, representing Chagnon, who declined to attend. Like Chagnon, Irons received his Ph.D. from Michigan and coedited *Evolutionary Biology and Human Social Behavior* with Chagnon (Chagnon & Irons, 1979).

Sitting side by side were historian Susan Lindee, a leading biographer of Neel, Magdalena Hurtado, an expert on the epidemiology of infectious diseases among South American Indians and Noeli Pocaterra, a native Wayuu Indian, leader of Venezuela's permanent commission for the protection of indigenous people, and a member of the National Assembly of Venezuela. The other two panelists were a specialist in medical ethics and a physician/epidemiologist (See Dalton, 2000; Geertz, 2001).

The session was scheduled for 6:15 pm but started late to accommodate the overflow crowd. AAA President Lamphere explained the decision to hold the special sessions and then turned the meeting over to the panelists. The panelists spoke one after the other with Tierney speaking last. Most questioned the charges against Neel and Chagnon in *Darkness in El Dorado*, with a few referencing statements by researchers at the University of California Santa Barbara, where Chagnon was on the faculty, the University of Michigan, where Neel was on the faculty, and the National Academy of Sciences. Irons asserted that the book was full of falsehoods, accused Tierney of being duped by Chagnon's enemics and urged boycotting the book (Dalton, 2000).

The exception was Pocaterra, wearing a traditional Wayuu dress, and speaking in Spanish. She announced that her government would investigate the scandalous affair. The investigation would ask Tierney for copies of all his interview notes and all his documents. She would "condemn those incidents which are so cruel and inhuman that they are hard to believe . . . And if any of Mr. Tierney's accusations are true . . . then such violations of human rights against indigenous people all over the world must never take place again" (Curran & Takata, 2000; Perlman, 2000). When Tierney finally spoke, he said he was not against vaccinations or science, but that many people would have difficulties coming to terms with his book. He hoped that the Santa Barbara and Michigan researchers would examine Chagnon's work as carefully has they had his book. He concluded by asking everyone to work together to address the issues raised in the book (Dalton, 2000; Geertz, 2001).

About 30 people spoke on Thursday evening during the open mike session. Each speaker was allocated 3–5 min. Tierney was not present since he had left to do promotional interviews for his book. Speakers include Turner and Sponsel who had read the galleys, but almost all the others had not read the book which was just being released. Some complained that several of the Wednesday panelists were arrogant in their attacks on Tierney's book, while others called for investigations and possible censure of anthropologists who had assisted him. A few thought the panel was overly focused on Neel and Chagnon and not on the vulnerable Yanomami. The session closed with the AAA president and the president-elect asking a past president to head up a commission to look into the question of whether an official committee of inquiry should be formed (Dalton, 2000; Geertz, 2001).

9.3.4 The Task Force Investigates the Controversy

At its February 2001 meeting, the AAA Executive Board appointed a six member El Dorado Task Force to assess the issues raised by the controversy and to recommend ways to improve anthropologists'practices in the field. Some complained that two of the task force members had publicly criticized Chagnon's conduct, and that a third, Raymond Hames, had worked with Chagnon (Glenn, 2006). The Task Force's charge required the posting of a preliminary report in time for the November 2001 Executive Board meeting.

Unfortunately, two Task Force members were unable to read the report in advance of the meeting. Since these two had not read the report and disagreed with some of the posted documents, they did not sign the report. The Task Force agreed to withdraw the document, replacing it with "Working Paper of the AAA El Dorado Task Force," and inviting association members, but not the public, to submit comments on the report and post them on AAA's website. Comments received as of April 19, 2002, were incorporated into the final report, but the website remained open for additional comments. The Task Force submitted its two-volume final report to the AAA Executive Board in May 2002 (Task Force, 2002a, b).

The Task Force (2002a:25–27) agreed with other investigations that Tierney was wrong and Neel had not initiated and exacerbated a measles epidemic and had not refused to provide medical care in order to observe the progression of the epidemic.

The Task Force found that Neel's vaccination program saved many lives and made research observations on the course of the disease and observed vaccination reaction.

In contrast, the Final Report (Task Force, 2002a:31, 38) was critical of Chagnon. It agreed with Tierney's claims that Chagnon's association with FUNDAFACI and Brewer-Carías unethically prioritized his own research over the well-being of the Yanomami and that his accounts and interpretations of the Yanomami way of life were damaging to them. The Report acknowledged that anthropological comparisons between contemporary human groups like the Yanomami and archeological evidence about people from earlier periods in human history are appropriate, but questioned Chagnon's characterization that the Yanomami needed warfare to survive.

9.3.5 The Referendum

The AAA Bylaws permit the Executive Board or a signed petition of 50 members in good standing to place a referendum before the membership. A majority of votes is needed to approve the referendum. In December 2004, Thomas Gregor, an anthropologist at Vanderbilt University interested in native peoples of South America and anthropological film, and Daniel Gross, a staff researcher at the World Bank, successfully initiated a referendum to rescind the AAA's acceptance of the Task Force Final Report.

They began with an article in *American Anthropologist* in which they laid out their case for the referendum (Gregor & Gross, 2004:687, 692–693). They contended that the inquiry did not follow the AAA policy prohibiting ethics adjudications and did not observe reasonable standards of evidence.

Overall, it reflected a culture of accusation and an anthropology uncertain of its ethical or scientific nature. They pointed out that three Task Force members had conflicts of interest and prejudgments, as touched on above. Fernando Coronil from the University of Michigan was appointed to the task force, despite the fact that his friend and thesis adviser, Terence Turner, had aggressively challenged Chagnon and Neel. Janet Chernela from the University of Maryland posted a paper on the AAA site months before the final report was issued which summarized the evidence against Chagnon and called for collective responsibility and reparations to the Yanomami. Hames, the only task force member with direct knowledge of Yanomami language and culture and who had worked with Chagnon, ultimately resigned to avoid the appearance of bias.

The Task Force (2005:28–29) collected comments on the referendum to rescind the El Dorado report, including the following:

> Leslie Sponsel from the University of Hawaii opposed the referendum. Along with Terence Turner, he had started the controversy when the two exchanged confidential emails about a possible scandal. Sponsel pointed out that early in the controversy, several organizations had conducted hasty investigations on a very narrow range of allegations, almost all of which were concerned with Neel instead of Chagnon, and which were not revised although glaring

discrepancies existed. Chagnon refused to participate on the panel dedicated to the matter at the AAA's 2000 annual meeting. He also refused to communicate with the Task Force to confront Tierney's allegations. Approval of the referendum would likely damage both the public and the self-image of the AAA and the profession, as well as weaken its Code of Ethics and future work of the Committee on Ethics. It would distract attention from the Yanomami; and alienate communities with whom anthropologists conduct research.

Dean Saitta, who taught Anthropological Theory and Evolutionary Anthropology at the University of Denver, was mostly against the referendum. He was concerned that the referendum advocates were incorrect in holding that the Yanomami would have been demonized by politicians and the press, regardless of the "fierce people" appellation, and that the alternative concept of the noble savage has never saved tribal folk from exploitation. Advocacy anthropology claims that it suffers from a lack of objectivity and other legitimate intellectual content. These trivializations don't help a discipline always at risk of marginalization in intellectual and public life.

Laura Graham at the University of Iowa supported the referendum. She wrote that it is a historic document and an attempt to shed light on the accusations reported in Tierney's book. It does not preclude other scholars from presenting other information on the accusations, either pro or con.

Jane Fajans at Cornell University argued against the referendum. She had carried out field work in two communities in Papua New Guinea, and was married to Turner. She thought that the proponents of the referendum focused on procedure, due process and fairness, rather than the findings that Chagnon, Neel and others had violated ethical standards. The referendum is designed to neutralize the substantive findings of unethical conduct against Chagnon and Neel and to make it all but impossible to undertake any subsequent investigation of the allegations against them.

Magdalena Hurtado (Task Force, 2005:8–9) at the University of New Mexico was a panelist at the special session at the 2000 San Francisco meeting. She wrote that the most serious problem with the report was its failure to consider the real needs of the Yanomamo. The Report had almost no examination of health and did not consider the crucial testimony of Venezuelan biomedical scientists who were spitefully attacked by Tierney. Rescinding the report was an essential step toward reclaiming anthropologists' own sense of purpose and directing our efforts toward the assistance of indigenous communities.

Paul Mattson (Task Force, 2005:10–11), who studied at UC Santa Barbara and taught courses in Biological Anthropology at Moorpark College in California, favored the referendum. He thought that the real issue was power. In his view, the scientist and humanist factions within anthropology are engaged in a conflict of worldviews. He personally hoped that anthropology would overcome this schismatic moment and try again to do comprehensive, multifaceted and interesting work.

Members voted on the referendum in April and May 2005, and the results were announced at the end of June. The referendum passed 846–338, with 54.7% in favor. As a result, the AAA was required to widely publicize the decision to rescind the report and to explain the reasons for doing so. The vote also affirmed that the association will follow its own policies prohibiting ethics adjudications.

After the vote, Gross suggested that the IRBs at UC Santa Barbara and the University of Michigan were in a better position to assess Tierney's allegations. Robert Borofsky, an anthropologist at Hawaii Pacific University, hoped that anthropology would move on to get a good sense of the place of ethics in the discipline and how to evaluate anthropologists fairly and honorably (Glenn, 2006).

9.4 Ethical Issues

Ethical issues surrounding this controversial work are as follows: the conduct of research during an epidemic, the collection of blood samples from the Yanomami, international ethics research codes, protecting Indigenous Peoples and the role of professional association codes of ethics with respect to research, practice and teaching.

According to Kurt Ruyter (2003), philosopher and Director General of the Regional Committees for Medical and Health Research Ethics at the University of Oslo, the conduct of research has been subject to some regulations since the beginning of the scientific revolution in the seventeenth century. The regulations reflect the normative system prevailing at a given time within a given research community. Researchers themselves have shown respect for general ethical rules and social norms. But over time, new scientific methods and areas of research generate calls for improving ethical guidelines, resulting in debates over the ethics of competing theories and practices. Some governments, organizations and individuals will observe more rigorous ethical standards and retrospectively impose them on previous studies, while others continue to hold and practice existing or even outmoded standards (Busch, 2011:240).

9.4.1 *Yanomami Blood Samples*

When Neel and Chagnon were with the Yanomami in the late 1960s and early 1970s, the major international ethical guidelines were the 1947 Nuremberg Code and the 1964 Declaration of Helsinki. Both addressed biomedical research conducted by physicians and encouraged informed consent. Neel and Chagnon collected blood samples from the Yanomami, who were promised that the blood would be used to learn more about the diseases ravaging them. They directly benefited when Neel brought a measles vaccine and inoculated them in early 1968. Neel retired in 1985 and sent his blood vials to Kenneth Weiss, a postdoctoral advisee at Pennsylvania State University.

Davi Kopenawa, the Yanomami leader, first learned about his relatives' blood samples being stored in the United States from Bruce Albert during a conversation about Tierney's book. In 2002, Albert wrote Weiss, including a note from Kopenawa that began years of negotiations on the reasons for and logistics of safely returning the samples. The Yanomami wanted the blood samples returned so that their surviving kinsmen could bury the blood according to Yanomami tradition. In 2015, blood samples from Penn State University, Binghamton University and the National Cancer Institute (NCI) were returned. The Brazilian Embassy in Washington, D.C. escorted them back to Brazil and the Yanomami. However, the Venezuelan government has not asked for samples taken from its Yanomamö tribes (Borofsky, n.d.; Couzin-Frankel, 2010).

9.4.2 International Ethics Research Codes

The development and acceptance of international codes of research ethics and practice got off to a very slow start. During the war crimes trials of Nazi doctors in 1947, several defendants asserted that no international law or informal statement distinguished between legal and illegal human experimentation. In response, Leo Alexander, an American physician working with the prosecution during the trial submitted a memorandum to Telford Taylor, the Counsel for the Prosecution, with six points defining legitimate research. These were incorporated into the verdict. Alexander and American physician Andrew Ivy then added four additional points, which became the ten points of the Nuremberg Code. Key points stated that there should be voluntary consent of the human subjects, that the degree of risk should never exceed that determined by the humanitarian importance of the problem and that the scientist in charge must be prepared to terminate the experiment at any stage.

These key points were included in subsequent ethical standards, but the Nuremberg Code was considered to be common law that could be cited in subsequent court decisions. The WMA's 1964 Declaration of Helsinki followed the attempts by the US Food and Drug Administration to standardize research on experimental drugs, following the thalidomide tragedy.

Thalidomide was a medication for morning sickness that was marketed without having been tested on pregnant women, and was soon linked to birth defects. The concern in this case was not criminal intent but rather establishing a set of guidelines for conducting clinical trials on potential therapeutic drugs. The Helsinki Declaration was, in essence, recommendations to physicians by physicians (Annas, 1991:21–28). As such, it did not directly impact nonclinical research or the social behavioral sciences.

In 1974, Congress passed the National Research Act in response to the exposé of the PHS Tuskegee Syphilis Study. The Department of Health, Education and Welfare (HEW) promulgated regulations requiring that biomedical and social science research protocols be reviewed and approved for meeting ethical standards approved by IRBs. Both Neel and Chagnon conducted their early research before rigorous and enforceable rules were legally in place.

9.4.3 Protecting Indigenous Peoples

Both the Nuremberg Code and Declaration of Helsinki addressed medical experiments. Marcia Angell (1997) was concerned about the temptation of researchers to subordinate the subjects' welfare when giving a control group a placebo or a local standard care in sub-Saharan Africa, instead of an existing effective treatment. Such ethical relativism treats human subjects as means to an end and could result in widespread exploitation of vulnerable Third World populations for research programs that could not be carried out in, and thus potentially benefit, the sponsoring country. In 1968, James Neel inoculated the Yanomami with the Edmonston B vaccine which, as readers will recall, was effective but was being replaced by the Schwarz vaccine, which had fewer side effects. It was not a placebo and not part of a controlled experiment.

Brazilian anthropologists Guedes and Guimarães (2020:213) contend that Neel and Chagnon should have been aware of and respected the Yanomami cultural prohibitions on blood collection. The Human Genome Project considered the Yanomami blood samples as good for humanity. But only recently has informed consent been broadened to include both individuals and the communities in which they live and interact. Kahn (2005) thought that risk and benefits can be assessed for individuals as well as communities and that the risk and benefits may differ. The question becomes who can give consent for the community? One answer is to partner with community organization and groups. Guedes and Guimarães encouraged researchers to invite indigenous people to serve as project advisors and evaluators.

In 2019, the Yanomami people produced a Consultation Protocol specifically aimed at government actions based on an article by Guedes and Guimarães (2020:213–214). The article states that in 2004, the Brazilian government signed the International Labour Organization Convent on the Indigenous and Tribal Peoples Convention, which preceded the United Nations Declaration on the Rights of Indigenous Peoples. This means that under Brazilian law, all peoples have the right to be consulted and to decide freely about everything that may impact their lives. Readers should note that this corresponds with forming a partnership between researchers and the community.

9.4.4 *Professional Codes of Ethics*

Sociologist Robert K. Merton (1958) wrote that professional associations provide individual members with social and moral support and services to help them perform their roles as professionals. They set rigorous standards for the education of potential members, for professional practice and for research to advance knowledge in the discipline. They also seek to improve the social standing of the profession, increase public understanding of the profession's practice and research and promote necessary licensure and certifications for individual and group practice, research and educational programs.

Professional codes of ethical practice are developed by academic disciplines (e.g., APA, AAA) and by professional practice associations (e.g., AMA, American Bar Association), in order to police the profession and avoid legal action. But professional codes of ethics are incomplete in the sense that it is impossible for a code to cover all possible situations that will arise (Kitchner & Kitchner, 2009:10–12). This means that ethical judgments about medical, public health and social/behavioral research and professional codes of practice will vary over time (See Busch, 2011:239–245; Failer, 2018).

As mentioned in Chap. 7, a major impetus for professional and legal ethics codes was the 1960s' controversy over Milgram's experiments on obedience to authority (Kitchner & Kitchner, 2009:10).

Another was the 1964 US Army-funded counterinsurgency study, code-named Project Camelot (see Horowitz, 1967). The study involved psychologists, sociologists, anthropologists and economists analyzing the society and culture of foreign countries and developing methods for predicting and influencing social change and potential wars. The issue of the purpose, methods and benefits of conducting research outside the United States resurfaced in anthropology in 2001, with the findings of the Eldorado Task Force. The social science disciplines have revised their professional codes of ethics several times since then.

9.5 Conclusion

Both social science research ethics and codes of professional ethics have continued to evolve since the end of World War II. Some disciplines have handled the ethical challenges better than others. One challenge is to address the problems confronting individual teachers, practitioners and researchers as well as the threats to the professions and society at large. Professional social science codes of ethics recognize a set of principles including integrity, respect for people's rights and dignity, fidelity and responsibility, and competence. In contrast to other research ethics, the social sciences permit deception under specific conditions.

A major principle of concern in the case of the Yanomami is respect for people's rights and dignity. Much of the controversy focused on the Yanomami's ability to understand the purposes and methods of the research and treatments they were subject to, who could represent and speak for them and what benefits they should receive from participating in the studies. The need to respect the rights and dignity of the Yanomami was clearly called for by Magdalena Hurtado, a panelist at the special session at the 2000 AAA meeting in San Francisco and an expert on the epidemiology of infectious diseases among South American Indians. She said that:

> the field of anthropology needs to make a concerted effort to put First World scientific research to good use by serving humanitarian ends among indigenous people ... Reporting mechanisms need to be established with international and national authorities that will be responsive to human rights abuses ... and research guidelines should ensure that natives can clearly identify fieldwork activities as positive for their communities. Anthropologists and medical scientists should not continue to respond to the plight of indigenous people with silence and complacency but rather with proactive plans of action that include carefully though-out research on indigenous health. (Task Force, 2005:8–9).

Acknowledgments I would like to thank Dianne Schaffer for her insightful comments.

References

AAA. (2002). American Anthropological Association. *Darkness in El Dorado* Controversy: Questions and Answers. Electronic document. http://www.aaanet.org/press/qa.htm

American Society of Human Genetics. (2002). Response to allegations against James V. Neel in *Darkness in El Dorado*, by Patrick Tierney. *American Journal of Human Genetics, 70*(1), 1–10. https://doi.org/10.1086/338147

Amnesty International. (1993, September 7). *Confirmation of killing of 18 Yanomami Indians from the village of Hazimu*. Index number: AMR 19/029/1993. Retrieved June 7, 2021, from https://www.amnesty.org/en/documents/AMR19/029/1993/en/

Angell, M. (1997). The ethics of clinical research in the third world (editorial). *New England Journal of Medicine, 337*(12), 847–849. https://doi.org/10.1056/NEJM199709183371209

Annas, G. (1991). Mengele's birthmark: The Nuremberg code in United States courts. *The Journal of Contemporary Health Law and Policy, 7*(1), 17–45.

Borofsky, R. (2004). Conceptualizing Public Anthropology. Electronic document. (http://www.publicanthropology.org/Defining/definingpa.htm). Accessed 15 July 2010. Google Scholar

Borofsky, R. (2005). *Yanomami the fierce controversy and what we can learn from it*. University of California Press.

Borofsky, R. (n.d.). *Returning blood samples to the Yanomami*. Retrieved March 21, 2022, from https://center-yanomami.publicanthropology.org

Brooke, J. (1993). Raids on Miners Follow Killings in Amazon. *New York Times*. September 19, 1993, Section 1, Page 10.

Brown, A. (2000). Sponsel and Turner assist Patrick Tierney. *The Darwin Wars*. Retrieved May 5, 2021, from http://www.darwinwars.com/cuts/oddsnsods/yanomamo/chagnon_uncut_5.html

Busch, L. (2011). *Standards: Recipes for reality*. MIT Press.

Cantor, N. (2001). A special message from University of Michigan Provost Nancy Cantor regarding the research of James V. Neel. *Medicine at Michigan, Winter, 2001*, 62–63. Retrieved May 14, 2021, from https://www.medicineatmichigan.org/sites/default/files/archives/v6cantor.pdf

CCPY. (n.d.). Comissão Pró Yanomami. Demarcation of Lands Manipulates the Future of the Yanomami. Available at: C C P Y - Comissão Pró-Yanomami (proyanomami.org.br). Accessed 9 August 2023.

Chagnon, N. A. (1968). *Yanomamö: The fierce people*. Holt, Rinehart and Winston.

Chagnon, N. A. (1988). Life histories, blood revenge, and warfare in a tribal population. *Science, 239*(4843), 985–992. https://doi.org/10.1126/science.239.4843.985

Chagnon, N. A. (1993, October 23). Covering up the Yanomamo massacre. *New York Times, 21*.

Chagnon, N. A. (2014). *Noble savages: My life among two dangerous tribes – The Yanomamo and the anthropologists*. Simon & Schuster Paperback.

Chagnon, N. A., & Irons, W. (1979). *Evolutionary biology and human social behavior: An anthropological perspective*. Duxbury Press.

Cooper, J. (2013, January 14). El Dorado: The truth behind the myth. *BBC News*. Retrieved April 30, 2021, from https://www.bbc.com/news/magazine-20964114

Couzin-Frankel, J. (2010). Researchers to Return Blood Samples to the Yanomamö. *Science, 328* (5983), 1218. https://en.wikipedia.org/wiki/Public_anthropology

Curran, J., & Takata, S. (2000). Research among the Yanomami. *American Anthropological Association*. Electronic document. http://www.scudh.edu/dearhaber,as/yanomamio2.htm

D'Antonio, M. (2000, January 30). Napoleon Chagnon's war of discovery. *LA Times Magazine* Retrieved June 6, 2021, from http://cogweb.ucla.edu/Abstracts/Chagnon_00.html

Dalton, R. (2000). Anthropologists in turmoil over allegations of misconduct. *Nature, 408*(6811), 391. https://doi.org/10.1038/35044222

Dreger, A. (2011). Darkness's descent on the American Anthropological Association. *Human Nature, 22*(3), 225–246. https://doi.org/10.1007/s12110-011-9103-y

Dreger, A. (2015). *Galileo's middle finger: Heretics, activists, and the search for justice in science*. Penguin Press.

Epatko, L. (2014, September 8). WHO: Many thousands of new cases of Ebola expected in Liberia. *PBS NewsHour-World*. Retrieved April 14, 2021, from https://www.pbs.org/newshour/world/many-thousands-new-cases-ebola-expected-liberia

Failer, J. L. (2018). Review of the book *Reasonableness and Fairness: A Historical Theory* by C. McMahon. *Notre Dame Philosophical Reviews.* Retrieved June 6, 2021, from https://ndpr.nd.edu/reviews/reasonableness-and-fairness-a-historical-theory/

Farmer, P. (1996). Social inequalities and emerging infectious diseases. *Emerging Infectious Diseases, 2*(4), 259–269. https://doi.org/10.3201/eid0204.960402

Frankel, J. C. (2010). Researchers to return blood samples to the Yanomamö. *Science, 328*(5983), 218. https://doi.org/10.1126/science.328.5983.1218

Geertz, C. (2001, February 8). Life among the Anthros: Review of the book *Darkness in El Dorado: How scientists and journalists devastated the Amazon* by P. Tierney. *The New York Review of Books, 48*(2).

Glenn, D. (2006, March 3). Blood feud: A controversy over South American DNA samples held in North American laboratories ripples through anthropology. *The Chronicle of Higher Education, 52*(26), A14–A6, A18.

Golden, T. (1991). Talk about culture shock: Ant people in sky-high huts. *New York Times*. 17 April, Section B, Page 1.

Gregor, T., & Gross, D. R. (2004). Guilt by association: The culture of accusation and the American Anthropological Association's investigation of *Darkness in El Dorado*. *American Anthropologist, 106*(4), 687–698.

Guedes, C., & Guimarães, S. (2020). Research ethics and indigenous peoples: Repercussions of returning Yanomami blood samples. *Developing World Bioethics, 20*(4), 209–215. https://doi.org/10.1111/dewb.12264

Hammer, J. (2013, March). Why was this man an outcast among anthropologists? *Innovation | Smithsonian Magazine*. Retrieved April 26, 2021, from https://www.smithsonianmag.com/innovation/why-was-this-man-an-outcast-among-anthropologists-22930097/

Horowitz, I. L. (1967). *The rise and fall of project Camelot: Studies in the relationship between social science and practical politics*. MIT Press.

Hurtado, A. M., & Salzano, F. M. (2004). Introduction. In F. M. Salzano & A. M. Hurtado (Eds.), *Lost paradises and the ethics of research and publication*. Oxford University Press.

Iannone, C. (2013). Darkness in anthropology: A conversation with Napoleon Chagnon. *Academic Questions, 26*(3), 256–269. https://doi.org/10.1007/s12129-013-9378-z

Kahn, J. (2005). Informed consent in the context of communities. *The Journal of Nutrition, 35*(40), 918–920. https://doi.org/10.1093/jn/135.4.918

Kellman, S. (1982). The Yanomamis: Their battle for survival. *Journal of International Affairs, 36*(1), 15–42. Retrieved April 14, 2021, from http://www.jstor.org/stable/24356398

Kitchner, R., & Kitchner, K. S. (2009). Social science research ethics: Historical and philosophical issues. In D. M. Mertens & P. E. Ginsberg (Eds.), *The handbook of social research ethics* (pp. 5–22). SAGE.

Leslie, M. (2000, January/February). Divided they stand. *Stanford Magazine*. Retrieved April 26, 2021, from https://stanfordmag.org/contents/divided-they-stand

Lindee, S. M. (2001). Review of Patrick Tierney: *Darkness in El Dorado*. *Current Anthropology, 42*(2), 272–274. https://doi.org/10.1086/320007

Mann, C. C. (2001). Anthropological warfare. *Science, 291*(5503), 416–421. https://doi.org/10.1126/science.291.5503.416

Merton, R. K. (1958). The functions of the professional association. *American Journal of Nursing, 58*(1), 50–54.

MEVA. (2023). *Evangelical mission of the Amazon*. Retrieved February 15, 2023, from https://meva.org.br/

Michigan News. (2000, February 1). James Neel, father of modern human genetics, died Feb. 1. *Michigan News*. University of Michigan, Ann Arbor. Retrieved April 14, 2021, from, https://news.umich.edu/james-neel-father-of-modern-human-genetics-died-feb-1/

Miller, D. W. (2001). Academic Scandal in the Internet Age. *Chronicle of Higher Education, 47* (18), A14–A17. 12 Jan 2021.
Monaghan, P. (1994, October 26). Bitter warfare in anthropology. *The Chronicle of Higher Education, A10*. 18, 19.
Neel, J. V. (1970). Lessons from a "primitive" people: Do recent data concerning South American Indians have relevance to problems of highly civilized communities? *Science, 170*(3960), 815–822. https://doi.org/10.1126/science.170.3960.81
Neel, J. V., Centerwalia, W. R., Chagnon, N. A., & Casey, H. L. (1970). Notes on the effect of measles vaccine in a virgin soil population of South American Indians. *American Journal of Epidemiology, 91*(4), 418–429. https://doi.org/10.1093/oxfordjournals.aje.a121152
Nichols, B. (1996). What really happened: The AX fight reconsidered. *Media International Australia, 82*(1), 6–11. https://doi.org/10.1177/1329878X9608200103
Perlman, D. (2000). Anthropology community upset over ethics scandal isolated Indians were corrupted, writer says. *San Francisco Chronicle*, November 16, 2000.
Peters, J. F. (1998). *Life among the Yanomami: The story of change among the Xilixana on the Mucajai River in Brazil*. Broadview Press.
Publishers Weekly. (1997, June 30). Review of the book *Last Tribes of El Dorado: The Gold Wars in the Amazon Rain Forest* by P. Tierney. Retrieved February 22, 2022, from https://www.amazon.com/Last-Tribes-El-Dorado-Amazon/dp/067083372X.
Ruyter, K. W. (2003). *Forskningsetikk. Beskyttelse av enkeltpersoner og samfunn. [Research ethics. Protection of individuals and society]*. Gyldendal Norsk Forlag. Retrieved February 22, 2022, from https://www.forskningsetikk.no/en/resources/the-research-ethics-library/systhematic-and-historical-perspectives/the-history-of-research-ethics
Sahlins, M. (2000). December 10). Jungle fever. *The Washington Post*. https://www.washingtonpost.com/archive/entertainment/books/2000/12/10/jungle-fever/e8b757ae-b365-4632-8f04-3d9e61371ed7/
Salzano, F. M. (2000). James V. Neel and Latin America – Or how scientific collaboration should be conducted. *Genetics and Molecular Biology, 23*, 557–561.
Santos, R. V., Lindee, S., & Sousa, V. S. (2014). Varieties of the primitive: Human biological diversity studies in cold war Brazil (1962–1970). *American Anthropologist, 116*(4), 723–735. https://doi.org/10.1111/aman.12150
Special Commission. (1991). *Special commission of the American Anthropological Association*. Retrieved May 3, 2021, from Report-of-the-Special-Commission-to-Investigate-the-Situation-of-the-Brazilian-Yanomami-rptyano2.pdf.
Sponsel, L. (2002). On reflections on *Darkness in El Dorado*. *Current Anthropology, 43*(1), 149–152. https://doi.org/10.1086/338288
Srikameswaran, A. (2000, November 15). Pittsburgh author's charges stir up anthropologists. *Pittsburgh Post-Gazette*.
Stellmach, D., Beshar, I., Bedford, J., du Cros, P., & Stringer, B. (2018). Anthropology in public health emergencies: What is anthropology good for? *British Medical Journal Global Health, 3*(2), e000534. https://doi.org/10.1136/bmjgh-2017-000534
Stoll, D. (2001). Science attacks Amazon tribe: Book review of P. Tierney, *Darkness in El Dorado*. *New Republic, 224*(12), 34–39.
Task Force. (2002a). *El Dorado task force final report vol I*. Retrieved June 7, 2021, from https://dwhume.com/darkness_documents/0598.pdf
Task Force. (2002b). *El Dorado task force final report vol II*. Retrieved June 7, 2021, from https://dwhume.com/darkness_documents/0599.pdf
Task Force. (2005). Comments on the referendum to rescind the AAA's acceptance of the El Dorado task force report. *Anthropology Newsletter, 46*(6), 28–29. Retrieved February22, 2022, from https://www.researchgate.net/publication/249457896. https://doi.org/10.1525/an.2005.46.6.28
Taylor, P. (2009). Retroactive ethics in rapidly developing scientific fields. *Cell Stem Cell, 4*(6), 479–482. https://doi.org/10.1016/j.stem.2009.05.002

The New Yorker. (2000, October 28). The New Yorker replies: Response of the editors of The New Yorker to Jungle Fever by J. Tooby. *Slate*. Retrieved June 8, 2021, from https://slate.com/news-and-politics/2000/10/the-new-yorker-replies.html

Tierney, P. (1997). *Last tribes of El Dorado: The gold wars in the Amazon rain forest*. Viking Press.

Tierney, P. (2000a, October 9). The fierce anthropologist. *The New Yorker*, 50.

Tierney, P. (2000b). *Darkness in El Dorado: How scientists and journalists devastated the Amazon*. W.W. Norton.

Tobin, J. (n.d.). *The fake news about James Neel*. University of Michigan Heritage Project. Retrieved January 6, 2023, from https://heritage.umich.edu/stories/the-fake-news-about-james-neel/

Tooby, J. (2000, October 25). Jungle Fever did two U.S. scientists start a genocidal epidemic in the Amazon, or was The New Yorker duped? *Slate*. Retrieved May 13, 2021, from https://slate.com/news-and-politics/2000/10/jungle-fever.html

Turner, T., & Sponsel, L. (2000). *Imminent anthropological scandal: Email to president and president- elect*. American Anthropological Association. Retrieved May 10, 2021, from https://dwhume.com/darkness_documents/0055.htm

Walsh, P. W., & Lehmann, D. (2021). Academic celebrity. *The International Journal of Politics, Culture, and Society, 34*(1), 21–46. https://doi.org/10.1007/s10767-019-09340-9

Weijer, C., & Emanuel, E. J. (2000). Protecting communities in biomedical research. *Science, 289*(5482), 1142–1144. https://doi.org/10.1126/science.289.5482.1142

Weiss, K. M., & Ward, R. H. (2000). James V. Neel, M.D., Ph.D. (March 22, 1915–January 31, 2000): Founder effect. *American Journal of Human Genetics, 66*(3), 755–760. https://doi.org/10.1086/302793

Wilson, E. O. (1975). *Sociobiology: The new synthesis*. Harvard University Press.

Wilson, E. O. (1978). *On human nature*. Harvard University Press.

Winkler, K. J. (1994). Parties in bitter dispute over Amazonian Indians reach a fragile peace. *The Chronicle of Higher Education*. Washington: Dec 14, 1994. 41(16):A18.

Wong, K. (2001). Fighting the darkness in *El Dorado*. *Scientific American, 284*(3), 26–28. https://doi.org/10.1038/scientificamerican0301-26

Index

A
Abu Ghraib, 183, 208
Accomplice, 132, 145, 146
Accountability, 33, 48, 49
Accreditation, x, 8, 29, 30, 42, 52, 55–59
Adequately debrief, 133, 149
Ad Hoc Advisory Panel, 95–96, 173
Adorno, T., 135
Advanced Notice of Proposed Rule Making (ANPRM), 33, 60, 62
Advertisement, 188
Africa, 142, 220, 228
African American, 3, 9, 71, 72, 74–84, 86, 87, 92, 95, 97, 98, 101, 102
Agentic Shift, 150
Aggression, 132, 184, 185, 188
Alabama State Health Department, 77
Alexander, L., 20, 228
Alport, G., 130
Amazon, 212, 218, 220–222
Amazon river, 211
Amdur, R.J., 54, 121, 122, 153, 176, 177
American Anthropological Association (AAA), 3, 11, 162, 177, 178, 212, 221–226, 230
American Association for Public Opinion Research (AAPOR), 165, 166
American Association of Political Consultants (AAPC), 4, 5
American Bar Association (ABA), 111, 114, 116, 118, 229
American Broadcasting Company (ABC), 118, 148, 172
American Civil Liberties Union (ACLU), 107
American Medical Association (AMA), 58, 92
American Philosophical Society (APS), 215
American Psychological Association (APA), 3, 6, 24, 99, 120, 149, 173
American Public Health Association (APHA), 79
American Social Hygiene Association (ASHA), 73, 74
American Society of Human Genetics (ASHG), 215
American Sociological Association (ASA), 3, 45, 109, 165, 173
Amnesty International, 219
Anderson, O., 87
Angell, M., 228
Anonymity, 26, 109, 174, 184
Anthropologist, 3, 11, 48, 211, 214–218, 220–226, 229, 230
Anthropology, x, 3, 24, 211, 215–217, 220, 222, 225, 226, 230
Antisocial action, 183
Anxiety, 27, 132, 137, 169
APA Code of Ethics, 6, 149
Appeal, x, 9, 25, 28, 32, 34, 35, 42, 43, 47, 50, 55, 59–64, 112, 114, 116, 172
Applied, 2, 4–5, 17, 22, 26, 29, 43, 51, 53, 54, 77, 100, 108, 109, 133, 167, 170, 175
Applied Sociology, 5
A priori theory, 134, 135, 150
Arbitrary, 60, 166, 202
Arendt, H., 135, 152
Arizona Supreme Court, 118
Asch, S., 130, 131
Asian American, 197, 202

H. Perlstadt, *Assessing Social Science Research Ethics and Integrity*, Clinical Sociology: Research and Practice, https://doi.org/10.1007/978-3-031-34538-8

Assess, 12, 44, 83, 96, 108, 110, 119, 165, 166, 206, 211, 212, 224, 226
Assessment, x, 3, 5, 24, 26, 27, 34, 96, 110, 138, 168, 173, 176, 214
Assign responsibility, 146
Association for Applied Clinical Sociology (AACS), 4, 5
Association of American Medical Colleges (AAMC), 56, 58
Atlanta, GA, 31, 76, 92, 94, 95, 100
Atomic, 213
Atomic Energy Commission (AEC), 213
Attica Prison, 183
Attorney, 4, 24, 97, 107, 109–111, 113, 115–117, 119–122, 125
Authoritarian, 130, 136, 144
Authoritative, 130, 136
Authority, 7–9, 23, 24, 27, 43, 45, 47, 49–51, 53, 55, 57, 60, 61, 63, 96, 121, 123, 130, 133, 135–139, 144–146, 148–151, 153, 173, 184, 192, 197, 199, 200, 205, 206, 219, 230
Authority figure, 10, 134, 135, 141, 147, 151, 152
Autonomous, 63, 150
Autonomy, 6, 7, 25, 54
Autopsy, 9, 19, 82, 84, 85, 87, 88, 93

B

Badhwar, N., 141, 143
Baker, J.N., 80, 81
Bales, R.F., 109, 110
Bankert, E.A., 42, 43, 121, 122, 153, 176, 177
Bar Association, 111, 114, 115
Barnard, C., 151
Bauman, Z., 153
Baumrind, D., 2, 10, 130, 136–139, 143, 146, 148, 149
Beauvois, J.-L., 144–146
Becker, H.S., 27, 169, 176
Beecher, H.K., 21, 90, 133
Behavioral, 2–4, 12, 17, 18, 21–26, 28, 29, 31–35, 41, 43, 44, 49–52, 54, 55, 62, 99, 117, 121, 133, 147, 149, 150, 159, 173, 175–177, 190, 208, 228, 229
Belmont Report, x, 1, 2, 6, 8, 12, 24–26, 28, 35, 41, 42, 47, 48, 54–56, 63, 95, 122, 159, 168, 170, 173–175
Beneficence, 6–8, 12, 25, 26, 41, 47, 54, 168
Benefits, 1, 6, 7, 17, 18, 22, 24, 26, 31, 41, 47, 50, 52–54, 63, 84, 88, 93, 94, 96, 97, 99, 101, 121, 138, 164, 166, 170, 171, 173–175, 213, 228–230
Binet, A., 131, 135
Biomedical, 1–3, 7, 12, 17, 18, 21–30, 33, 35, 41, 43, 49, 50, 52, 54, 55, 98, 121, 124, 133, 159, 173, 175, 176, 226–228
Biosphere, 219, 220
Blau, P.M., 151
Blood, 23, 72, 75, 83, 84, 86, 87, 99, 212, 214, 227
Blood sample, 212, 214, 215, 223, 227, 229
Boise, ID, 160
Borofsky, R., 226
Brazil, 11, 211, 212, 214, 215, 218, 220, 221, 227
Brazilian, 214, 217, 218, 221, 229
Brewer-Carías, C., 218, 219, 225
Bridgeport, CT, 134, 136, 150
British Broadcasting Company (BBC), 144
Brown v. Board of Education of Topeka, 112
Brownell, H. Jr., 116
Browning, C., 152
Bureaucracy, 8, 18, 30, 35, 42, 43, 46, 52–53, 151
Burger, J., 142, 143
Busch, L., 18, 32
Buxtun, P.J., 93–95

C

California, 47, 50, 74, 142, 171, 226
Canada, 43, 58, 61, 62
Canadian Tri-Council Policy (TCPS), x, 28
Cartwright, D., 135
Case, 4, 6–9, 11, 27, 43, 54, 74, 77, 79, 82, 83, 87, 88, 97, 108–112, 116, 118–122, 124, 159, 163, 172, 173, 177, 198, 225
Case Western Reserve University, 97
Chagnon, N.A., 11, 211, 212, 214, 215, 220–229
Chain gang, 11, 185, 194
Charcot, J.-M., 135
Charitable, 74, 217
Charity, 6, 77
Chicago Board of Health, 86
Chicago Commission on Race Relations, 76
Chicago, IL, 57, 76, 86–88, 110, 112–114, 121
Chicago Syphilis Control Program, 86–87
Chicago Tribune, 86
Circuit Court of Appeals, 111, 112
Civil trial, 107, 108, 119, 122
Clark, T., 73, 78–83, 85
Class, 6, 145, 152, 163
Class action law suit, 71, 99
Class experiment, 132

Clinical, 2–6, 12, 19, 21, 22, 24, 25, 31, 34, 52, 62, 71, 79, 80, 85, 89, 90, 109, 133, 136, 144, 148, 178
Clinical practice, 19
Clinical Sociology, 4
Clinical Study Oversight Committee (CSOC), 206
Clinical trial, 52, 57, 228
Clinton, B., 30, 95, 98
Clinton, H., 101
Code, ix, 3, 18, 35, 48, 54, 58, 61, 122, 172, 173, 222, 227–230
Code of ethics, 3–6, 92, 93, 149, 172, 177, 226
Cohort, 87, 97
Colbert, J.B., 49
Collegial, 1, 8, 22, 44, 53–54
Colonization, 194, 197–198
Colonizer, 197, 202
Columbia Broadcasting System (CBS), 118, 119
Columbia University, 50, 78
Commission, 8, 24, 25, 29, 32, 57, 76, 95, 100, 173, 174, 219, 221, 223, 224
Common Man Authority, 140
Common Rule (*45 CFR 46*), 2, 8, 18, 24, 26–35, 42–45, 47, 48, 50, 51, 57–59, 62, 63, 99, 122, 125, 162, 173, 178, 206
Communal self-censorship, 196
Community, 5, 8, 19, 26, 35, 42, 44, 46, 50–52, 55, 63, 64, 72, 75–77, 79, 84, 85, 87, 92, 93, 98, 101, 111, 159–162, 166, 170–172, 174–177, 191, 211–215, 226, 227, 229, 230
Comparison group, 9, 82, 163
Confidence, 5, 72, 83, 123
Confidentiality, 31, 54, 56, 74, 112, 122, 167, 171, 173, 174, 189
Conflict of interest, 54, 206
Conformity, 130, 131, 140, 141
Consent, ix, 1, 6, 8, 9, 12, 20–22, 25, 31, 45, 52, 54, 85, 95, 98, 107, 108, 111, 116–118, 121, 123, 124, 149, 162, 168, 175, 212, 222, 228, 229
Consequence, 18, 49, 63, 132, 136, 150, 153, 169, 174
Consortium of Social Science Associations (COSSA), 24
Construct validity, 139
Contractual agreement, 190
Control group, 9, 80, 84, 89, 99, 164, 186, 203, 228
Controversial, x, 1, 7–12, 125, 169, 171, 205, 219, 227
Conversion, 194, 198–199
County, ix, 46, 49, 50, 75, 77–81, 83–85, 88, 95, 191
Criminal trial, 118, 121
Critic, 91–94, 133, 139, 167, 216, 217, 219
Culture, 8, 11, 17, 27, 43–45, 48, 49, 134, 216, 217, 225, 230
Cutler, J.C., 88, 89, 94, 100, 101

D

Data and Safety Monitoring Board (DSMB), 99, 206
Davis, M.M., 78, 79
Death camp, 130, 136, 152
Debrief, 138, 139, 189
Debriefing, 134, 138, 139, 149, 187, 200
Deception, 7, 9, 10, 12, 27, 33, 34, 100, 123, 136, 138–140, 148–150, 153, 168–170, 177, 178, 189, 196, 206, 230
Deceptive debriefing, 132, 133
Declaration of Helsinki, 18, 19, 21, 22, 227, 228
Defer to authority, 152
Deibert, A.V., 88, 91
Deindividualized group, 184, 185
Deindividuation, 184, 185
Delamare, N., 49–51
Delegating, 120, 121
Demand, 26, 44, 142, 143, 197, 203
Denver, CO, 111
Department of Health and Human Services (DHHS), ix, 2, 8, 18, 28, 29, 33, 34, 44, 45, 51, 56, 60, 62, 63, 98, 173
Department of Health, Education and Welfare (DHEW), 8, 12, 23, 26, 55, 57, 82, 92, 95, 148, 162, 164, 177, 188, 228
Design, 31, 42, 96, 134, 139, 161–162, 174, 184
Destructive obedience, 136, 148, 152
Deviance, 160
Deviant, 27, 46, 161, 170, 171, 174
Dibble, E.H. Jr., 81–83
Dingwall, R., 20, 52, 167, 168
Disadvantaged, 20, 99
Discouraged from quitting, 189
Disease, 9, 19, 22, 52, 71, 74–75, 79–86, 90, 92, 96, 100, 211, 212, 214, 223, 225, 227, 230
Disobedient, 146, 190
Documentary, 85, 100, 108, 117, 118, 138, 144, 146, 218
Doyle v. Miller, 110, 114, 119, 122
Dreger, A., 215, 222
Duke University, 20, 57

E

Eastland, J., 117
Economics, 3, 4, 24, 32, 51, 78, 87, 96, 149, 211
Ehrenreich, B., 167, 168
Ehrlich, P., 73
Eichmann, A., 130, 152, 153
El Dorado, 11, 220–225
Electric shock, 2, 10, 132, 141, 145, 184
Emory University, 91
Emotional stress, 137, 188
Empirical, 19, 25, 125, 220
  ethics, 152
  findings, 193
  research, 25, 77, 108, 109
  studies, 135
England, 19, 108, 144
Epidemic, 11, 72, 212, 215, 220, 222, 224, 227
Erikson, K.T., 27, 169, 171, 172
Ethical dilemma, 99, 152, 178
Ethical guideline, x, 227
Ethical issue, x, 9, 22, 55, 59, 90, 91, 99, 123, 149, 168, 176–178, 205–206, 227–230
Ethical principle, 2, 5–8, 12, 18, 19, 21, 24, 25, 28, 42, 43, 47, 48, 50, 53, 58, 59, 63, 125, 168, 173, 174
Ethical research, 1, 6–7, 18, 30, 35, 43, 98, 99, 136, 175
Ethical standards, 18, 23, 44, 53, 54, 100, 137, 212, 226–228
Ethicist, 24, 27, 63, 120, 125, 141, 147, 213
Ethnographer, 172, 178
Ethnographic, 161, 178, 215
Ethnography, 211
Ethnomethodology, 48, 52
Europe, 49, 81, 92
Evaluation, ix, 3, 5, 18, 19, 34, 35, 79, 80, 133, 201, 204
Evidence, 25, 42, 63, 85, 95, 96, 109, 110, 123, 160, 166, 207, 225
Executive Board, 11, 212, 222, 224, 225
Exempt, 4, 24, 32, 49, 62
Exempt research, 48, 56, 62, 178
Experiment, x, 2, 6, 7, 10, 11, 17–21, 27, 28, 32, 55, 57, 72, 84, 89, 90, 94, 96, 99–101, 109, 115, 129–147, 149, 150, 152–154, 183–198, 203–209, 212, 228–230
Experimental condition, 10, 132, 135, 136, 138, 141, 142
Experimental design, 95, 110, 205
Experimenter, 129, 131–137, 140, 141, 143–147, 151, 184–187, 203
Exploratory experimentation, 134
Exploratory study, 188
Exposé, 9, 18, 71, 90–98, 101, 228

F

Fajans, J., 226
Farkas, M.A., 200
Father McDermott, 195, 201, 209
Federal, ix, x, 1–3, 7–9, 12, 18, 21, 22, 24, 27, 28, 30–35, 41, 43–48, 50–53, 55–61, 63, 95, 107, 108, 110, 111, 113, 116, 121, 122, 124, 125, 148, 153, 162, 164, 166, 171, 173
Federalwide Assurance (FWA), 29, 51
Female, 73, 78, 133, 142–145, 147, 184, 186, 187, 200, 202
Festinger, L., 100
Fidelity, 7, 230
Field visit, 220
Field, S.J., 49
Film, 108, 117–119, 189, 213, 215, 216, 218, 219, 225
Fisk University, 76, 79
Folkways, 45–49, 52
Food and Drug Administration (FDA), 57, 173, 228
Food Lion v. Capital Cities/ABC, Inc., 172
Ford Foundation, 9, 108, 109, 117, 122, 124
Frame of reference, 137
France, 19, 49, 74, 130
Frank, J., 131, 135
Friedrich, C.J., 135
Fritz, J.M., 3, 5
Full debriefing, 132, 133
Funding, 1, 8, 12, 24, 28, 51, 53, 55, 56, 61, 76, 77, 79, 80, 82, 83, 108, 124, 139, 159, 172, 177, 213

G

Galliher, J.F., 159, 160, 164, 165
Geertz, C., 223, 224
General Counsel, 134
Genetics, 11, 211, 213–216
Germany, 19, 20
Gibson, C.D. Jr., 91, 92
Giddings, F.H., 78
Glazer, M., 164, 165, 171
Goffman, E., 169, 191, 194
Gold, 217, 219–221
Gold rush, 217–221

Government, x, 1, 3–5, 7, 8, 22, 25, 28, 29, 32, 33, 35, 43, 46, 49–52, 55, 57–59, 62, 71, 74, 76, 80, 83, 84, 89, 95–98, 102, 107, 109, 113, 116, 120, 122, 124, 136, 149, 169, 198, 213, 215, 217–220, 223, 227, 229
Graham, L., 226
Gray, F.D., 73, 79–81, 83–85, 87, 88, 92, 97, 98
Gregor, T., 225
Grievance committee, 201, 203
Gross, D., 225, 226
Group pressure, 130
Group Pressure to Disobey, 140, 143, 146
Group Pressure to Obey, 140
Guards, 11, 46, 148, 183, 185, 187–201, 203–205, 207–209
Guatemala, 89, 94, 100, 101
Guedes, C., 229
Guideline, 1–3, 8, 12, 20, 22–24, 28, 32–34, 41, 51, 55, 63, 113, 125, 162, 171–173, 228, 230
Guimarães, S., 229

H

Haney, C., 196, 197, 202, 204
Harm, 6, 9, 17–20, 26, 27, 31, 32, 56, 99, 122, 131, 137, 138, 148, 149, 152, 153, 162, 170, 171, 173, 174, 194, 205, 207, 216
Hartshorne, R., 116
Harvard University, 20
Hastings Center, 96
Hastings Center Report, 94
Hawthorne Effect, 112
Health care system, 72, 102, 167
Health promotion, 21, 79
Hearing, 2, 22, 25, 62, 95, 107, 108, 110, 117, 121, 197, 202, 204
Heller, J., 55, 71, 90, 94, 95, 100
Heller, J.R., 84
Helpless, 141, 204
Helsinki Declaration, 21, 22, 48, 54, 133, 228
Henri, V., 131, 132
Herrera, C., 173
Hill, D.C., 112–116, 122, 124
Historian, 26, 89, 152, 215, 223
History, 1–3, 7–8, 12, 17–35, 42, 49, 71–73, 80, 82, 90, 93, 96, 97, 121, 130, 138, 154, 163, 176, 202, 212, 214, 217, 225
Hoax, 137, 148
Hobbes, T., 217
Holocaust, 20, 26, 148, 151–153
Homosexual, x, 10, 159–162, 164, 168, 169, 174, 176–178
Homosexuality, 27, 160, 169, 171
Horowitz, I.L., 161, 165, 167, 174
Humanitarian, 212, 214, 228, 230
Humanities, 12, 28–30, 61, 137, 217, 229
Human Rights, 218, 220, 221, 224, 230
Human Subjects Research Review Committee, 183, 188
Humphreys, L., x, 7, 10, 27, 159–171, 173–178
Hunger strike, 193, 197
Hurtado, M., 223, 226, 230
Hutchins, R., 108, 109
Hypnosis, 184–188, 193
Hypotheses, x, 44, 125, 134–136, 143, 150, 178, 193

I

Identifiers, ix, 10, 34, 62, 115, 122, 160, 164
Identifying information, 62, 112, 176
Illinois White Paper, 29
Improvised adjustment, 203
Independent variable, 136, 203
Indigenous, 212, 213, 218, 219, 221, 223, 224, 226–230
Individual, x, 3–7, 11, 12, 19, 25, 29, 30, 32–35, 41–44, 46, 49, 51, 52, 62, 63, 71–73, 79, 84, 85, 87, 88, 94, 99, 122, 123, 131, 134, 144, 146, 147, 149–153, 160, 161, 168, 169, 171, 174, 175, 183, 184, 186–188, 193, 197, 207, 208, 211–213, 215, 227, 229, 230
Individualized group, 184, 185
Individuate, 11
Individuation, 185, 188
Inducement, 72, 84, 99, 212
Informed, 7, 9, 85, 89, 112, 113, 118, 121, 137, 141, 142, 145, 150, 164, 168, 197, 222
Informed consent, ix, 2, 6, 12, 17, 20–22, 24–26, 29, 31, 32, 42, 44, 47, 52, 54, 63, 72, 84, 97, 99, 120, 122, 124, 133, 138, 139, 145, 148, 149, 161, 162, 164, 166, 171, 173–175, 177, 178, 189, 205, 212, 213, 227, 229
Institute of Medicine (IOM), 57, 58
Institutional Review Board (IRB), ix, x, 4, 7, 8, 12, 24, 29–35, 41–45, 48–63, 120–122, 125, 149, 153, 159, 167, 168, 172, 173, 176, 178, 206, 213
Institutional Review Board Member Handbook, 54, 121, 176, 177

Integrity, 5, 32, 58, 64, 108, 120, 122–124, 170, 171, 230
International, 3, 4, 21, 33, 34, 74, 123, 227, 228, 230
International law, 21, 228
Interpersonal process analysis (IPA), 109, 110
Intervention, 3–7, 18, 33, 34, 62, 80, 211–213
Intransigent, 194, 195, 199
Irrational, 18, 46–48, 50, 63
Iskrant, A.P., 91

J
Japan, 213
Jenkins, B., 92, 93
Jerusalem, 130
Johns Hopkins University, 60, 78
Johnson, C.S., 76, 77, 79, 84
Jones, J.H., 78, 79, 83, 84, 91, 97, 98
Journalism, 34, 172–173
Journalist, 10, 26, 27, 90, 109, 124, 138, 166–168, 172, 178, 212, 215
Journal of the American Medical Association (JAMA), 73, 89
Judge, 4, 9, 25, 41, 46, 47, 53, 107–118, 120–125, 186
Juror, 9, 107–125
Jury, 9, 12, 27, 28, 107–123, 125, 167, 169
Jury selection, 4, 108, 117, 119, 125
Jury system, 9, 108, 109, 111, 114–116, 120, 121, 123, 125
Justice, ix, 6–8, 12, 25, 26, 28, 41, 47, 54, 97, 108, 111, 114–116, 122–124, 168, 175
Justify, 6, 122, 137, 138, 146

K
Kahn, J., 213, 229
Kaiser Family Foundation (KFF), 101
Kalven, H. Jr., 107, 109, 116, 122, 124
Kant, I., 147
Katz, J., 1, 22, 98, 107, 120–122, 133, 173, 174
Kinsey reports, 2, 22, 117
Kitch, P., 111
Kitchner, K.S., 6, 7
Kitchner, R.F., 6, 7
Knowledge, 4, 10, 19, 31, 32, 34, 48, 51, 53, 61, 90, 99, 115–117, 123, 144, 145, 153, 166, 169, 183, 192, 225, 229
Kopenawa, D., 218, 221, 227

L
Laboratory, 6, 10, 19, 27, 86, 92, 132, 134–137, 139, 143–145, 203
Lacks, H., 98
Lamphere, L., 221–223
Law, 4, 5, 9, 18, 19, 24, 27, 28, 35, 41–64, 91, 94, 95, 97, 108–110, 113, 116, 117, 120–123, 147, 164, 172–174, 212, 228, 229
Lawyer, 9, 109, 111, 113, 118, 119, 122–125, 191
Learner, 129, 132–135, 139–143, 145–147, 185
Legacy Committee, 98
Legislation, 23, 24, 47, 63, 96, 117
Legitimate, 7, 20, 57, 63, 150, 205, 226, 228
Legitimize, 20, 197
Levels of shock, 132, 135
Levi, E.H., 107, 109, 111, 113, 115, 116, 121, 122, 124
Levine, R.J., 24, 42, 174, 175
Lewin, K., x, 131
Lewis, A., 26
Local, ix, 4, 8, 29, 31, 33, 35, 42, 43, 46, 49–55, 63, 71, 77, 79, 82, 84, 102, 111, 121, 124, 134, 165, 166, 185, 201, 211, 228
Lock and key, 10, 112, 113, 164, 177
Longitudinal study, 9, 23, 78, 87–90
Los Angeles Times, 9, 116

M
Macon County, AL, 23, 55, 72, 75–77, 79, 80, 82, 83, 88, 97
Maslach, C., 193, 204, 209
Mathes, I.B., 160
Matos, C., 219
Mattson, P., 226
Mauss, A., 90, 94, 96
Measles, 11, 212, 214–215, 222, 224, 227
Memorial Sloan Kettering Cancer Center, 100
Memory, 27, 129, 131, 133, 138, 149
Mental breakdown, 183, 207
Merton, R.K., 52
Method, x, 4, 7, 12, 20, 30, 52, 55, 77, 87, 109–111, 125, 131, 135, 138, 161–162, 166, 170, 172, 212, 220, 227, 230
Methodology, 42, 44, 78, 79, 109, 125, 142, 160, 167, 208
Mikva, A., 111, 113, 114
Milbank Foundation, 84, 94
Milbank Memorial Fund, 85

Milgram, S., x, 2, 7, 9, 10, 18, 27, 129–139, 141–153, 184, 185, 187, 205, 208, 230
Military, 20, 73, 74, 164, 183, 191, 198, 208, 215, 219
Miller, A.G., 152, 153
Mills, C.W., 44, 73, 165
Mind control experiment, 204
Mischel, W., 151
Missionary, 212, 214, 215, 218, 219, 223
Mock jury, 110, 111, 114, 119, 122, 125
Moore, J.E., 82, 88, 89, 92
Moral, x, 7, 19, 27, 32, 35, 46, 49, 50, 63, 90, 92, 168, 176, 177, 229
  actions, 125, 149
  compass, 35, 63, 141–143
  imperative, 147
  responsibility, 98–101, 150, 198
Morality, 27, 73, 94, 177
Mores, 45–49
Multi-site study, 29, 31, 44, 45, 60

N
National Academy of Medicine (NAM), 213
National Bioethics Advisory Commission (NBAC), 29–31
National Cancer Institute (NCI), 100, 227
National Commission, 2, 6, 8, 12, 18, 24–26, 41, 42, 55, 56, 173
National Institute of Mental Health (NIMH), 10, 164
National Institutes of Health (NIH), 1, 2, 22, 23, 29, 101
National Research Act, 24, 43, 54, 55, 95, 173, 228
National Research Council (NRC), 32, 33
National Science Foundation (NSF), 61, 133, 134, 139, 149
National Urban League, 76
Neel, J.V., 11, 211–215, 218, 222–229
Neighborhood, 3, 87, 163, 202
New England Journal of Medicine (ENJM), 21, 90, 133
Newspaper ads, 11, 138, 149
New York City, 78, 79, 119
New York Times, 26, 55, 100, 135, 168, 222
Nonlaboratory replication, 10, 143–148
Nonprofit, 24, 50, 52, 96, 122, 124, 212, 217
Normative, 63, 141, 227
Norms, 3, 9, 19, 47, 53, 57, 189, 208
Notice of Proposed Rulemaking (NPRM), 34, 62, 178
Nuremberg Code, 18, 20, 22, 48, 54, 227, 228
Nurse, 10, 79, 81, 83, 144

O
Obama, B., 101
Obedience, x, 2, 7–10, 18, 27, 129–154, 199, 205, 213, 230
Obedient, 129, 132, 135, 137, 140, 141, 146, 184, 198, 199
Obey, 10, 129, 131, 132, 134, 135, 137, 141, 146–148, 153, 192
Observation, 6, 19, 34, 48, 52, 62, 80, 82, 83, 85, 99, 161, 167, 169–173, 175, 177, 178, 188, 190, 205, 215, 225
Office for Human Research Protections (OHRP), ix, 29, 33, 51, 58
Office for Protection from Research Risks (OPRR), ix, 27, 56, 57
Office of Naval Research (ONR), 186
Office of Social Sciences, 133
Olansky, S., 76, 77, 88–92
Oral history, 26, 34, 62
Organization, 3–6, 17–19, 24, 30, 32, 42, 49–53, 57, 58, 96, 107, 122, 141, 151, 171, 177, 197, 217, 218, 222, 225, 227, 229
Organization of American States (OAS), 218
Oronoco River, 211
Oslo study, 73, 80, 91

P
Pan American Sanitary Bureau, 89
Parent, ix, 45, 86, 184, 193, 195, 203–204
Parental control, 136
Parental permission, 86
Paris, France, 19, 76
Park, R.E., 76, 167
Parks, R., 97
Parole, 11, 118, 197, 199, 201, 202, 204
Parole board, 11, 89, 197, 199, 202–204, 206, 209
Parran, T. Jr., 78–81, 86, 89, 100
Passive observation, 71, 72, 80
Penicillin, 9, 19, 23, 71, 72, 88–97, 99–101
Pennsylvania State University, 227
Perry, G., 132, 134, 135, 138–139, 144
Personality, 2, 4, 134, 151, 183, 187, 189, 208
Personally responsible, 205
Personal power, 205

Personal responsibility, 137, 152
Persuasion, 46, 131, 132
Philanthropic foundation, 124
Phillips, O.L., 111, 112, 114–116
Pilot study, 79, 132
Play acting, 196
Pocaterra, N., 223
Police, 8, 10, 41–64, 101, 102, 144, 147, 148, 152, 160, 166, 168, 170, 174, 187, 188, 190, 191, 195, 198, 229
Policemen, 60, 152, 162
Policy, 2, 4, 5, 7, 8, 11, 12, 22–24, 28, 30–32, 42–44, 47, 49, 55–62, 149, 164, 166, 178, 212, 225, 226
Political, 3–5, 35, 47, 51, 53, 54, 61, 86, 100, 107, 117, 148, 167, 196, 211, 216, 217, 219, 221
Political Science, 3, 4, 23, 24, 26, 50, 55, 93, 130
Political Scientist, 4, 32, 49, 123–125, 151, 160
Pollard, C., 97, 98
Potential harm, 121
Power, 8, 12, 20, 31, 32, 41–64, 120, 121, 135, 145, 146, 151, 152, 183, 192, 197, 199, 205, 207, 208, 212, 226
Practice, 1, 3, 5–7, 17, 21, 35, 43, 46, 48, 55, 56, 59, 64, 77, 79, 92, 97, 99, 109, 119, 137, 163, 169, 171, 172, 212, 213, 224, 227–229
Practitioner, 19, 81, 230
Prank, 10, 130, 144, 147–148
Precedent, x, 8, 30, 47, 59, 63, 116
Prescott, C., 11, 191, 197, 201, 204, 209
Prevent, 5, 23, 34, 43, 50, 51, 55, 80, 86, 116, 151, 176, 212
Principle, 1, 3, 5–8, 12, 21, 25–27, 41, 42, 47, 48, 52–54, 63, 75, 159, 175, 176, 199, 230
Principlism, 6, 7
Prior review, 2, 21, 22, 34, 133, 166
Prison, 11, 21, 25, 47, 89, 148, 183, 187–199, 201–208
Prison chaplain, 11, 193, 195, 201, 203, 209
Prisoner, 6, 11, 19, 44, 89, 101, 183, 185, 187–209
Privileges, 108, 192, 194
Problem, 1, 3, 5, 10, 17, 19, 22, 52, 57, 58, 73–74, 77, 78, 80–84, 89, 92, 95, 96, 99, 100, 119, 121, 136, 137, 139, 145, 149, 151, 167, 178, 195, 206, 218, 226, 228, 230
Prodding, 145
Prods, 129, 131, 143, 145
Professional, 4, 5, 7, 18, 19, 24, 30, 44, 52, 58, 99, 118, 134, 145, 149, 152, 169–172, 188, 200, 213, 216, 229, 230
Professional association, 33, 35, 52, 62, 171, 213, 227, 229
Professional ethics, 1, 7, 171, 230
Program, ix, 1, 3, 5, 8, 22, 25, 29, 30, 52, 57, 58, 72, 74, 76–80, 83, 85–87, 91, 93, 98, 100, 114, 115, 118, 124, 130, 139, 144–146, 187, 202, 218–220, 225, 228, 229
Project Camelot, 230
Protecting vulnerable subjects, 205
Protocol, x, 8, 9, 18, 21, 22, 31, 42–45, 47, 52–54, 59, 60, 63, 80, 95, 97, 112, 133, 175, 177, 178, 213, 228, 229
Proximity, 131, 134, 152, 185
Proximity variations, 135
Psychiatrist, 20, 131, 135
Psychological stress, 150
Psychologist, 2, 4, 6, 10, 12, 24, 32, 48, 109, 130, 131, 137, 142, 144, 148, 149, 151, 152, 178, 195, 207, 230
Psychology, x, 3, 4, 24, 27, 119, 130, 132, 134–136, 141, 144, 148, 152, 153, 173, 183, 184, 186, 188, 190–192, 201, 203, 204, 207, 208
Public Broadcasting System (PBS), 117
Public health, 22, 49, 50, 73–74, 78, 79, 83, 86, 89, 99, 100, 172, 214, 215, 229
Public Health Service (PHS), 2, 21–23, 56, 78–80, 86, 91, 133, 166
Public hearing, 96, 108, 148
Public relations, 76, 111, 222
Punishment, 46, 49, 129, 133, 147, 191, 192, 194, 200

Q

Queens College, City University of New York (CUNY), 130
Questionnaire, 2, 6, 23, 111, 114, 119, 123, 133–135, 138–140, 142, 144, 160, 163, 178, 186, 189, 190

R

Race, 76, 77, 79, 80, 86, 90, 101, 162, 163, 202
Racism, 5, 23, 71, 72, 90, 92, 98, 101–102
Rainwater, L., 160–162, 164, 167, 174
Random assignment, 187
Rationally, 147, 153
Raven, B., 205

Rebellion, 188–197, 201, 203
Recording, 9, 28, 34, 48, 86, 108–117, 120, 121, 123, 125, 161, 186
Referendum, 11, 225–226
Regulation, x, 2, 3, 7–9, 12, 17–35, 41–52, 54–56, 58–62, 122, 133, 148, 153, 159, 164, 166, 173, 177, 188, 192, 213, 227, 228
Religion, 95, 170
Religious, 11, 35, 45–47, 107, 163, 195, 201–203
Replicate, 10, 142, 205, 207
Research, 1, 17, 41, 71, 129, 159, 183, 212
  design, 80, 82, 125, 137, 162, 203, 208
  ethics, 1–3, 6–8, 12, 18–30, 35, 42, 43, 52, 54, 55, 57, 90, 95, 96, 99, 108, 120–122, 148, 149, 159, 168, 173, 176–177, 199, 208, 228, 230
  hypothesis, 188
Respect, 7, 8, 12, 19, 25, 30, 31, 33, 41, 47, 54, 61, 63, 168, 175, 192, 230
Respect for people, 230
Response rate, 114, 123, 135, 139
Responsibility, 29, 43, 44, 50, 53, 54, 89, 119, 121, 125, 133, 138, 146, 152, 165, 166, 171, 176, 177, 184, 205, 225, 230
Responsibility to Participant, 132, 149
Retroactive, 213
Retroactively, 133
Reverby, S.M., 77, 80, 81, 84, 89–92, 98, 100, 101
Review panel, 44
Rights, ix, 8, 21, 22, 26, 31, 41, 43, 44, 46, 48, 49, 90, 92, 94, 97, 100, 101, 113, 121, 124, 133, 139, 141, 143, 149, 153, 164–166, 170, 176, 185, 195, 198, 217, 218, 221, 229, 230
Risk, 1, 2, 6, 8, 18, 19, 22, 24, 26, 27, 31, 33, 34, 41, 42, 47, 48, 52–54, 56, 57, 59, 62, 72, 89, 97, 111, 122, 124, 152, 162, 164, 166, 173–175, 206, 213, 226, 228, 229
Rivers, E., 81, 83, 85, 87, 88, 94, 99
Rockefeller Foundation, 75, 78
Rocky Mountain News, 115
Rokeach, M., 135
Role, 10, 27, 30, 44, 48, 56, 71, 100, 101, 119, 129, 132, 159–161, 169, 170, 174, 187–189, 191, 193, 196, 197, 201, 203, 206, 207, 213, 227, 229
  expectation, 187, 188, 208
  play, 142, 153
  playing, 142
  reversal, 202
Rose, R., 118, 119
Rosenwald Foundation, 9, 76–80, 82, 83
Rosenwald, J., 75–76
Rosenwald School, 75
Rule, 11, 18, 25, 27, 28, 30, 32–35, 41, 43–47, 50, 52, 56, 60, 62, 63, 71, 95, 108, 115, 133, 143, 145, 173, 176, 187–189, 191–193, 197–200, 205, 206, 208, 217, 227, 228
Ruyter, Kurt, 227

S
Safeguard, 47, 50, 109, 115, 166
Safety, 24, 46, 59, 62, 99, 102, 151, 206
Sahlins, M., 216, 219
Saitta, D., 226
Salamone, F.A., 220
Salesian, 214, 218–220
Salesian missionary, 214, 218
Sample, 6, 10, 31, 132, 133, 146, 160, 162–164, 168, 184, 214, 227
San Francisco, CA, 31, 93, 94, 221, 223, 230
San Quentin State Prison, 183, 191, 201
Santa Clara University, 142
Scalia, A., 55
Schatz, I.J., 92
Schrag, Z., 2, 22, 23, 26, 55, 56, 62, 162
Science [journal], 11
Scientific, 3, 4, 29, 30, 32, 41, 44, 53, 54, 61, 64, 73, 78, 79, 81–83, 95, 98, 99, 108, 116, 125, 130, 134, 137, 144, 145, 149, 165, 169, 172, 189, 217–219, 221, 225, 227, 230
Scientific replication, 142–143, 150
Segregation, 84, 90, 97
Senate, 75, 95, 109, 111–115, 117
Senate hearing, 12, 122
Sexual, 2, 22, 72, 73, 84, 159–161, 163, 164, 166, 167, 171, 208
Simon, H., 53, 151
Simulation, 192, 193, 196, 201–204, 206, 213
Site visit, 25, 57, 133, 139, 149
Situation, 3, 25, 111, 131, 132, 137, 141, 146–148, 151, 153, 170, 172, 176, 178, 184, 186, 188, 189, 201–203, 205–208, 221, 229
Situation ethics, 168, 170
Skilled worker, 134, 145
Sleep deprivation, 190
Snow, C.P., 130
Social condition, 5, 152
Social constraint, 197

Social distance, 90, 153
Social emotional contagion, 187
Social issue, 4, 216
Social movement, 90, 96
Social norm, 53, 197, 227
Social pressure, 131
Social problem, 71, 90, 96, 109, 159–178
Social science, x, 1–5, 7, 8, 12, 17–35, 49, 52, 55, 61, 77, 108, 120, 124, 125, 133, 153, 159, 166, 167, 169–173, 175, 176, 178, 208, 213, 228, 230
Social scientist, 2, 4, 8, 12, 23, 26, 28, 29, 52, 55, 108, 112, 120, 123, 166–169, 173, 176, 178, 211, 216
Social Security Act, 79, 84, 86
Social support condition, 146
Sociobiology, 217
Sociologist, 3, 5, 6, 12, 17, 19, 20, 24, 27, 32, 48, 52, 53, 63, 71, 73, 79, 87, 90, 108, 123–125, 148, 151, 153, 160, 167–172, 178, 191, 215, 229, 230
Sociology, 3, 4, 10, 17, 24, 27, 45, 76, 78, 90, 109, 120, 159, 160, 164, 165, 167, 168, 171–173, 220
Solitary confinement, 190, 194, 196
South America, 220, 225
Sponsel, L.E., 221, 224, 225
Standard, 2, 5, 7, 12, 18, 29, 30, 32, 33, 35, 47, 48, 50–52, 57, 58, 62, 63, 73, 92, 95, 96, 132, 160, 167, 168, 173, 177, 189, 190, 207, 225, 227–229
Stanford Prison Experiment, x, 7, 9, 11, 148, 183
Stanford University, 79, 183, 187, 188, 190
St Louis Post Dispatch, 10, 136, 165
Strategy, ix, 5, 24, 136, 175, 211, 214, 222
Strodtbeck, F., x, 109–111, 113–115, 119, 122
Student, x, 5, 11, 12, 46, 61, 76, 77, 79, 86, 92, 96, 130–133, 136, 142, 153, 160, 163, 171, 172, 176, 178, 184, 185, 187–188, 190–192, 198, 201, 202, 205–207
Suggestion, 59, 110, 114, 131, 135, 162, 186
Sumner, W.G., 45, 46, 49, 51, 52
Supreme Court, 116
Supreme Court Justice, 49, 113
Surgeon General, 1, 2, 22, 79, 81–83, 85, 86, 91, 94, 100, 133, 166
Survey, 2, 6, 17, 18, 24, 31, 33, 34, 48, 49, 53, 56, 62, 71, 77–82, 86, 87, 89, 101, 114–116, 123, 125, 134, 138, 140, 160, 163, 164, 166, 168, 170, 177, 204, 215
Syphilis, x, 7–9, 18, 19, 21, 23, 24, 55, 71–102, 173, 228
Syphilitics, 73, 80–83, 85, 87–89, 92, 94, 96, 97, 99
Systemic forces, 148

T

Taboo, 192, 212, 223
Tape recording, 114, 136, 184
Task Force, 11, 212, 224–226, 230
Teacher, 129, 131–135, 139–143, 145–147, 151, 185, 230
Television, 10, 108, 117–119, 124, 130, 143–146, 205
Tertiary syphilis, 74, 78, 79, 93
The New Yorker, 11, 221–223
Theory, x, 4–6, 17, 49, 94, 132, 134, 135, 150, 151, 160, 170, 216, 217, 227
Therapy, 19, 28, 57, 79, 85, 88, 92, 94, 202
Thomas, D.S., 108
Tierney, P., 11, 212, 215, 221–227
Time magazine, 160, 167, 222
Tooby, J., 222
Total institution, 191–193, 207
Traditional, 17, 18, 20, 35, 45, 63, 172, 183, 212, 223
Tri-Council Policy Statement (TCPS), x, 28
Trust, 8, 27, 44, 48, 49, 54, 56, 101, 107–125, 137, 149
Tuskegee, x, 7–9, 18, 19, 21, 23, 24, 71–102, 173, 228
Twelve Angry Men, 119

U

Unable to quit, 197
Unethical, 3, 20, 43, 55, 60, 100, 133, 177, 226
United Kingdom (UK), 43
United Nations (UN), 218
United States (US), x, 1–3, 7–8, 10, 12, 17–35, 42, 43, 45, 49–55, 58, 61–64, 71–102, 107, 115–117, 120, 121, 124, 125, 133, 141, 142, 149, 167, 172, 183, 187, 188, 213, 219, 222, 227, 228, 230
University of California, Berkeley, 136
University of California, Santa Barbara, 223
University of Chicago, x, 9, 50, 55, 75–77, 107–109, 111, 112, 114, 115, 123, 221
University of Hawaii, 221, 225
University of Kansas, 175
University of Michigan, 91, 211, 213, 223, 225, 226

University of Oregon, 93, 207
University of Pittsburgh, 89, 100, 101
University of Virginia, 98
University of Wisconsin, 117
US Court of Appeals, 113
US Public Health Service, 1, 173
US Supreme Court, 49, 50, 55, 108, 113, 116

V
Vaccination, 19, 212, 214, 223–225
Vaccine, 11, 19, 89, 98, 102, 212, 214, 215, 222, 223, 227, 229
Validity, 44, 95, 177
Value, 3, 7, 17, 18, 26, 27, 35, 44, 45, 53, 61, 63, 83, 85, 90, 95, 100, 120, 137, 149, 174, 176, 178, 189, 198, 199, 208
Vanderbilt University, 225
Variation, 10, 54, 134–136, 139, 140, 143, 145, 198, 207, 211
Velásquez, R.J., 219
Venereal disease, 19, 73, 74, 77, 78, 81, 86, 89, 94, 100
Venezuela, 11, 211, 212, 218–221, 223
Verdict, 20, 47, 109–111, 118, 119, 121, 122, 228
Videotaping, 108, 118, 190
Virginia, 57, 78
Virtue, 8, 18, 42, 46, 50, 52–53, 63
Voice feedback, 140–143, 145, 146
Volt, 129, 135, 140–142, 145
Voluntary, 2, 20, 22, 58, 197, 228
Volunteer, 6, 63, 84, 91, 93, 94, 137, 142, 188, 190, 193, 198, 207, 213
Vonderlehr, R.A., 81–87, 91, 100
Von Hoffman, N., 166–169, 174
Von Wassermann, A.P., 73

W
Warner, L., 77
Warren, C.A.B., 170, 171
Warren, E., 116
Warwick, D.P., 27, 164, 168, 169
Washington, B.T., 75, 76, 81
Washington Post, 10, 93, 166, 167
Washington University in St. Louis, 171
Wassermann test, 73
Watch queen, 10, 161, 163, 164, 168, 174, 176
Weber, M., 18, 43, 46, 47, 52, 53, 59, 63, 135, 151
Wenger, O.C., 78, 79, 81–83, 85–87
Western Reserve University, 78, 89
Whistleblower, 71, 90, 93–95
Wichita, KS, 9, 12, 107, 111, 120–122
Wilson, E.O., 217
Withdraw, 44, 142, 190, 194, 205, 224
Withdrawal, 193–195
Women, 3, 10, 24, 25, 73, 77, 83, 86, 109, 119, 134, 141–143, 145, 147, 153, 168, 170, 171, 185, 188, 191, 214, 215, 219, 228
Work, ix, 3–5, 17, 18, 26–30, 42, 44, 45, 50, 57, 58, 61, 63, 75–77, 80, 81, 86, 90, 93–95, 101, 108, 117, 119, 120, 130, 133, 144, 148, 160, 165, 168–171, 173, 177, 185, 186, 189, 190, 192, 199–201, 207, 208, 213–216, 218, 219, 221, 224, 226, 227
Workers, 46, 93, 94, 96, 112, 120, 134, 145, 148, 151, 200, 201
World Bank, 4, 218, 225
World Health Organization (WHO), 61, 64, 211
World Medical Association (WMA), 19, 21
World War I, 74, 77
World War II, 19, 101, 130, 131, 152, 213, 230

Y
Yale University, 134, 150
Yanomami, x, 7, 9, 11, 211–227, 229, 230
Young Men's Christian Association (YMCA), 74

Z
Zimbardo, P.G., x, 7, 11, 27, 148, 183–185, 188 193, 195, 198, 201, 203–205, 207–209

The manufacturer's authorised representative in the EU is Springer Nature Customer Service Centre GmbH, Europaplatz 3, 69115 Heidelberg, Germany. If you have any concerns regarding our products, please contact ProductSafety@springernature.com

Printed and bound by CPI Group (UK) Ltd, Croydon, CR0 4YY
30/09/2026
02225296-0007